THE PEDIATRIC CLINICS OF NORTH AMERICA

VOLUME 35 / NUMBER 6
DECEMBER 1988

CHILDREN AT RISK: CURRENT SOCIAL AND MEDICAL CHALLENGES

Barry Zuckerman, MD, Michael Weitzman, MD, and Joel J. Alpert, MD, *Guest Editors*

W. B. SAUNDERS COMPANY
Harcourt Brace Jovanovich, Inc.

Philadelphia London Toronto
Montreal Sydney Tokyo

W. B. SAUNDERS COMPANY
Harcourt Brace Jovanovich, Inc.

The Curtis Center
Independence Square West
Philadelphia, PA 19106–3399

The *Pediatric Clinics* are also published in translated editions by the following:

Spanish   Nueva Editorial Interamericana, S.A. de C.V., Cedro 512,
            Apartado 26370, Mexico 4, D.F., Mexico

Italian   Piccin Editore, Via Brunacci, 12, 35100 Padava, Italy

Portuguese Interlivros Edicoes Ltda.
            Rio de Janeiro, Brazil

The Pediatric Clinics of North America are covered in *Index Medicus, Excerpta Medica, Current Contents, Science Citation Index, ASCA, ISI/BIOMED,* and *BIOSIS.*

THE PEDIATRIC CLINICS OF NORTH AMERICA   ISSN 0031-3955
December 1988   Volume 35—Number 6

The Pediatric Clinics of North America (USPH 424-660) is published bimonthly by W. B. Saunders Company, The Curtis Center, Independence Square West, Philadelphia, PA 19106–3399. Subscription price is $53.00 per year. Second class postage paid at Philadelphia, PA 19106–3399, and additional mailing offices. POSTMASTER: Send address changes to W. B. Saunders Company, The Curtis Center, Independence Square West, Philadelphia, PA 19106–3399. There is a postage charge of $12.00 for subscriptions billed to U.S. addresses and shipped outside the U.S.

This issue is Volume 35, Number 6.

The editor of this publication is Mary K. Smith, W. B. Saunders Company, The Curtis Center, Independence Square West, Philadelphia, Pennsylvania 19106–3399.

Printed by the Maple-Vale Book Manufacturing Group, York, Pennsylvania.

Contributors

ROBIN ADAIR, MD, Fellow in Behavioral Pediatrics, Boston City Hospital and the Boston University School of Medicine, Boston, Massachusetts

GARTH ALPERSTEIN, MB, CHB, MPH, Medical Consultant, Bureau for Families with Special Needs, New York City Department of Health; Attending Pediatrician, St. Luke's-Roosevelt Hospital Center, New York; Assistant Clinical Professor of Pediatrics, College of Physicians and Surgeons, Columbia University, New York, New York

JOEL J. ALPERT, MD, Professor and Chairman, Department of Pediatrics, Boston University School of Medicine, Boston City Hospital, Boston, Massachusetts

ELLIS ARNSTEIN, MD, Director, Bureau for Families with Special Needs, New York City Department of Health, New York, New York

HOWARD BAUCHNER, MD, Assistant Professor of Pediatrics, Boston University School of Medicine; Boston City Hospital, Division of Developmental and Behavioral Pediatrics, Boston, Massachusetts

ELIZABETH BROWN, MD, Associate Professor of Pediatrics, Boston University School of Medicine; Director, Division of Neonatology, Boston City Hospital, Boston, Massachusetts

IRA J. CHASNOFF, MD, Associate Professor of Pediatrics and Psychiatry, Northwestern University Medical School; Director, Perinatal Center for Chemical Dependence, Northwestern Memorial Hospital, Chicago, Illinois

ELLEN R. COOPER, MD, Assistant Professor of Pediatrics, Division of Infectious Diseases, Boston University School of Medicine; Clinical Director of Pediatric AIDS Program, Boston City Hospital, Boston, Massachusetts

EFSTRATIOS DEMETRIOU, MD, Clinical Assistant Professor of Pediatrics, Boston University School of Medicine, Boston, Massachusetts

HOWARD DUBOWITZ, MD, Assistant Professor of Pediatrics, University of Maryland Medical School; Co-Director, Child Protection Team, University Hospital, Division of Pediatric Medicine, Baltimore, Maryland

DEBORAH A. FRANK, MD, Assistant Professor of Pediatrics and Public Health, Boston University Schools of Medicine and Public Health; Director, Failure to Thrive Program, Division of Developmental and Behavioral Pediatrics, Boston City Hospital, Boston, Massachusetts

LINDA M. GRANT, MD, MPH, Assistant Professor of Pediatrics, Boston University School of Medicine, Boston, Massachusetts

STEVEN GREER, MD, Instructor in Pediatrics, Boston University School of Medicine; Fellow in Developmental and Behavioral Pediatrics, Boston City Hospital, Boston, Massachusetts

MICHAEL A. GRODIN, MD, Director, Program in Medical Ethics; Associate Professor of Pediatrics and Sociomedical Sciences (Ethics), Boston University Schools of Medicine and Public Health; Chairman, Institutional Review Board, Associate Visiting Physician (Pediatrics), Medical Ethicist, Boston City Hospital, Boston, Massachusetts

ALICE HAUSMAN, PhD, MPH, Assistant Professor, Boston University School of Public Health, Boston, Massachusetts

NEELA P. JOSHI, MBBS, MPH, DCH, Assistant Professor, Pediatrics, Boston University School of Medicine, Boston, Massachusetts

LORRAINE V. KLERMAN, DrPH, Professor, Public Health, Department of Epidemiology and Public Health, Yale School of Medicine, New Haven, Connecticut

MIREILLE LeMAY, MD, Research Fellow, Pediatric Infectious Diseases, Boston University School of Medicine, Boston, Massachusetts

LORA H. MELNICOE, MD, Medical Director, Las Animas-Huerfano Counties District Health Department, Trinidad, Colorado

ALAN MEYERS, MD, MPH, Assistant Professor, Boston University School of Medicine; Department of Pediatrics, Boston City Hospital, Boston, Massachusetts

WILLIAM E. MACLEAN, JR, PhD, Assistant Professor of Psychology, George Peabody College, Vanderbilt University, Nashville, Tennessee

CAROLYN MOORE NEWBERGER, ED D, Instructor in Psychology, Department of Psychiatry, Harvard Medical School; Director, Victim Recovery Study and Associate in Medicine and Psychiatry, The Children's Hospital, Boston, Massachusetts

ELI H. NEWBERGER, MD, Assistant Professor of Pediatrics, Harvard Medical School; Director, Family Development Study; Senior Associate in Medicine, The Children's Hospital, Boston, Massachusetts

STEVEN PARKER, MD, Assistant Professor of Pediatrics, Boston University School of Medicine; Director, Developmental Assessment Clinic, Boston City Hospital, Boston, Massachusetts

STEPHEN I. PELTON, MD, Associate Professor of Pediatrics, Vice Chairman of Department of Pediatrics, Division of Infectious Diseases, Boston University School of Medicine, Boston, Massachusetts

JAMES M. PERRIN, MD, Associate Professor of Pediatrics, Harvard Medical School, Boston, Massachusetts

JOY PESKIN, MD, Fellow, Division of Developmental and Behavioral Pediatrics, Boston University School of Medicine, Boston City Hospital, Boston, Massachusetts

DEBORAH PROTHROW-STITH, MD, Assistant Professor, Boston University School of Medicine; Commissioner, Department of Public Health, The Commonweath of Massachusetts, Boston, Massachusetts

EDWARD L. SCHOR, MD, Clinical Associate Professor, Department of Pediatrics, Stanford University Medical School; Program Officer, The Henry J. Kaiser Family Foundation, Menlo Park, California

MARCIA SCOTT, MD, Assistant Professor, Psychiatry, Boston University School of Medicine, Boston, Massachusetts

HOWARD SPIVAK, MD, Assistant Professor of Pediatrics, Boston University School of Medicine; Director, Adolescent Services, Boston Department of Health and Hospitals, Boston, Massachusetts

MICHAEL WEITZMAN, MD, MPH, Associate Professor of Pediatrics and Public Health, Boston City Hospital and the Boston University School of Medicine and Public Health, Boston, Massachusetts

PAUL H. WISE, MD, Assistant Professor, Department of Pediatrics, Harvard Medical School; Research Fellow, Division of Health Policy Research and Education, Harvard University; Joint Program in Neonatology, Brigham and Women's Hospital, Boston, Massachusetts

STEVEN H. ZEISEL, MD, PhD, Associate Professor of Pathology and Pediatrics, Nutrient Metabolism Laboratory, Boston University School of Medicine and Boston City Hospital, Boston, Massachusetts

BARRY ZUCKERMAN, MD, Professor of Pediatrics, Boston University School of Medicine; Director, Division of Developmental and Behavioral Pediatrics, Boston City Hospital, Boston, Massachusetts

Contents

        Poverty is now more heavily concentrated in children than
at any other time in U.S. history. Poverty's influence on
child health is pervasive and creates a variety of clinical
challenges. This discussion reviews the clinical expression
of poverty in childhood and assesses our clinical and
political capacity to reduce its tragic impact.

        Malnutrition is the primary biologic insult in most cases of
failure to thrive. A transactional model of infant development provides a framework for understanding the psychosocial context in which such malnutrition occurs. Each
child who fails to thrive should receive a multidisciplinary
evaluation to address the diagnostic and therapeutic implications of nutritional, medical, psychosocial, and developmental factors contributing to growth failure.

        Approximately 40,000 infants weighing less than 1500
grams are born in the United States each year. Caring for
these infants after their discharge from the newborn intensive care unit is complex and difficult. The survival, growth,
routine health care maintenance, neurologic and develop-

risk factors related to adverse outcomes of such behavior, and potential interventions that practitioners working with their adolescent patients may undertake are reviewed.

Howard Dubowitz, Carolyn Moore Newberger,
Lora H. Melnicoe, and Eli H. Newberger

The increase in single-parent families, step-families, maternal employment, and young children in substitute care are among several important changes in the American family in recent decades. Although it is not clear that these changes necessarily lead to negative outcomes in children, it is apparent that a variety of potential risks and challenges confront many families today. Pediatricians can play a valuable role by helping families to adjust and cope with certain difficulties, such as divorce. However, in other areas such as child care, changes in public policies and programs are needed to better support families to optimally nurture their children.

Michael Weitzman and Robin Adair

Divorce is a common event in the United States today, affecting approximately one million children per year. This makes divorce a problem that frequently appears in a pediatrician's patient population. These children and families tend to suffer stresses and difficulties that vary from the mundane and shortlived to profound, long-term problems. The pediatrician can be helpful by serving as the child's advocate, offering anticipatory guidance, helping the family weather the turmoil of the acute stage, screening for maladjustment or maladaptive behavior of children and parents, providing counseling, and referring the children and family for more specialized mental health input where indicated.

The Prevention of Dysfunction

James M. Perrin and William E. MacLean, Jr.

This article reviews the consequences of dysfunction that results from chronic illness. This dysfunction may be manifest in several ways, from a knee that functions poorly, to a long-term illness that affects other aspects of the child's development. The goal of services for these children is to diminish the impact of the illness and to prevent dysfunction wherever possible.

Adolescents, Violence, and Intentional Injury

> *Howard Spivak, Deborah Prothrow-Stith, and*
> *Alice J. Hausman*

> Violence and its consequences of injury and death are a
> major issue confronting the public health community. An
> understanding of the characteristics and contributing factors
> of violence provide insights for both preventive and treat-
> ment strategies. Interventions at the societal, public health,
> and clinical levels are possible and evidence is being
> accumulated that suggests these interventions are an im-
> portant component to addressing this complex and serious
> problem.

> *Neela P. Joshi and Marcia Scott*

> This article reviews use and depression in adolescents and
> explores the thesis that depressed mood and deviant actions
> represent deviant modes of coping and are the result of
> failed efforts to handle different and sometimes overlapping
> constitutional and social risk factors. Theories of drug use
> and depression and various studies in support of the
> theoretical framework are examined. Implications are sug-
> gested for public health interventions and clinical manage-
> ment as derived from the theoretic background and empiric
> evidence. Also provided are guidelines for assessment and
> intervention that can be useful for primary care physicians
> and other professionals working with troubled teenagers.

> *Ellen R. Cooper, Stephen I. Pelton, and Mireille LeMay*

> Cases of AIDS in children have been described since 1982.
> Diagnosis is more complex in children than in adults owing
> to the more varied clinical presentations and the difficulty
> in interpretation of laboratory tests. Our current under-
> standing of HIV infection in children is reviewed, as well
> as the controversies regarding medical, psychosocial, and
> public health issues.

> *Michael A. Grodin and Joel J. Alpert*

> The use of children in research raises the questions about
> proper justification, assessment of benefit in relation to
> risk, ability to consent, compensation, and the just selection

of subjects. Although substantive and procedural standards have evolved, subpopulations of vulnerable children created new challenges and concerns.

With the increasing use of cocaine and other illicit drugs by women of childbearing age, increasing numbers of children are being born affected by substance exposure. The infant delivered to a drug-addicted woman is at risk for problems of growth and development often compounded by environmental factors that can negatively influence long-term outcome. Early intervention by the health care community will be necessary to ensure the best prognosis for these children.

The health status of homeless children has become of major concern as the numbers of homeless families and children has dramatically increased in the United States over the past decade. There is some evidence to suggest that the health problems of homeless children are of greater frequency and of greater severity than those of poor children with homes. It is imperative that pediatricians begin to play a major role in handling this problem before the health status of this disenfranchised group of children is jeopardized even further.

RECENT ISSUES

October 1988
PEDIATRIC ALLERGIC DISEASE
Philip Fireman, MD, *Guest Editor*

August 1988
THE LEUKEMIAS
David G. Poplack, MD, *Guest Editor*

June 1988
NEW TOPICS IN PEDIATRIC INFECTIOUS DISEASE
Sheldon L. Kaplan, MD, *Guest Editor*

April 1988
PEDIATRIC GASTROENTEROLOGY II
Emanuel Lebenthal, MD, *Guest Editor*

FORTHCOMING ISSUES

February 1989
PEDIATRIC LABORATORY TESTING
John J. Buchino, MD, and Beverly Dahms, MD, *Guest Editors*

April 1989
SEIZURE DISORDERS
John M. Pellock, MD, *Guest Editor*

June 1989
ACUTE PAIN IN CHILDREN
Neil Schechter, MD, *Guest Editor*

Preface

In many respects, children have never been healthier than they are today. For a significant proportion of American children, however, this picture is highly inaccurate. Children are at risk because of high rates of poverty, divorce, single-parent households, chronic illness, school failure, teenage pregnancy, drug abuse, suicide, homicide, injuries, and problems relating to learning and behavior. The higher infant mortality rate among blacks compared to whites and the higher school failure rates experienced by Hispanics are further evidence of children being at high risk because of race and ethnicity. Concern regarding these statistics has gone beyond the health and education communities that traditionally have been the main forces addressing problems of children and youth. In a recent report, the committee for Economic Development, made up of leaders in the business community, issued a statement emphasizing the need to bolster the health, education, and well-being of the whole child, beginning with the formative years.[1] Impetus for this statement is concern from the business community regarding the need for a qualified and competitive work force.

Although pediatricians are trained to handle changes associated with growth and development of their patients, their training and knowledge also must encompass change in the traditional problems addressed. It is not enough to treat the biologic or medical aspects of an illness alone, but treatment should ensure the child's functioning and appropriate adaptation to his or her environment. A great many families now experience stress because of a wide array of factors. In the report, "Stress and Human Health," the Institute of Medicine concluded that persons experiencing stress are at an increased risk for developing a physical or mental problem.[2] This conclusion is well known to pediatricians, who daily see the relationship between illness and disadvantage. We know that children living in poverty experience significantly higher rates of reported health problems than do their nonpoor peers. Pediatricians cannot adequately meet or understand children's needs in the limited framework of traditional medical problems but rather must understand the broader relationship between health and social factors.

This edition of *The Pediatric Clinics of North America* provides the clinician with information regarding the social context that places children at risk for not only poor health but also an unhappy and unproductive life. Solutions to these problems must be addressed at many different levels. Clinical roles such as identification, management, or referral are a first level for helping children. A second level includes expansion of knowledge through research. A third level includes advocacy as well as sharing knowledge with parents, service providers.

and policy makers to develop and implement programs and policies that affect children and their parents. Services need not only to be expanded but also must be comprehensive and integrated, emphasizing both medical need and the social context of children's lives. It is only through efforts of all these levels that improved health and development of American children will be achieved.

REFERENCES

1. Children in Need: Investment Strategies for the Educationally Disadvantaged. New York, A Committee for Economic Development.
2. Stress and Human Health; Report from the Institute of Medicine, 1986

BARRY ZUCKERMAN, MD, MICHAEL WEITZMAN, MD, AND JOEL J. ALPERT, MD

Guest Editors

Boston City Hospital
818 Harrison Avenue
Boston, Massachusetts 02118

Poverty and Child Health

Paul H. Wise, MD, MPH,* and Alan Meyers, MD, MPH†

A child growing up in poverty remains one of the great tragedies of our time. Regardless of political perspective, few accept widespread childhood poverty as a necessary element of their vision of a vibrant and just society. Despite this apparent concensus, profound poverty afflicts millions of America's children, stifling the vitality of their daily lives and reshaping forever the promise of their collective future. This seeming inconsistency between societal intent and social reality confronts pediatricians with a profound dilemma: how can optimal child health be realized if our clinical capability to improve health is challenged by the pervasive power of poverty to destroy it? This dilemma is played out both in the broad and fractious deliberation of public policy as well as in the many daily frustrations of clinical practice. This discussion attempts to give form to the elements and complexities of these tensions, and to assess poverty's influence on child health in relation to our clinical and political capacity to reduce its detrimental impact.

RECENT TRENDS IN CHILDHOOD POVERTY

Despite the common belief that childhood poverty has remained a relatively stable phenomenon in recent American history, rates of childhood poverty have undergone considerable change over the past three decades (Fig. 1). In 1960, slightly more than one quarter of all children under the age of 18 years were living in families with reported incomes less than the officially designated poverty level (approximately three times the income needed to meet a federal estimate of minimal nutritional subsistence).[12] Beginning in the mid-1960s this percentage began to fall, reaching a low point of 14.4 per cent in 1974. The early 1980s witnessed a disturbing increase in the percentage of children living in poverty, the rate climbing to over 22 per cent in 1983, from which it has dropped only slightly. At present, it is estimated that approximately one in five children residing in the United States lives in poverty.[121] Almost one half of all black children and more than one third of Hispanic children live in families with incomes below the poverty line.

The recent increase in childhood poverty is even more alarming when it is

*Assistant Professor, Department of Pediatrics, Harvard Medical School; Research Fellow, Division of Health Policy Research and Education, Harvard University; Joint Program in Neonatology, Brigham and Women's Hospital, Boston, Massachusetts

†Assistant Professor, Boston University School of Medicine; Department of Pediatrics, Boston City Hospital, Boston, Massachusetts

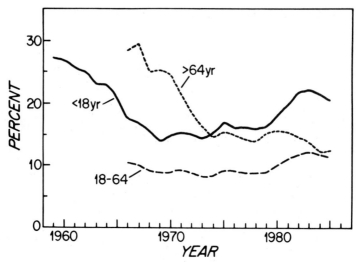

Figure 1. Percentage of Persons Living Below Federal Poverty Level By Age: United States 1959 Through 1985. Bureau of the Census. Current Population Reports. Series P-60. U.S. Department of Commerce. Washington, D.C., U.S. Government Printing Office.

viewed in relation to poverty trends in other segments of the American population.[89] Among the elderly, approximately 25 per cent were living in poverty in 1970.[11] However, by 1985, this percentage had fallen to just 12.6 per cent. Thus, over the period that witnessed a 37 per cent increase in childhood poverty, the rate for the elderly fell a dramatic 49 per cent. When noncash transfers, such as Medicare are included, this divergence is even more profound. These trends have left childhood in a precarious position: the concentration of poverty rates in children has never been as great as it is today.

THE CHANGING ROLE OF THE FAMILY

The departure of fathers from the typical American family has been noted for some time.[64] Between 1959 and 1985, the number of female-headed households with children more than tripled, whereas the number of male-present families with children rose less than 10 per cent over this same period.[11, 12] At present, approximately one in five families in the United States is headed by a woman; in 1959, it was one in eleven. Moreover, approximately half of all poor children now live in female-headed households. This clearly represents a disproportionately high rate of childhood poverty in these female-headed households.[11, 12, 121] This observation has been popularly labeled the "feminization of poverty" and has dominated the public discussion of poverty in America.[66] However, a singular focus on this one issue obscures a deeper complexity of determinants. There is a renewed appreciation of the role of economic change and persistent male unemployment in generating these trends.[125] In addition, the presence of a working father is no guarantee that a child will not grow up in poverty. More than 70 per cent of the increase in the number of poor children that occurred in the early 1980s was due to rising poverty in families with a man present. In addition, approximately one fourth of children in families with married parents would be poor if they depended on their father's income alone. Although these trends have complex origins, they document the growing inability of the American family to provide the economic essentials all children need.

THE CHANGING ROLE OF THE STATE

For children, the alternative to the family for income distribution is the state. Here, the distinction between how the elderly and children have been treated is striking. In 1960 the ratio of government spending on the elderly relative to that spent on children was about three to one.[86] Expenditures for both groups rose substantially during subsequent years so that by 1979 the ratio remained roughly three to one, even though in actual dollars, spending for the elderly had increased far more, since their level of funding was so much higher than that of children to begin with. After 1979, this relationship changed. The policies that provided stability in the generational ratio of government spending for children and the elderly were altered radically. The primary government programs supporting children were reduced, whereas those of greatest benefit to the elderly continued to expand. For example, the major child support program, Aid to Families with Dependent Children (AFDC) has been changed such that only about half the children presently living in poverty are enrolled in the program.[12] In 1979, almost three out of four were enrolled. Health care, child nutrition, food stamps, and aid to education have experienced disproportionately the pressures of severe spending restraints.[13, 89, 121] For every one dollar the federal government spends on children, it now spends ten dollars on the elderly.

The intent of this discussion is not to pit the needs of children against those of the elderly. To the contrary, the needs of the elderly and children have far more in common than in conflict, and it would be a conceptual and practical error to portray the interests of these two groups of Americans as being inherently at odds. Rather, these data are useful in documenting the deteriorating relative status of childhood in America, while at the same time underscoring this society's capacity to improve the conditions of life for large sectors of our society.

THE MECHANISMS OF POVERTY'S INFLUENCE ON CHILD HEALTH

The power of poverty lies as much in its pervasiveness as it does in its deadening persistence. It is not surprising, therefore, that childhood poverty has been linked to a variety of specific health problems.[15, 24, 55, 106] Recognition of their common elements can help facilitate the development of an effective clinical response. Poverty can be seen as elevating the likelihood of poor health by two possible mechanisms: the enhancement of risk for poor health and the reduction of access to those interventions effective at minimizing the impact of elevated risk.

Elevated risk can affect health by increasing the probability that an illness or traumatic event will occur, or by increasing the severity with which the illness or injury affects the child.[110, 111] Enhanced risk can take the form of an increased duration or intensity of exposure, or the suppression of protective mechanisms that reduce the capacity of any given exposure to inflict symptomatic harm. However, risk can be modulated by intervention. Indeed, the clinician's primary task is to modify how risk ultimately affects the occurrence or severity of illness. Therefore, where a capacity to alter a risk's impact exists, then disparities in access to this capacity can create inequities in outcome.

Reduced access to effective interventions can affect the health of children by increasing the occurrence of illness or trauma, or by increasing the severity with which such conditions affect their health and well-being.[110, 111] Interventions that reduce the occurrence of illness or injury relate to primary prevention.[128] The classic example of primary prevention is immunization, an intervention that reduces the child's risk of being harmed by specific infective organisms. Interventions that are directed at reducing the severity of illness and injury relate to secondary and tertiary prevention. Secondary prevention is directed toward altering the impact of a pathologic condition after it has begun but prior to its actual expression as recognized symptoms.[128] An example of secondary prevention is newborn screening for phenylketonuria (PKU). Tertiary prevention confronts the failures of primary and secondary prevention. It is directed at limiting the disability and suffering associated with chronic illness. Here, the pathologic process has produced symptoms, and the task becomes the reduction of suffering and the promotion of adaptation.[128] Be it in the arena of primary, secondary, or tertiary prevention, reduced access to effective interventions for poor children ultimately can find expression in elevated rates of morbidity and mortality.

DISPARITIES IN MORTALITY

The starkest manifestation of poverty's influence on child health lies in its power to create disparities in survival. Social differences in mortality are troubling for several important reasons. First, the outcome to be measured (death) is not likely to be misdiagnosed and usually is well documented in public records. Second, death is the ultimate expression of poor health, representing the final common pathway of what is usually a complex interaction of causes and mediating events. Third, death has social meaning; it is perceived societally as final, tragic, and when preventable, as the ultimate failure of our societal capacity to assure subsistence and opportunity. Although poverty influences child mortality from a variety of causes, several illustrative categories are discussed below.

Poverty and Infant Mortality

Infant mortality has long been recognized as a sensitive indicator of social conditions.[3, 31, 46, 115, 119] However, the mechanisms by which poverty exerts its influence on infant survival are complex and dynamic, since the infant mortality rate represents a composite of a series of contributing rates, each with its own relationship to socioeconomic status.[126] In the United States most infant deaths occur in the neonatal period. By far the most powerful determinant of neonatal mortality is birth weight. In general, the lower the birth weight the higher the mortality. Therefore, disparities in neonatal mortality can be created through two basic mechanisms: differences in the distribution of birth weights (e.g., elevated rates of low birthweight), and differences in the mortality rates of neonates of comparable birth weights.

Poverty increases the probability that a pregnancy will end in the delivery of a low birth weight baby (less than 2500 gm).[48, 52, 127] This appears to be due to increased rates of both prematurity and intrauterine growth retardation.[48, 127] As the fundamental causes of these conditions remain unclear, the precise mechanisms of poverty's effects are difficult to define. However, there is some evidence that they are related to both elevated risk and reduced access to medical care. The risks associated with low birth weight have received significant recent attention.[40] However, of significance to this discussion are those risks that mediate poverty's influence. Poor nutrition, small stature, increased stress, and obstetric complications can all affect birth weight and are more common among poor women.[37, 40, 143] A risk often overlooked is the state of a women's health prior to conception.[37, 43, 57] In this context, the effect of poverty on birth outcome may represent in part a legacy of inferior health status of poor women both before and during their child-bearing years. Poverty also affects behaviors in pregnancy. Of particular concern are cigarette smoking, heavy alcohol consumption, and illicit drug use.[30, 45, 113] However, the challenge in deciphering poverty's ability to alter birth outcome lies less in compiling lists of associated risks than it does in determining the relative contribution these risks make to the important clinical problems experienced by poor women in pregnancy. To date, there remains a striking paucity of data that address this issue.

There are clear disparities between poor and nonpoor women in the utilization of prenatal care services.[40, 69, 120] National data suggest that approximately one in five women giving birth in the United States begins prenatal care later than the first trimester, and that this failure to begin care early is concentrated heavily among women of low socioeconomic status. The barriers to care for these women vary considerably. However, in one recent survey of poor women, approximately half reported multiple barriers to the receipt of adequate prenatal care. The most commonly reported factors were the lack of money to pay for care, lack of transportation to the provider of care, and an unawareness of pregnancy.[120]

Although there is little argument over the existence of profound inequities in prenatal care utilization, there is considerable controversy surrounding their relative impact on birth outcomes. A recent review of this literature by a committee convened by the Institute of Medicine concluded that the evidence for the positive effects of prenatal care was sufficient to support a national effort to improve access to prenatal care.[40] However, other reviewers have been more cautious in their appraisal, concerned with the methodologic difficulties inherent in this work and the variability of specific outcome findings.[54, 109] Nevertheless, the thrust of these cautions has been to focus on the need to improve the content of prenatal care and the analytic utility of its evaluation, not to undermine calls for greater equity of prenatal care utilization.

Less controversy exists regarding the effectiveness of interventions related to birth weight–specific outcome. Improved survival of high-risk newborns has been generally attributed to interventions associated with neonatal intensive care.[82, 123] Indeed, technical innovation and programs affording access to this innovation have played a powerful role in reshaping the epidemiology of neonatal mortality in recent years. Poverty does not appear to influence the survival of low birth weight infants as long as it does not reduce their access to perinatal intensive care services.[83, 127] However, the survival of normal birth weight neonates is considerably reduced by poverty.[6, 127] It would appear that social factors conveying elevated risk in pregnancy and the inadequate use of medical interventions, particularly near term, could be important contributors to mortality in this group of newborns. Nevertheless, the importance of regionalized perinatal services to the survival of poor infants of all birth weights cannot be overstated. This highlights the fear that without purposeful action, changing hospital reimbursement policy could signal the unraveling of regionalized perinatal care. This "deregionalization" based on the ability to pay could have a devastating impact on the survival of poor, high-risk infants.[88]

Despite major reductions in postneonatal mortality since the mid-1960s, major social class effects persist.[47, 74] Historically, infectious diseases have been the major contributors to elevated mortality in this period.[85] However, the sudden infant death syndrome (SIDS) also occurs more frequently among poor infants,[7] and this entity makes a significant contribution to disparities in postneonatal mortality. Since the etiology of SIDS remains unclear, explanations for this observed social effect is difficult to assess.[5] Despite the uncertainties regarding SIDS, the large contribution of conditions known to be amenable to medical intervention continues to make the postneonatal period an important arena for preventive efforts.[2]

The Contribution of Trauma

Since the occurrence of life-threatening injury is tied so deeply to the activities of daily life, social conditions play an important role in shaping childhood patterns of trauma and mortality. Indeed, from a diverse empirical literature, traumatic causes appear to be the largest contributors to social disparities in childhood mortality beyond infancy in the United States.[15, 55, 127]

Fire Mortality. In two recent reports from urban and rural populations, the disparity between poor and nonpoor children was greater for fire mortality than for any other cause of unintentional trauma.[15, 127] Housefires are the source of the overwhelming portion of childhood fire deaths.[4, 58] The leading cause of fatal housefires is the adult use of cigarettes, accounting for approximately 30 per cent of all such fires. However, the second and third leading causes are related directly to the adequacy of housing, especially heating and electrical equipment. In addition to malfunctioning equipment, heating systems that are not functioning, either because of defects or the lack of fuel, force residents to use alternative and often dangerous sources of heat.[63] Space heaters, makeshift wood stoves, and kitchen ovens too often become the primary heating sources for poor families, and increase the risk of fire. Arson also may be an important contributor to fire mortality in poor communities. The determinants of arson are diverse. However, when the market value of housing falls appreciably below its insured value or its potential value as remodeled or "gentrified" housing, then arson can devastate whole low income neighborhoods and cost the lives of many residents.[9, 60]

There is good evidence that the presence of a working smoke detector can reduce the likelihood of mortality once a fire has begun.[4, 58] In many communities, education and legislation have increased the number of homes in which smoke detectors have been installed. However, access to working smoke detectors may be hindered by several factors common to poor families. First, the cost of the units may be prohibitive. Second, legislation mandating the installation of detection equipment by landlords tends to focus on new construction and may ignore the need in older housing.[104] Third, in communities where housing is scarce, the fear of eviction tends to overpower incentives to report violations of housing standards; therefore inspection and enforcement may be insufficient to ensure optimal detector utilization. Also, detectors require the periodic replacement of batteries, a task that may be less commonly performed in poor neighborhoods.[58, 104]

Mortality and Motor Vehicles. Injury associated with the use of motor vehicles, either as occupants or pedestrians, represents the largest contributor to traumatic mortality in childhood.[75] In general, motor vehicle occupant mortality is higher in children living in poverty.[55] This tends to occur both as passenger and as vehicle operator. The reasons for this association have not been well defined. However, differing rates of alcohol consumption by social class could be contributory, as it is estimated that approximately half of all drivers involved in fatal motor vehicle collisions are legally intoxicated.[27] The impact of instability and strife in the family also may influence driving behavior. Also, social conditions may ultimately enhance the risk for injury or death[62, 65] through poverty's influence on the development of health-related and risk-taking behaviors.[94]

Despite this general association between poverty and occupant mortality, local conditions may alter this relationship considerably. For example, a recent report from Boston documented significantly higher occupant mortality among wealthier children.[127] This finding was apparently due to the urban nature of the population and the reliance of poor families on a well-developed mass transit system. In this setting, the exposure of poor children to motor vehicle occupancy is likely to be lower in those areas where the ownership of a motor vehicle is essential.[15] Where motor vehicles are used by families of all incomes, then the impact of poverty probably will be expressed in elevated mortality.

Over the past decade, the importance of restraint systems in reducing injury and death from motor vehicle collisons has become widely appreciated.[96] Therefore, in addition to an elevated risk of being in a car involved in a serious crash, the reduced utilization of appropriate child restraint systems by poor families also could be contributing to the elevated occupant mortality of poor children. This underscores the importance of educational and low cost car seat programs, as well as the potential significance of airbags in reducing occupant mortality in poor children.[96]

Pedestrian mortality is heavily influenced by social status.[15, 98] However, as for occupant mortality, the precise mechanisms of effect are not well understood. Pedestrian death is concentrated in urban areas, and for children, strongly related to place of residence.[75] Because poor neighborhoods are often located in seriously congested, inner-city areas, the risk of pedestrian injury to children in this setting is likely to be elevated substantially.[108] The importance of the street as a play area, and the lack of barriers separating children from motor vehicle thoroughfares contribute to the functional proximity of young children and moving vehicles, an association that virtually ensures high rates of pedestrian injury and death.[25, 77]

Homicide. The tragedy of homicide in children has defied clear understanding; however, its concentration in poor communities has been documented repeatedly.[15, 55, 127] The empirical literature has shown a number of demographic, social, and psychological factors to be associated with child homicide.[18, 42, 78, 85, 93] For infanticide and young child homicide, the focus of attention has been placed on parental attributes, including social isolation, a history of familial violence, and high levels of stress.[78, 93] In older children, the focus has centered on the learned appreciation of violence as an unavoidable, if not acceptable, method of conflict resolution and social advancement. However, a common element in this fabric of homicide causation is poverty. A variety of disciplines have defined potential pathways by which poverty may surface as a specific risk factor for child homicide (e.g., stress, limited opportunity, availability of weapons, drugs and alcohol abuse).[18, 42, 78, 85, 93] However, poverty also may act by drastically increasing the likelihood that these multiple risks converge in the course of daily life.

DISPARITIES IN MORBIDITY

Through death, poverty eliminates the promise that childhood traditionally affords. However, poverty also can create a range of less severe effects, altering risk and access such that the occurrence and severity of conditions affecting child health may increase profoundly.[111] Children of poor families experience more time lost from school and more days of restricted activity due to illness than do those of the nonpoor.[24, 101] The inadequacy of their diet has produced significantly elevated rates of iron deficiency anemia and failure to thrive among poor children.[24, 129] Inadequate housing conditions also can affect morbidity, as lead poisoning is heavily concentrated in poor children.[91] Poverty's influence on childhood morbidity also can be conveyed by the reduced utilization of effective clinical interventions. For example, poor children suffering from appendicitis are more likely to experience perforation and peritonitis than are wealthier children with this condition.[107]

Chronic Conditions

Evidence for disparities in the prevalence of chronic conditions in childhood is quite variable. In general, surveys of parent-reported diagnoses among the poor and nonpoor are similar. However, when the prevalence of severe chronic illness is examined, poor children appear to be significantly more affected. For example, household surveys of childhood asthma suggest that while poor children may have a lower prevalence of this condition,[32, 59] they have a higher rate of severe asthma.[61, 86] Attacks occur more often and are more likely to reduce activity and require hospitalization. These observations could be due to a reduced prevalence but greater severity of asthma in poor children. However, it seems more likely that this phenomenon reflects the under-reporting of less severe asthma by poor families. For many conditions such as asthma, diagnosis requires the receipt of medical care. One might expect therefore, that minor cases of these conditions would go without specific diagnosis in children traditionally underserved by the medical care system.[24]

Hearing loss is more prevalent among poor children.[68] Although the precise etiology of this finding is not clear, it is important to note that poor children experience significantly more otitis media than do their nonpoor counterparts.[84] Recurrent chronic otitis media is also more common in poor children, and it is more likely to be associated with subsequent hearing loss.[8, 39, 81] Although these findings could be due to an increased occurrence of otitis media or a reduced ability to combat ongoing middle ear disease, it seems probable that a reduced access to early diagnosis and comprehensive followup services could play an important role in generating social disparities in complicated otitis media, hearing loss, and its serious developmental sequelae.[37–39] Vision acuity tends to be slightly better in poor children than in nonpoor children.[67] However, nonpoor children are far more likely to have these problems diagnosed and adequately corrected, leaving poor children with a greater functional burden of impaired vision.[72, 73]

The Legacy of Low Birth Weight

The survival of low birth weight infants has improved dramatically over the past two decades.[123] The emerging population of high-risk survivors has focused attention on the complex spectrum of morbidity associated with low birth weight.[50] Estimates of adverse neurodevelopmental outcomes have varied widely, although in general the risk for serious handicap is inversely related to birth weight. Low birth weight survivors (<2500 gm) experience approximately three times the rate of significant neurologic sequelae than do infants of normal birth weight.[118] Very low birth weight survivors (<1500 gm) are at even greater risk, with between 12 and 25 per cent experiencing serious neurodevelopmental handicaps.[28, 33, 114] Although less well studied, there is mounting evidence that low birth weight may be associated with learning difficulties and school failure.[92] Low birth weight infants are also at increased risk for several other serious conditions, including lower respiratory tract illnesses, chronic pulmonary disease, and the adverse sequelae of medications and techniques used in an intensive care setting.[56]

In light of this profound morbidity, poverty's influence on the distribution of low birth weight not only implies elevated neonatal mortality but also conveys an increased burden of illness and physical challenge. The transition from the intensive care unit to home links the probability of optimal outcome to the adequacy of the social environment. The clinical task lies in providing a range of medical, educational, and social services to all infants with high-risk conditions.[19] However, the diversity of needed services can overwhelm standard health care delivery systems, and the financial barriers to such care are profound. Indeed, the conditions that heighten an infant's risk of being born at low birth weight also heighten its risk for poor outcome subsequent to hospital discharge. When compared to nonpoor survivors of comparable birth weight, poor infants have greater postneonatal mortality, lower IQ scores, and are more likely to exhibit problems in school.[26, 92] This "double jeopardy"[26] underscores the pervasive nature of poverty's influence and embodies the common clinical frustration of sending an obviously high-risk infant into an obviously high-risk environment.

The Impact of the Acquired Immunodeficiency Syndrome

Of great and pressing concern is the emerging problem of the acquired immunodeficiency syndrome (AIDS) in young children. Primarily the product of maternal transmission,[49, 90] AIDS implies significant morbidity in early childhood. Recent data suggest that in areas where drug abuse is relatively common, as many as 1 in 50 women giving birth test positive for the human immunodeficiency virus (HIV). Based on an estimated perinatal transmission rate of between 30 and 50 per cent, the number of newborns that ultimately will acquire HIV approaches 1 in 150 births.[51] There is some preliminary evidence that in particularly impoverished communities the rate of HIV seropositivity among newborns has reached approximately 1 in 60.[51]

Clearly, the direct effects of AIDS on chronic childhood illness in these disadvantaged communities will be profound. The potential for powerful indirect effects on the broader population of poor children also can be dramatic, however. These effects are related to the transfer of public resources from traditional, but effective, maternal and child health programs for poor children to those dealing with the immense challenges of AIDS. In areas where the impact of AIDS has been greatest, there has been a tendency to finance AIDS-related services by the redistribution of public resources within the public health domain. Judging from the recent experience of Los Angeles,[53] the public provision of prenatal and infant care services may be particularly vulnerable to such pressures.

Morbidity and the Importance of Medical Care

The purpose of medical care in the setting of poverty is to uncouple poverty from its implications for health. It is a common misconception that medical care has little to offer children in poverty. However, in view of the relentless increase in health care costs and the current retrenchment of public spending for social programs, addressing this mistaken view has taken on new importance.

In an early controlled experiment in the effects of comprehensive pediatric primary care, low-income families using a hospital emergency department and lacking a regular source of care were randomly assigned to a group offering comprehensive pediatric care or to one of two control groups.[97] The comprehensive care group had significantly more preventive health visits than the control group, better immunization records, fewer illness visits, lower rates of hospitalization and surgery, and fewer laboratory tests than the controls.[97] The Rand Health Insurance Experiment similarly assigned families randomly to differing health insurance plans.[122] Although increased cost sharing led to a reduced use of ambulatory services, the investigators did not demonstrate significant differences in health status between those receiving free care and those in cost-sharing plans. Other analysts have pointed out that the power of the study to detect differences of outcome within high-risk subpopulations of children was small, the outcome measures chosen were relatively insensitive to the effects of differential utilization, and that among poor children there was a trend toward improved outcomes in six of the eight measures of health status studied that might have achieved statistic significance with larger samples.[35, 112]

A population-based survey conducted in Washington, D.C., in 1971 found that whereas adverse living conditions constituted the major link between low income and higher morbidity among poor children, access to physician care was consistently and independently related to a lower likelihood of health problems.[22] Differences in the quality of ambulatory care were positively associated with differences in child health outcome.[23] Another study of medical care effectiveness confirmed improved infant outcomes with increased utilization of medical care between 1969 and 1978.[34]

A review of the available literature on the effectiveness of child health care by

Shadish found that among 38 controlled studies, a clear positive effect was demonstrated in 19, mixed effects in 15, and no effect in only 4 studies.[105] Starfield has reviewed the evidence for the effectiveness of medical care for children.[109] Analyses of national data indicate that the availability of legal abortion, family planning services, and Medicaid coverage of prenatal care also are related to improved birth outcome. Postneonatal mortality rates underwent an abrupt and large decline associated with the War on Poverty programs of the mid-1960s, in part due to improved access to medical services.[109] Similarly, programs oriented toward adolescents, including family planning and abortion services, have been associated with substantial decreases in teenage fertility rates. Furthermore, preventive and therapeutic medical care has been shown to be effective in preventing the occurrence, or ameliorating the effects, of many child health problems, including anemia, lead poisoning, primary and recurrent acute rheumatic fever, diabetes, seizure disorder, bacterial meningitis, appendicitis, and asthma.[109, 127]

LIMITING POVERTY'S IMPACT: ASSURING ACCESS TO CARE

Medicaid

The single most important health program for low-income children is Medicaid.[10] It accounts for over 55 per cent of all public expenditures for child health, 26 per cent of all (public and private) hospital payments for children under age 6 years, 30 per cent of all payments for hospital deliveries of teenage mothers, and 10 per cent of all payments for pediatric ambulatory care.[16] In 1984, Medicaid served some 10.5 million children,[16] or 16 per cent of the total child population.[14]

Medicaid was created in 1966 as a joint federal–state grant-in-aid program under the Title XIX amendment to the Social Security Act, with the goal of removing the financial barriers that stood between low-income people and appropriate medical care. In 1967, Congress amended the program to include early and periodic screening, diagnosis, and treatment (EPSDT), which finances a broad range of primary and preventive services. EPSDT provides for screening, assessment, and comprehensive care of pediatric medical, dental, developmental, and sensory disorders, and mandates outreach activities to reach the population in need.

Medicaid funds provide reimbursement for care delivered to eligible children; individual state Medicaid agencies administer the program, and determine, with substantial flexibility, eligibility criteria and reimbursement rates. Although certain basic services are mandated, states may choose to limit their scope and duration.[10] The major test by which the states determine Medicaid eligibility is the Aid to Families with Dependent Children (AFDC) program.[100] However, because of the flexibility with which the individual states determine financial eligibility for AFDC, eligibility for Medicaid varies greatly from state to state. For example, in 1985 a family of three living in Alaska qualified for Medicaid at or below a monthly income of $719 (97 per cent of the federal poverty level), while in Alabama or Mississippi, the same family would qualify only at incomes of $120 or less (16 per cent of the poverty level).[100] For the 50 states, the median eligibility is 45 per cent of the federal poverty level. At their discretion, states also may extend Medicaid to children and pregnant women with incomes of 100 to 133 per cent of the states' AFDC payment level. At present, only 36 states do so.[100]

There is no doubt that the Medicaid program has improved access to medical care for poor children.[20, 21, 99, 110] In one study, the proportion of poor children who had not seen a physician in the year prior to Medicaid declined from 33.2 per cent to 18.7 per cent after the institution of Medicaid. This compared with a decline from 15 per cent to 12 per cent for nonpoor children.[124] Average annual number of physician visits rose from 2.3 to 3.8 for poor children, an increase of 65 per cent, whereas for nonpoor children it rose from 4.0 to 4.3, a 7 per cent increase. Findings of local studies are consistent with these national data. The EPSDT program has been shown to be effective in its goal of improving the health status of low-income children by screening, identification, and followup care of potential health problems.[41, 44]

Despite this positive record, changes in government funding of AFDC during the 1980s have had a dramatic impact on Medicaid's availability to poor children. The income level at which a poor family qualifies for AFDC has decreased significantly during this decade, resulting in an estimated half-million families losing their AFDC benefits. In 1985, only 51 per cent of children living in families below the federal poverty standard report Medicaid coverage, compared to a high of 83.6 per cent in 1973.[11, 12] Among children of near-poor families (100–125 per cent of the poverty line), only 13 per cent receive Medicaid benefits.[11, 12]

In addition to its failure to cover all children in need, there have been other shortcomings of the Medicaid program. Due to frequent changes in program regulations and families' status, many children on Medicaid do not receive consistent coverage; in 1980, one third of all children on Medicaid were not covered for the entire year.[80] Medicaid also was intended to "provide the poor with the same access as the rich to mainstream medical care," in the words of the enabling legislation.[80] Evidence suggests that this goal has not been achieved. Low-income children are less likely to use private practitioners or group practices than are high-income children.[50] One detailed study showed that a greater percentage of children covered by Medicaid did not identify a physician as a regular source of care than did those not on Medicaid, and fewer Medicaid children had pediatricians as their regular source of care.[30] In addition, the disparity in physician use between white and minority children with Medicaid coverage persists.[20]

Children Without Medical Insurance

Data from the Current Population Survey of the U.S. Bureau of the Census show that in 1985, 17 per cent of the population under age 65 years—nearly 37 million people—lacked any insurance for medical care, public or private.[17] There has been an increase of nearly 15 per cent in the number of people in civilian, nonagricultural families without health insurance since 1982.[17] During this period, coverage has declined most rapidly for children and employed adults (see Fig. 2). One third of the uninsured are children; nearly 20 per cent of all children under age 18 years had no health insurance coverage from any source in 1985, an increase of 1.5 million, or 15.6 per cent, since 1982. Two thirds of uninsured adults are employed.[17]

Among uninsured children, 38.9 per cent live below the federal poverty line, 10.2 per cent live at 100 to 124 per cent of poverty, and 22.2 per cent live at 125 to 199 per cent of poverty. Those most likely to lack health insurance are the children of the working poor: two thirds of uninsured children live in families headed by a worker; roughly half these families are single-parent households. The proportion of children covered by employer-based health plans declined from 64.3 per cent in 1982 to 61.9 per cent in 1985, and that covered by private health insurance fell from 9 to 7 per cent. In fact, in 1985, nearly 20 per cent of uninsured children lived with a working, insured parent whose employer-based health insurance did not extend to the child. Thus, the growth in the number and proportion of uninsured children is probably due to the rising rates of children in poverty, the rising cost of health insurance, and the erosion of Medicaid coverage among the poor.[17]

Butler et al. have shown that for 1980, 22 per cent of sampled children lacked health insurance for the full year, 14 per cent were covered for only part of the

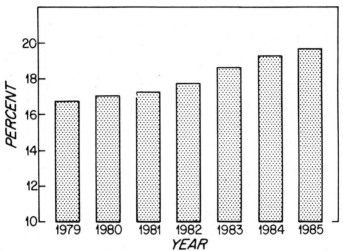

Figure 2. Percentage of Children (18 years of Age) without Health Insurance: United States 1979 Through 1985. U.S. Bureau of the Census. Current Population Reports. Series P-70, No. 8. Disability, function limitation, and health insurance coverage: 1984/85. Washington, D.C., U.S. Government Printing Office, 1986.

year, and 8 per cent had no coverage at all.[14] The children most likely to be without full-year coverage were the near-poor (36.7 per cent), poor (33.1 per cent), Hispanic/Latino (31.1 per cent), and black (26 per cent). The youngest children (0–2 years) were the age group most likely to lack full-year coverage (26.4 per cent). In addition, health insurance coverage appears to be little better among children with disabilities, with approximately 11 per cent lacking coverage. However, special-needs children in one study were more likely to be uninsured if they were low income or Hispanic.[13]

Persistent Disparities in Health Care Utilization

There can be little question that Medicaid has played a profound role in improving the health care of poor children. However, given the lack of health care insurance among poor children and the limitations of care for those with Medicaid coverage, it is not surprising that the disparity in access to medical care between poor and nonpoor children persists 20 years after the enactment of Medicaid.[110] One third of poor children surveyed by the Robert Wood Johnson Foundation in its National Access to Health Care Survey in 1986 had no ambulatory visit in the prior year, a rate 40 per cent higher than that for nonpoor children. Fifteen per cent of poor children had no regular source of care, twice the rate of their nonpoor counterparts.[95] Moreover, within the same income strata, black children had 23 per cent fewer visits than did white children. When children of comparable need for medical care are compared, these differences increase: poor children reported to be in fair or poor health have 47 per cent fewer visits to a physician than high-income children, and black children have 38 per cent fewer visits than white children at each income level.[95] National data suggest this pattern of inequity persists.[76, 77] Medicaid coverage nearly eliminates this inequity, but 56 per cent of low-income children in fair or poor health, and 58 per cent of those with chronic activity limitations, lack Medicaid coverage.[76, 77]

National data suggest a relationship between health insurance coverage and health care utilization. Among uninsured children, 17 per cent lacked a regular source of pediatric care, compared to 10 per cent of those with full-year public insurance and 5 per cent of those with full-year private insurance.[14] Among poor children, the uninsured had 38 per cent fewer medical care visits than those with insurance, and children less than 2 years of age were almost 2.5 times more likely to have gone without a medical visit if they had no coverage. These disparities may be magnified for some subpopulations. In one survey of five metropolitan areas, only 20 per cent of uninsured Hispanic children with disabilities had seen a physician in the prior year, compared to 58 per cent of those with insurance.[13] In fact, the effect of health insurance on use was seen within all demographic subgroups of disabled children, and within all access patterns. In this study, having health insurance and a regular source of care both exerted an independent effect on the likelihood of a disabled child seeing a physician; taken together, the disabled child with all of these elements of health care access was nine times more likely to have seen a physician in the prior year than the disabled child with none.[13]

In addition to suffering poorer health and less access to health care, low-income families bear a greater burden of the direct costs of health care for their children. Newacheck and Halfon found that families living below the poverty line without full-year Medicaid coverage incurred out-of-pocket expenses for child health care that were 15 times higher (as a percentage of family income) than that of poor families with Medicaid coverage, and more than 10 times the relative expenditures of families living at three times the poverty level. These survey data also showed that 19 per cent of poor families, and 36 per cent of the near-poor, paid out-of-pocket expenses for all the care their children received.[76, 77]

CONFRONTING SOCIAL DISPARITIES IN CHILD HEALTH: THE ROLE OF THE CLINICIAN

Ultimately, it is the clinician who provides health services to poor children. However, the needs of these children can never fully be met by clinical management alone. In this setting, the role of the clinician is defined by the dual appreciation of medicine's efficacy and its inherent limitations. The emphasis of one to the exclusion of the other can be problematic. A total dependence on the provision of direct clinical service will not address the larger social forces that shape clinical need. Rejecting the importance of clinical contributions could preclude their many ameliorative effects and undermine efforts to bring about greater equity to their effective availability.

Alternatively, three related avenues for clinician activity are required. First, and perhaps most fundamental, is the provision of care to all children in need. This involves the effort to ensure access to all relevant clinical services. Given the many barriers to the clinician's ability to provide such access, this may involve advocating for improvements in the content or administration of public programs for poor children. It also may involve the refinement of clinical practices to meet the specific health problems of poor children in local communities. Community-based epidemiology and structured needs assessments may prove useful in this regard.

A second area of clinician involvement lies in the shaping of local, community-based programs. The clinician can play a powerful role as a local advocate, conveying both the purpose and expertise needed to assure the success of community-based programs. The power of local efforts to confront serious health problems is often underestimated.

The third arena of involvement is the need to address the primary determinants of childhood poverty. The successful implementation of public policies designed to reduce the number of children living in poverty will require the expertise, political strength, and energy of the pediatric community. It is likely that present social welfare policies affecting children will undergo considerable change in the near future. Undoubtedly, the development of these new policies will stimulate considerable controversy and national debate. In this setting, the challenge lies in ensuring that these emerging policies reflect faithfully the experience and concern of all those who directly care for children. For in the end, it will be these practitioners who inherit the clinical legacy of yet another generation shaped by the tragic sequelae of preventable illness and profound social injustice.

REFERENCES

1. Alan Guttmacher Institute: Blessed Events and the Bottom Line: Financing Maternity Care in the United States. New York, Alan Guttmacher Institute, 1987
2. Amler RW, Dull BH: Closing the Gap: The Burden of Unnecessary Illness. New York, Oxford University Press, 1987
3. Antonovsky A, Bernstein J: Social class and infant mortality. Soc Sci Med 11:453–470, 1977
4. Baker SP, O'Neill B, Karpf R: Burns and fire deaths in The Injury Fact Book. Lexington, Massachusetts, Lexington Books, 1984, pp 139–154
5. Bass M, Kravath RE, Glass L: Death-scene investigation in sudden infant death. N Engl J Med 315:100–105, 1986
6. Binkin NJ, Williams RL, Hogue CJR et al: Reducing black neonatal mortality: Will improvement in birthweight be enough? JAMA 253:372–375, 1985
7. Black L, David RJ, Brouilette RT et al: Effects of birth weight and ethnicity on incidence of sudden infant death syndrome. J Pediatr 108:209–214, 1986
8. Bluestone CD, Shurin PA: Middle ear disease in children: Pathogenesis, diagnosis and management. Pediatr Clin North Am 21:379, 1974
9. Brady J: Arson, urban economy, and organized crime: The case of Boston. Soc Problems 31:1–27, 1983
10. Budetti PP, Butler J, McManus P: Federal health program reforms: Implications for child health care. Milbank Mem Fund Q 60:155–181, 1982
11. Bureau of the Census. Current Population Reports. Series P-60. U.S. Department of Commerce. Washington, D.C., U.S. Government Printing Office, 1987
12. Bureau of the Census. Receipt of Selected Non-cash Benefits. Series P-60. U.S. Department of Commerce. Washington, D.C., U.S. Government Printing Office, 1986
13. Butler JA, Singer JD, Palfrey JS et al: Health insurance coverage and physician use among children with disabilities: Findings from probability samples in five metropolitan areas. Pediatrics 79:89–98, 1987
14. Butler JA, Winter ED, Singer JD et al: Medical care use and expenditure among children and youth in the United States: Analysis of a national probability sample. Pediatrics 76:495–507, 1985
15. Children's deaths in Maine: 1976–1980. Augusta, Maine Department of Human Services, 1983
16. Children's Defense Fund. A Children's Defense Budget: An Analysis of the FY1987 Budget and Children. Washington, D.C., Children's Defense Fund, 1986
17. Chollet DF: Uninsured in the United States: The Nonelderly Population Without Health Insurance. Washington, D.C., Employee Benefit Research Institute, 1987
18. Christoffel K: Homicide in childhood: A public health problem in need of attention. Am J Public Health 74:68–70, 1984
19. Colangelo AL, Vento TB, Taeusch HW: Discharge planning. In Taeusch HW, Yogman MW (eds): Follow-up Management of the High-Risk Infant. Boston, Little, Brown & Co., 1987
20. Davis K, Gold M, Makuc D: Access to health care for the poor: Does the gap remain? Ann Rev Public Health 2:159–182, 1981
21. Donabedian A: Effects of Medicare and Medicaid on access to and quality of health care. Public Health Rep 91:322–331, 1976
22. Dutton DB, Silber RS: Children's health outcomes in six different ambulatory care delivery systems. Med Care 18:693–714, 1981
23. Dutton DB: Socioeconomic status and children's health. Med Care 23:142–154, 1985

24. Egbuonu L, Starfield B: Child health and social status. Pediatrics 69:550–557, 1982
25. Embry D, Malletti S: Safe playing. Falls Church, VA, AAA Foundation for Traffic Safety, 1982
26. Escalona SK: Babies at double hazard: Early development of infants at biologic and social risk. Pediatrics 70:670–676, 1982
27. Fell JC: Alcohol involvement in traffic accidents: Recent estimates from the National Center for Statistics and Analysis. Report DOT HS 806 265. Springfield, VA, NHTSA, 1982
28. Fitzhardinge PM: Follow-up studies of the low birth weight infant. Clin Perinatol 3:503–516, 1976
29. Fitzhardinge PM, Steven EM: The small-for-date infant. II. Neurologic and intellectual sequelae. Pediatrics 50:50–57, 1972
30. Gortmaker SL: Medicaid and the health care of children in poverty and near poverty: Some successes and failures. Med Care 19:567–582, 1981
31. Gortmaker SL: Poverty and infant mortality in the United States. Am Sociol Rev 44:280–297, 1979
32. Graham PJ, Rutter ML, Yule M et al: Childhood asthma: A psychosomatic disorder? Br J Prev Soc Med 21:78–94, 1967
33. Hack M, Fanaroff AA, Merkatz IR: The low birth-weight infant—evolution of a changing outlook. N Engl J Med 301:1162–1165, 1979
34. Hadley J: More Medical Care, Better Health? An Economic Analysis of Mortality Rates. Washington, D.C., The Urban Institute Press, 1982
35. Haggerty RJ: The Rand Health Insurance Experiment for children. Pediatrics 75:969–971, 1985
36. Harvey D, Prince J, Bunton J, Parkinson C et al: Abilities of children who were small-for-gestational-age babies. Pediatrics 69:296–300, 1982
37. Hemminki E, Starfield B: Prevention of low birth weight and pre-term birth. Milbank Mem Fund Q 56:339–361, 1978
38. Hingson R, Alpert JJ, Day N et al: Effects on maternal drinking and marijuana use on fetal growth and development. Pediatrics 70:539–546, 1982
39. Holm VA, Kunze LH: Effect of chronic otitis media on language and speech development. Pediatrics 43:833, 1969
40. Institute of Medicine. Preventing Low Birthweight. Washington, D.C., National Academy Press, 1985
41. Irwin PH, Conroy-Hughes, R: EPSDT impact on health status: Estimates based on secondary analysis of administratively generated data. Med Care 20:216–234, 1982
42. Jason J: Child Homicide Spectrum. Am J Dis Child 137:578–581, 1983
43. Kaltreider DF, Kohl S: Epidemiology of preterm delivery. Clin Obstet Gynecol 23:27–31, 1980
44. Keller WJ: Study of selected outcomes of the Early and Periodic Screening, Diagnosis, and Treatment Program in Michigan. Public Health Rep 98:110–119, 1983
45. Kelly J, O'Conner M: Smoking in pregnancy: Effects on mother and fetus. Br J Obstet Gynecol 91:111–117, 1984
46. Kessner D: Infant death: An Analysis by Maternal Risk and Health Care. Washington, D.C., Institute of Medicine, 1973
47. Khoury MJ, Erickson JD, Adams MJ: Trends in postneonatal mortality in the United States: 1962 through 1978. JAMA 252:367–372, 1984
48. Kleinman JC, Kessel SS: Racial differences in low birth weight: Trends and risk factors. N Engl J Med 317:749–754, 1987
49. La Pointe N, Michaud J, Perkovic D et al: Trans-placental transmission of HTLV-III virus. N Engl J Med 312:1325–1326, 1985
50. Ladenheim KE, Wilensky G: Trends in the number and characteristics of the uninsured. Presented at the American Public Health Association Annual Meeting, New Orleans, October, 1987
51. Landesman S, Minkoff H, Holman S et al: Serosurvey of human immunodeficiency virus infection in parturients. JAMA 258:2701–2703, 1987
52. Lieberman E, Ryan KJ, Monson RR et al: Risk factors accounting for racial differences in the rate of premature birth. N Engl J Med 317:743–748, 1987
53. Los Angeles Times, May 14, 1987
54. Main DM, Richardson D, Gable S et al: Prospective evaluation of a risk scoring system

for predicting preterm births in indigent inner city women. Am J Obstet Gynecol 153:562–568, 1986

55. Mare RD: Socioeconomic effects on child mortality in the United States. Am J Public Health 72:539–547, 1982

56. McCormick MC: The contribution of low birthweight to infant mortality and childhood morbidity. N Engl J Med 312:81–90, 1985

57. McDonald P, Alexander D, Catz C, Edelman R: Summary of a workshop on maternal genitourinary infections and the outcome of pregnancy. J Infect Dis 147:596–605, 1983

58. McLoughlin E, Crawford JD: Burns. Pediatr Clin North Am 32:61–76, 1985

59. McNichol KN, Williams HE, Allan J, et al: Spectrum of asthma in children III: Psychological and social components. Br Med J 4:16–25, 1973

60. Mierley MC, Baker SP: Fatal house fires in an urban population. JAMA 249:1466–1468, 1983

61. Mitchell RG, Dawson B: Educational and social characteristics of children with asthma. Arch Dis Child 48:467, 1973

62. Morgan MC, Wingard DL, Felice ME: Subcultural differences in alcohol use among youth. J Adolesc Health Care 5:191–195, 1984

63. Moyer CA: The sociologic aspects of trauma. Am J Surg 87:421–430, 1954

64. Moynihan P: The Negro Family: The Case for National Action. Washington, D.C., Office of Policy Planning and Research, U.S. Department of Labor, 1965

65. Muhlin GL: Ethnic differences in alcohol misuse: A striking reaffirmation. J Stud Alcohol 46:172–173, 1985

66. Murray C: Losing ground: American social policy, 1950–1980. New York, Basic Books, 1984

67. National Center for Health Statistics: Binocular Visual Acuity of Children: Demographic and Socioeconomic Characteristics, United States. DHEW Pub. No. (HSM) 72–1031. (Vital and health statistics. Series 11: Data from National Health Survey, No. 112.) Rockville, Maryland, National Center for Health Statistics, 1972

68. National Center for Health Statistics: Examination and Health History Findings among Children and Youths 6–17 Years, United States. DHEW Pub. No. (HRA) 74–1611. (Vital and health statistics. Series 11: Data from National Health Survey, No. 129.) Rockville, Maryland, National Center for Health Statistics, 1975, pp 17, 50–51

69. National Center for Health Statistics: Health: United States, 1985. Rockville, Maryland, National Center for Health Statistics, 1986

70. National Center for Health Statistics: Hearing Levels of Children by Demographic and Socioeconomic Characteristics, United States. DHEW Pub. No. (HSM) 72–1025. (Vital and health statistics. Series 11: Data from National Health Survey, No. 111.) Rockville, MD, National Center for Health Statistics, 1972, p 9

71. National Center for Health Statistics: Hearing Levels of Youths 12–17 Years, United States. DHEW Pub. No. (HRA) 75–1627. (Vital and health statistics. Series 11: Data from the National Health Survey, No. 145.) Rockville, Maryland, National Center for Health Statistics, 1975, p 17

72. National Center for Health Statistics: Monocular Visual Acuity of Persons 4–74 Years, United States 1971–72. DHEW Pub. No. (HRA) 77–1646. (Vital and health statistics. Series 11: Data from National Health Survey, No. 201.) Rockville, Maryland, National Center for Health Statistics, 1977, p 43

73. National Center for Health Statistics: Visual Acuity of Youths 12–17 Years, United States. DHEW Pub. No. (HSM) 73–1609. (Vital and health statistics. Series 11: Data from National Health Survey, No. 127.) Rockville, Maryland, National Center for Health Statistics, 1973, pp 18–19

74. National Center for Health Statistics: Vital Statistics Reports. Rockville, Maryland, National Center for Health Statistics, 1987

75. National Safety Council: Accident Facts, 1985. Chicago, National Safety Council, 1987

76. Newacheck PW, Halfon N: Access to ambulatory care services for economically disadvantaged children. Pediatrics 78:813–819, 1986

77. Newacheck PW, Halfon N: The financial burden of medical care expenses for children. Med Care 24:1110–1117, 1986

78. Newberger CM, Newberger EH: The etiology of child abuse. In Ellerstein NS (ed): Child Abuse and Neglect. New York, John Wiley & Sons, 1981

79. Organization for Economic Cooperation and Development: Traffic Safety of Children. Paris, 1983
80. Orr ST, Miller CA: Utilization of health services by poor children since advent of Medicaid. Med Care 19:583–590, 1981
81. Palfrey JS, Hansen MA, Pleszczynska C et al: Selective hearing screening for young children. Clin Pediatr 19:725, 1979
82. Paneth N, Kiely JL, Wallenstein S et al: Newborn intensive care and neonatal mortality in low-birthweight infants: A population study. N Engl J Med 307:149–155, 1982
83. Paneth N, Wallenstein S, Kiely JL et al: Social class indicators and mortality of low birthweight infants. Am J Epidemiol 116:364–375, 1982
84. Paradise JL: Otitis media in infants and children. Pediatrics 65:917, 1980
85. Paulson JA, Rushforth NB: Violent death in children in a metropolitan country: Changing patterns of homicide, 1958 to 1982. Pediatrics 78:1013–1020, 1986
86. Peckham C, Butler N: A national study of asthma in childhood. J Epidemiol Comm Health 32:79–86, 1978
87. Pharoah POD, Morris JN: Postneonatal mortality. Epidemiol Rev 1:178–183, 1979
88. Poland RL, Bollinger RO, Bedard MP et al: Analysis of the effects of applying federal diagnosis-related grouping (DRG) guidelines to a population of high-risk newborn infants. Pediatrics 76:104–109, 1985
89. Preston SH: Children and the elderly: Divergent paths for America's dependents. Demography 21:435–457, 1984
90. Pyun KH, Ochs HD, Dufford MTW et al: Perinatal infection with human immunodeficiency virus. N Engl J Med 317:611–614, 1987
91. Quah R, Stark A, Meigs JW: Children blood lead levels in New Haven: A population-based demographic profile. Environ Health Perspect 5:128–134, 1982
92. Ramey CT, Stedman DJ, Borders-Patterson A et al: Predicting school failure from information available at birth. Am J Ment Defic 82:525–534, 1978
93. Resnick PJ: Child murder by parents: A psychiatric review of felicide. Am J Psychiatry 126:325–334, 1969
94. Richmond JB, Kotelchuck M: Personal health maintenance for children. West J Med 141:816–823, 1984
95. Robert Wood Johnson Foundation: Access to Health Care in the United States: Results of a 1986 Survey. Princeton, New Jersey, Robert Wood Johnson Foundation, 1987
96. Robertson LS: Motor vehicles. Pediatr Clin North Am 2:87–94, 1985
97. Robertson LS, Kosa J, Heagarty M et al: Changing the Medical Care System: A Controlled Experiment in Comprehensive Care. New York, Praeger, 1974
98. Rivara FP: Demographic analysis of childhood pedestrian injuries. Pediatrics 76:375–381, 1985
99. Rogers DE, Blendon RJ, Moloney TW: Who needs Medicaid? N Engl J Med 307:13–18, 1982
100. Rosenbaum S, Johnson K: Providing health care for low-income children: Reconciling child health goals with child health financing realties. Milbank Mem Fund Q 64:442–478, 1986
101. Rudov MH, Santangelo N: Health Status of Minorities and Low Income Groups. DHEW Pub. No. (HRA) 77–628. Washington, D.C., U.S. Government Printing Office, 1977
102. Sabel KG, Olegard R, Victoria L: Remaining sequelae with modern perinatal care. Pediatrics 57:652–658, 1976
103. Scott A, Moar V, Ounsted M: The relative contribution of different maternal factors in small-for-gestational-age pregnancies. Eur J Obstet Gynecol Reprod Biol 12:157–265, 1981
104. Senate Special Committee on Aging. Home Fire Deaths: A Preventable Tragedy. Hearings before the Special Committee on Aging. Washington, D.C., 1983
105. Shadish WR: A review and critique of controlled studies on the effectiveness of preventive child health care. Health Policy Q 2:24, 1982
106. Shapiro S, Schlesinger ER, Nesbitt REL Jr: Infant, perinatal, maternal, and childhood mortality in the United States. Cambridge, MA, Harvard University Press, 1986
107. Sher K, Coil J: Appendicitis: Factors that influence the frequency of perforation. South Med J 73:1561–1563, 1980
108. Sondels S: Young children in traffic. Br J Educ Psychol 40:111–115, 1970

109. Starfield B: The Effectiveness of Medical Care: Validating Clinical Wisdom. Baltimore, Maryland, The Johns Hopkins University Press, 1985
110. Starfield B: Family income, ill health, and medical care of U.S. children. J Pub Health Policy 3:244–259, 1982
111. Starfield B, Budetti PP: Child health status and risk factors. Health Services Res 19:817–886, 1985
112. Starfield B, Dutton D: Care, costs and health: Reactions to and reinterpretations of the Rand findings. Pediatrics 76:614–621, 1985
113. Stein Z, Kline J: Smoking, alcohol, and reproduction. Am J Public Health 73:1154–1156, 1983
114. Stewart A, Turcaro D, Rawlings S et al: Outcome for infants at high risk of major handicap. In Major Mental Handicap: Methods and Costs of Prevention, CIBA Foundation Symposium 59. Amsterdam, Elsevier/North Holland, 1973
115. Stockwell EG: Infant mortality and socioeconomic status: A changing relationship. Milbank Mem Fund Q 40:101–111, 1962
116. U.S. Bureau of the Census: Current Population Reports. Series P-70, No. 8. Disability, function limitation, and health insurance coverage: 1984/85. Washington, D.C., U.S. Government Printing Office, 1986
117. U.S. Bureau of the Census: Money, Income and Poverty Status of Families and Persons in the U.S. Series P-60. U.S. Department of Commerce. Washington, D.C., U.S. Government Printing Office, 1987
118. U.S. Congress: Office of Technology Assessment. Neonatal Intensive Care for Low Birthweight Infants: Costs and Effectiveness. Washington, D.C., U.S. Congress, 1987
119. U.S. Department of Health, Education and Welfare: Infant Mortality Rate: Socioeconomic Factors. Vital and Health Statistics, Series 22, No. 14. Washington, D.C., U.S. Government Printing Office, 1972
120. U.S. General Accounting Office: Prenatal Care: Medicaid Recipients and Uninsured Women Obtain Insufficient Care. Washington, D.C., U.S. Government Printing Office, 1987
121. U.S. House of Representatives: Children in Poverty. U.S. Congress. Washington, D.C., U.S. Government Printing Office, 1985
122. Valdez RB, Brook RH, Rogers WH et al: Consequences of cost-sharing for children's health. Pediatrics 75:952–961, 1985
123. Williams RL, Chen DM: Identifying the sources of the recent decline in perinatal mortality rates in California. N Engl J Med 306:207–214, 1982
124. Wilson RW, White EL: Changes in morbidity, disability, and utilization differentials between the poor and nonpoor: Data from the Health Interview Survey: 1964 and 1973. Med Care 15:636–646, 1977
125. Wilson WJ: The truly disadvantaged. Chicago, The University of Chicago Press, 1987
126. Wise PH, First LR, Kotelchuck M et al: An increase in infant mortality despite high access to tertiary care. Pediatrics (in press)
127. Wise PH, Kotelchuck M, Wilson ML et al: Racial and socioeconomic disparities in childhood mortality in Boston. N Engl J Med 313:360–366, 1985
128. Wise PH, Richmond JB: Preventive services in maternal and child health. In Wallace H (ed): Maternal and Child Health Practices. Third Edition. Oakland, Third Party Publishing Company (in press)
129. Yip R, Binkin NJ, Fleshood L, et al: Declining prevalence of anemia among low-income children in the United States. JAMA 258:1619–1623, 1987

Division of Health Policy, Research, and Education
Harvard University
641 Huntington Avenue
Boston, Massachusetts 02115

0031-3955/88 $0.00 + .20

Failure to Thrive

Deborah A. Frank, MD, and Steven H. Zeisel, MD, PhD†*

Failure to thrive in infancy and early childhood challenges the diagnostic and therapeutic skills of the most experienced pediatrician. In broadest terms, failure to thrive refers to infants and children whose growth deviates from the norms for their age and sex. Berwick reported that failure to thrive accounts for 3 to 5 per cent of admissions to academic pediatric hospitals.[14] In outpatient settings, growth failure is even more common. Several surveys of low-income children in primary care suggest that nearly 10 per cent show weight or length below the fifth percentile for age.[85, 101, 144] Clinical audits in inner city emergency departments reveal a 15 to 30 per cent rate of growth deficits among young children brought in for acute care.[19, 89, 108] This common condition is of great concern to clinicians because failure to thrive in early life identifies children who are at high risk for lasting deficits in growth, cognition, and socioemotional functioning.[14, 38, 41, 63, 105-107, 130] While pediatricians have struggled to care for children who fail to thrive for nearly a century,[64] the past decade has witnessed a number of theoretical and practical advances in diagnosis and treatment.

Traditionally, the causes of failure to thrive were dichotomized as organic or nonorganic. *Organic* failure to thrive was ascribed to a major illness or organ system dysfunction, thought to be sufficient to account for growth failure. In contrast, *nonorganic* failure to thrive was attributed to "maternal deprivation," an insufficiently nurturing environment in home or institution.[20, 30, 109, 139] It was thought that "anaclitic depression"[139] and psychosocial stress created neuroendocrine disturbances that accounted for growth failure, despite adequate food intake.[119] In 1981, Homer and Ludwig suggested a third category based on the recognition that in many cases of failure to thrive the effects of organic disease were compounded by psychosocial difficulties.[75] Subsequent writers have termed this *mixed* failure to thrive.[21]

Theoretic advances in pediatrics and child development have recently transformed the conceptualization of failure to thrive and made the traditional classification scheme obsolete. Pediatricians now realize that in all cases of nonorganic failure to thrive and in many cases of organic failure to thrive, the primary biologic insult is malnutrition.[17, 21, 53, 64, 136, 150] Thus, all children with nonorganic failure to thrive suffer from a serious organic insult: primary malnutrition.[17] Moreover, for

*Assistant Professor of Pediatrics and Public Health, Boston University Schools of Medicine and Public Health; Director, Failure to Thrive Program, Division of Developmental and Behavioral Pediatrics, Boston City Hospital, Boston, Massachusetts

†Associate Professor of Pathology and Pediatrics, Nutrient Metabolism Laboratory, Boston University School of Medicine and Boston City Hospital, Boston, Massachusetts

many children with serious medical illnesses associated with failure to thrive (e.g., congenital heart disease, cerebral palsy, gastrointestinal disorders),[15, 42, 70, 124, 134] malnutrition secondary to the disease is a major cause of growth failure.[78] Malnutrition, whether primary or secondary, not only impairs growth and health but contributes to disordered behavior and development both at the time of acute malnutrition and in later life.[4, 9, 26, 28, 34, 54, 58–63, 76, 141] Therefore, the therapeutic and diagnostic focus in medical management of failure to thrive has shifted from detection of occult disease to assessment and treatment of malnutrition and its complications, using techniques initially evolved for treating malnourished children in the developing world.[112, 122, 152]

At the same time that malnutrition was identified as the critical biologic factor in most cases of failure to thrive, a transactional model of infant development[127] superseded the simplistic concept of "maternal deprivation" as a framework for understanding the psychosocial correlates and socioemotional consequences of failure to thrive.[17, 21, 122] The transactional model of failure to thrive suggests that the quality of parental care reflects not only individual psychodynamics, but also the ecological conditions impinging on the family. These conditions include economic forces,[55, 80] social networks,[2, 104] and health beliefs.[120] Parents may have difficulty meeting the needs of some children and not others, depending on their own history of nurturance as children and the current stresses in their lives.

Moreover, the transactional model[127] recognizes that the quality of the parent–child relationship reflects characteristics of the child as well as the parent. Not all children effectively elicit parental care. Children who become malnourished may be difficult to nurture for many reasons, including temperamental characteristics, disorganized behavioral responses associated with prematurity or intrauterine growth retardation, or underlying illnesses or handicaps that make them burdensome to caretakers.[3, 17, 122, 126] Undemanding infants who are breastfed are at particular risk, since mothers may not offer them the breast often enough for adequate growth.[126] Once malnutrition occurs, the lethargy and irritability typical of the malnourished child may further compound the interactive breakdown between parent and child.[23, 28, 54, 56, 118] Stresses in the caretaking environment and the parent–child relationship create the context in which malnutrition leading to failure to thrive occurs and exacerbate the developmental and behavioral effects of malnutrition.

Rather than attempting to diagnose each case of failure to thrive as organic or nonorganic, current practice is to evaluate the diagnostic and therapeutic implications of nutritional, medical, psychosocial, and developmental factors.[122] To address effectively the complex interaction of these factors, a multidisciplinary team approach is recommended.[1, 13, 17, 24, 112, 122] Such a team typically consists of a pediatrician, a social worker, a nurse, and a nutritionist, with consultation as needed from specialists such as mental health professionals and physical and occupational therapists. Team management usually involves consultation to inpatient services, close outpatient followup, and home visits.

While the efficacy of multidisciplinary team treatment has not been established in controlled trials, uncontrolled studies have found improved growth within a year of diagnosis in roughly 50 per cent of treated patients and stabilization of growth in another 40 per cent.[24, 85] Ten per cent of children deteriorate despite multidisciplinary treatment.

In clinical settings, nutritional, medical, psychosocial, and developmental issues must be handled simultaneously in the care of children with failure to thrive. Current thinking about the management of each area will now be discussed.

NUTRITIONAL FACTORS

In management of failure to thrive, three nutritional issues must be considered: (1) interpretation of anthropometric assessments; (2) evaluation of dietary intake; and (3) nutritional rehabilitation for catch-up growth (Table 1).

Table 1. *Nutritional Management*

Anthropometric evaluation
Dietary assessment
1.5 to 2 times RDA of calories and protein for catch-up growth
Multivitamin supplement with iron and zinc

DIAGNOSTIC AND THERAPEUTIC IMPLICATIONS OF ANTHROPOMETRIC ASSESSMENTS

Historically, the label of failure to thrive implied not only growth deficit, but disordered behavior and development as well.[125, 150] Recently, a consensus has emerged that failure to thrive should be diagnosed on the basis of anthropometric criteria alone.[36] Protocols for obtaining accurate and reproducible anthropometric measurements have been well described and will not be repeated here.[17, 122, 154]

While anthropometric evaluation is the cornerstone of diagnosing failure to thrive, there are no universally accepted anthropometric diagnostic criteria for either clinical or research purposes. Two types of criteria are used in the literature: those based on growth velocity and those based on attained growth below a specified percentile on a growth grid. Within these categories, the severity of growth failure required for diagnosis varies considerably. Published velocity criteria differ in the period beyond which a depressed rate of weight gain is considered failure to thrive. They vary from 10 or more days,[147] to 56 days for children under 5 months of age,[50] or 90 days for children over 5 months of age.[50] The crossing of two major percentiles on a growth grid over any period is also used as a velocity criterion of failure to thrive.[17] Velocity criteria are clinically useful in primary care settings where serial measurements are available. Documented weight loss over time is an even clearer indicator of pathology because normally there is steady incremental growth of weight from infancy to adulthood.

Common criteria for attained growth are also variable, from weight below the tenth percentile for age[107] to height and weight below the third percentile for age.[41]

When attained growth criteria are selected for the diagnosis of failure to thrive, the relationship of weight and height to standard norms and to each other may be used to identify the chronicity of nutritional deficit and growth failure. By international consensus, the National Center for Health Statistics (NCHS) growth charts are used to evaluate the growth of children regardless of ethnic or racial background.[69, 153] Weight for age represents a composite measure of past and present nutrition and growth, reflecting both current and previous insults.[82] Although weight fluctuates with short-term changes in nutritional status, height does not. Height does not decrease with nutritional deprivation but fails to increase once the period of deprivation has extended to weeks and months. Thus, when genetic and constitutional causes can be ruled out, depressed height for age is considered evidence of chronic malnutrition.[148] In contrast, depressed weight for height indicates acute and recent nutritional deprivation.[148] A recent review of children referred for tertiary care for failure to thrive found that 95 per cent showed depressed weight for age and 64 per cent showed depressed height for age, while 68 per cent showed depressed weight for height.[111] Children at highest risk are those for whom both weight for height and height for age are deficient, indicating acute malnutrition superimposed upon chronic.[148]

Because by definition most children identified as having failure to thrive have weights or heights at or below the lower percentiles on the NCHS charts, additional calculations are necessary to determine the severity of nutritional risk as a guide to clinical care. Categorizing growth according to standard deviation units (*z scores*) is the most accurate technique for classifying growth deficits for research purposes but proves unwieldy in clinical settings.[111, 154] A more useful clinical technique is the evaluation of the child's growth as a percentage of the median for age: taking the actual measurement and dividing it by the median value for that age. According to this scheme, initially developed by Gomez[66] and Waterlow,[148] weights for age or for height above 90 per cent of the median are considered within normal limits. Children whose weights are less than 60 per cent of the median for age or less than 70 per cent of the median for height are in acute danger of severe morbidity and possible mortality from their undernutrition and uniformly should be hospitalized.[82] Children whose weight for age falls between 61 and 75 per cent of median or whose weight for height is between 70 and 80 per cent of median are at moderate risk and warrant intensive outpatient monitoring. If such children are suffering from infection or there is any doubt about the family's ability to follow through with outpatient care, hospitalization should be seriously considered. Children whose weight for age is 76 to 90 per cent of median for age or 80 to 90 per cent of median for height are not in acute jeopardy but should be treated actively as outpatients to restore normal growth and to protect development.

EVALUATION OF DIETARY PRACTICES

Children who fail to thrive have been found to have less adequate dietary intake, when compared to controls.[113] Ascertainment of dietary practices by history, and ideally by observation, is a crucial component of the evaluation of every child with failure to thrive. The results of a 24-hour dietary recall and a 7-day food frequency should be obtained and evaluated by a nutritionist for the adequacy of calories, protein, and micronutrients.[103] The schedule of feedings should be determined. Many children who fail to thrive constantly sip milk, juice, or carbonated beverages.[112, 127] Thus, they have no opportunity to develop an appetite for scheduled meals.

Caretakers' knowledge and health beliefs about child nutrition should be elicited as critical determinants of dietary practices. Over- and underconcentration of formula has been found in 11 per cent of infants under 6 months of age who visit a primary care clinic.[99] Intellectually limited mothers may not understand appropriate food choices for children.[131] Newly arrived immigrant families frequently are bewildered by American markets and do not know how to find culturally appropriate foods for their children. Parents may offer children an inadequate diet because of adherence to unusual dietary practices prescribed by nontraditional religions.[156] Failure to thrive also has been observed following overzealous application to the diets of toddlers of dietary principles appropriate for preventing cardiovascular disease and obesity in adults.[120]

PRINCIPLES OF NUTRITIONAL TREATMENT IN FAILURE TO THRIVE

The goal of nutritional treatment in failure to thrive is to promote compensatory "catch-up" growth, which restores deficits in weight and height.[22, 112] To achieve an accelerated growth rate, the child must receive nutrients in excess of the normal age-specific requirements of recommended daily allowances.[49] Daily caloric needs for catch-up growth in calories per kilogram are estimated as follows:[96]

$$\text{kcal/kg} = \frac{120 \text{ kcal/kg} \times \text{median weight for current height}}{\text{current weight (kg)}}$$

In most cases, according to this calculation, children will require 1.5 to 2 times the expected intake for their age to achieve optimal catch-up growth.[22, 96, 112] Protein intake must be enhanced in similar proportions to permit maximal growth.[96, 103, 112]

Nutritional rehabilitation must address the child's needs for micronutrients as well as calories and protein. Iron deficiency, with or without associated anemia, is seen in as many as half of all children presenting with failure to thrive.[16] Vitamin D deficiency rickets also has been described.[73] The role of zinc deficiency in failure to thrive is not as clearly delineated but has been implicated in impaired linear growth among low-income children.[25] The demand of rapid tissue synthesis during catch-up growth may produce deficiencies in micronutrient stores that were adequate when the child was growing slowly. A multivitamin supplement containing iron and zinc should therefore be prescribed routinely for children with failure to thrive during nutritional rehabilitation. Additional iron or vitamin D supplements should be provided if iron deficiency or rickets has been diagnosed.

In general, it is not possible for a child to eat twice the normal volume of food to obtain the nutrient levels necessary for catch-up growth. Instead, the child's usual diet must be fortified to increase nutrient density. For example, this may be achieved by providing formula of 24 to 30 calories per ounce rather than the standard 20 calories per ounce. Detailed protocols for dietary supplementation have been published elsewhere.[103, 122] The participation of an experienced pediatric nutritionist is critical in developing a dietary regimen appropriate for each child.

The process of refeeding to promote catch-up growth must be undertaken with caution. If high intakes are provided at the beginning of nutritional resuscitation, severely malnourished children may develop vomiting, diarrhea, and circulatory decompensation.[147] To minimize these complications, such children should be restricted to the normal dietary intake for age for the first 7 to 10 days of treatment.[147] Feedings during this period should consist of small, frequently offered portions. Over the next week, the child may be gradually advanced to a diet that meets the calculated requirements for catch-up growth. In contrast, moderately and mildly malnourished children may be offered food *ad libitum* while calorie counts are obtained. Once a baseline of spontaneous intake is established, preferred foods may be enriched to bring dietary intake to catch-up levels.

Depending on the severity of initial deficit, 2 days to 2 weeks of refeeding are generally required to initiate catch-up growth.[22, 39] Accelerated growth must then be maintained for 4 to 9 months to restore a child's weight for height.[22, 146] Intake and rates of growth spontaneously decelerate toward normal levels for age as deficits are repleted.[22, 146] Because weight will be restored more rapidly than height, caretakers may become alarmed that the child is becoming obese. They should be reassured that the catch-up growth in height lags behind that in weight by several months but will occur if dietary treatment is not prematurely terminated.[17]

MEDICAL FACTORS

Multiple medical issues arise during the diagnosis and management of failure to thrive. They include (1) assessing the impact of perinatal risk factors, (2) recognizing and treating the infection/malnutrition cycle, (3) identifying intercurrent lead poisoning, (4) evaluating the role of chronic illness as a potential contributor to growth failure, and (5) obtaining appropriate laboratory evaluations (Table 2).

Perinatal Factors

Perinatal factors exert a powerful influence on patterns of postnatal growth. Ten to forty per cent of children diagnosed as failure to thrive have birth weights below 2500 gm, compared to approximately 7 per cent of the general popula-

Table 2. *Medical Management*

Emphasize history and physical examination.	Look for elevated blood lead levels.
Assess perinatal risk factors.	Evaluate chronic illness.
Interrupt infection/malnutrition cycle.	Minimize laboratory assessment.

tion.[55, 85, 101, 107, 130] Even when researchers exclude low birth weight infants from their samples, infants with failure to thrive have significantly lower birth weights than controls.[145]

For accurate evaluation of a child's growth, it is important to ascertain not only the child's birth weight, but gestational age, birth length, and head circumference.[18] Unless growth parameters are corrected for gestational age, children born prematurely may be inappropriately labeled as failure to thrive. The age used to evaluate height and weight should be calculated by subtracting the number of weeks a child was premature from the number of weeks since birth. Such corrections should be made for head circumference until 18 months after birth, for weight until 24 months, and for height until 40 months.[18] A child whose growth is abnormal after correcting for prematurity deserves careful evaluation because the neurologic, cardiorespiratory, and gastrointestinal sequelae of prematurity, as well as the behavioral disorganization characteristic of some premature infants, may lead to postnatal malnutrition.[126] Such potentially correctable growth failure should not be ignored on the grounds that the child was "born small."

Intrauterine growth retardation (IUGR; birth weight less than the tenth percentile for gestational age), as well as prematurity, places children at risk for failure to thrive. The growth prognosis for children with a history of IUGR varies with the nature of the prenatal insult. Asymmetric IUGR, in which birth weight is disproportionately more depressed than length or head circumference, has the best prognosis for later growth. Asymmetrically growth-retarded infants are at risk for failure to thrive because they are often behaviorally difficult.[3] However, with enhanced postnatal nutrition, they are capable of significant catch-up growth in the first 6 to 8 months of life.[3, 146] In contrast, infants who are symmetrically growth retarded at birth have a poor prognosis for later growth and later may present as cases of failure to thrive relatively resistant to treatment.[46] These infants often suffer from intrauterine infections, chromosomal abnormalities, or prenatal exposure to teratogens such as opiates,[46] alcohol,[71] or anticonvulsants.[72] A careful search for dysmorphic features in such infants may provide clues to diagnosis.[17] In spite of the limited growth potential of infants with symmetric IUGR, clinicians should be alert to potentially treatable postnatal medical and psychosocial factors that may compound the effects of prenatal deficits. For example, many of the causes of symmetric IUGR are associated with neurologically based oral motor dysfunction. In cases in which symmetrical growth retardation reflects prenatal alcohol or substance abuse, clinicians should be aware that if mothers continue to use these substances postpartum, they may not provide adequate care to allow symmetrically growth-retarded children to realize even their limited growth potential.

Infection-Malnutrition Cycle

Children who fail to thrive often suffer from recurring infections, since malnutrition severe enough to produce growth failure also may impair immune function.[142] Cell-mediated immunity and the production of complement and secretory IgA are particularly vulnerable to malnutrition.[142] Otitis media and gastrointestinal and respiratory infections are more common among children who fail to thrive than among their well-nourished peers.[84, 101, 132] With each infection, the child's appetite and nutrient intake decrease, while nutrient requirements are increased by fever, diarrhea, and vomiting.[142, 147] Unless attention is paid to restoring the child's nutritional status, as well as treating the acute illness, cumulative nutritional deficits will occur, leaving the child increasingly vulnerable to more severe and prolonged infections and to even less adequate growth. To interrupt this infection–malnutrition cycle, full immunization and aggressive workup and treatment of suspected infections are critical. In addition, management of acute illness should include specific instruction about appropriate diet during and after illness.

Most immune dysfunction seen in children who fail to thrive is secondary to malnutrition and resolves when the child's nutritional status is restored to normal. A depressed absolute lymphocyte count (<1500) and anergy to common skin tests are useful functional indicators of the severity of the child's malnutrition.[138] More elaborate evaluations of immune function are usually not indicated. However, clinicians should be aware that failure to thrive is considered a potential symptom of HIV infection in children under 15 months with positive test results for HIV antibody and evidence of cellular and humoral immune deficiency.[8] HIV antibody screening is indicated for children who fail to thrive when their mothers are intravenous drug users or partners of intravenous drug users or bisexual men, or when mother or child has a history of receiving a blood transfusion.[8]

Correlation of Elevated Lead Levels with Failure to Thrive

Nutritional deficiencies of iron and calcium found in children with failure to thrive may enhance the absorption of lead and other toxic heavy metals. In the Second National Health and Nutrition Examination Survey, increasing blood lead levels in the range of 5 to 35 mg per dl correlated strongly with impaired growth.[129] A recent clinical study demonstrated that blood lead levels in children with failure to thrive were significantly higher than those of children matched for age, sex, and socioeconomic status.[16] Sixteen per cent of the failure to thrive children in this sample had lead levels high enough to warrant chelation.[16] In areas where lead intoxication is endemic,[97] all children with failure to thrive should be screened for elevated blood lead and treated as necessary.

Role of Chronic Illness

Growth disturbances occur in almost all severe and chronic childhood illnesses. The enzymatic, metabolic, and endocrine mechanisms of growth failure in chronically ill children, which have been recently reviewed,[78] are beyond the scope of this article. Clinicians should be aware, however, that growth failure in chronic illness may reflect nutritional and psychosocial difficulties, as well as the underlying disease process.

Chronic illnesses entail multiple barriers to adequate nutrition.[1] Such barriers may be structural, as in the case of oral facial malformations, or functional, as in the oral–motor discoordination typical of children with neurologic diseases. Similarly, exhaustion and tachypnea during feeding may lead to inadequate dietary intake among children suffering from cardiorespiratory diseases. Untreated dental caries and abscesses also interfere with food intake. Children with tonsillar-adenoidal hypertrophy may also manifest poor feeding and growth that may be partly secondary to mechanical difficulties with eating and partly secondary to hypoxia.[128] In contrast, although some children with gastrointestinal illnesses show marked anorexia, most take food without difficulty, but do not retain sufficient nutrients for adequate growth because of vomiting (e.g., gastroesophageal reflux) or diarrhea and malabsorption (e.g., celiac disease, cystic fibrosis).[15, 17, 42, 70, 130]

ROLE OF THE LABORATORY IN MEDICAL ASSESSMENTS

Acute or chronic illnesses that lead to growth failure are rarely occult. Unless an illness other than primary malnutrition is suggested by history or physical

Table 3. *Psychosocial Management*

Assess economic circumstances.	Rule out active maltreatment.
Identify family dysfunction.	Individualize intervention.
Evaluate feeding disorder.	

examination, the yield of extensive laboratory workup in children who fail to thrive is almost nil.[15, 34] Several investigators have recommended a minimal initial laboratory evaluation, consisting of a complete blood count, lead and free erthryocyte protoporphyrin, urinalysis and urine culture, PPD, and, in genetically at risk populations, a sweat test.[17, 31, 122] In children with history of diarrhea or malodorous stools, or those attending congregate day care, stool cultures and evaluation for ova and parasites are warranted. Giardiasis, in particular, has been implicated in growth failure.[68] More extensive laboratory workups should be guided by the results of these initial tests and the history and physical findings of the child.

The laboratory should be used to assess the degree of nutritional risk as well as evaluating illnesses other than malnutrition. For example, in more severely malnourished children, an albumin level is useful in evaluating visceral protein stores. Alkaline phosphatase will be elevated with rickets and depressed in severe zinc deficiency.[138]

PSYCHOSOCIAL FACTORS

The psychosocial management of children who fail to thrive includes (1) evaluating the role of poverty and material deprivation, (2) identifying sources of family dysfunction, (3) determining the nature of the feeding disorder, (4) ruling out active maltreatment, and (5) providing psychosocial interventions (Table 3).

Poverty and Malnutrition

Poverty is the most important single social risk factor for failure to thrive, because of the close association between poverty and childhood malnutrition.[19, 55, 93, 108] Although failure to thrive may occur in children of all social classes, most clinical cases come from low-income families.[55, 113] Economic dislocations and changes in social policy have placed many children at risk.[137] In 1985, 23 per cent of American children under the age of 5 years lived below the federal poverty level.[29] These children are by definition at high risk for failure to thrive, since the poverty level is set at three times the purchase cost of a marginally adequate diet.[19, 55] Nutritional deprivation linked to poverty has been described both in children whose parents are welfare dependent and those whose parents are unemployed or employed at or near the minimum wage.[19, 26, 93]

Federal nutrition programs serving families and children have not kept pace with rising need.[19] Many impoverished families do not receive benefits. Even when benefits are available, they are often insufficient for a diet adequate for a healthy child and fall far below the enhanced requirements for catch-up growth. Food stamps, for example, allow approximately 49 cents per meal per person.[19] The WIC program reaches fewer than half the eligible families with pregnant women and young children.[29] Even when WIC is available, parents report difficulty in paying for infant formula once the child's needs outstrip the 26 ounces per day provided by the program.[99]

In addition to nutritional deprivation children in poverty suffer other forms of material deprivation that may contribute to failure to thrive. In our setting, 13 per cent of children presenting with failure to thrive are homeless, lodged in shelters or hotels without facilities for food storage or preparation. More than one third of children living below poverty also lack health insurance.[29] Thus they may have limited access to treatment of intercurrent infections and other medical conditions contributing to failure to thrive.

Family Dysfunction and Disordered Parent–Child Interaction

In all social classes, failure to thrive usually indicates that the family system is not functioning adaptively to meet the child's needs.[2, 36, 90, 122] Chronically ill children may overwhelm the caretaking abilities of families that could provide adequate care for healthy children. Contrary to the popular belief that weight gain during hospitalization rules out major organic disease, such children often grow in the hospital where many trained personnel are available to share the burden of their care.[15, 84] Parents require aid and respite if such children are to sustain growth following hospital discharge.

In addition to poverty and the difficulty of caring for a chronically ill child, a wide variety of stresses impinge on the parents of children who fail to thrive. These include marital discord, chronic physical illness, depression, intellectual impairment, recent death of a family member, abuse of alcohol and other substances, and isolation from relatives and the wider community.[2, 5, 13, 17, 20, 27, 30, 36, 44, 47, 51, 57, 80, 84, 88, 90, 104, 106, 109, 122, 131, 143] Parents of children who fail to thrive often were deprived or actively abused themselves as children.[104, 115, 145] Painful and unresolved issues from their own childhood, referred to by Fraiberg[52] as "ghosts in the nursery," may impede their ability to recognize and respond to their children's needs.

Current and past stresses, including the condition of the child who is failing to thrive,[56] interact to produce a breakdown of parent–child interaction. On the one hand, parents of children who fail to thrive manifest decreased responsiveness to and acceptance of the child, and impaired ability to organize the home environment to meet the child's needs.[23, 26, 113, 149] On the other hand, the listless irritability of the malnourished child alienates caretakers, giving them little satisfaction in their attempts to provide nurturance.[23, 28, 118, 125]

Assessment of Feeding Disorders

Growth is affected when the interactive breakdown within the family and between parent and child encompasses the feeding situation. Children who fail to thrive have a higher incidence of behavioral feeding problems than controls.[114] The nature of the interactive feeding disorder is most readily ascertained by direct observation of a meal, ideally during a home visit. The observer should ascertain whether the child is adaptively positioned for feeding, whether there are inappropriate distractions, whether feedings are constantly interrupted for cleaning by an overfastidious caretaker, or whether there are multiple and inconsistent feeders.[57, 112] Parents may engage in open conflict with each other during meals, frightening and distracting the child.[57]

Lethargic, ill, or hypersensitive infants may frustrate the increasingly frantic attempts of parents to feed and comfort them, withdrawing into sleep or vomiting and appearing inconsolable.[122] Depressed, physically ill, or substance-abusing caretakers may be unresponsive to a child's hunger signals.[122] Chatoor and colleagues have noted that when parents have difficulty in accepting the child's drive for autonomy, which emerges in the second half of the first year, a feeding disorder may result.[27] The child's need to gain attention, assert independence, or express anger by refusing to eat overides the need to satisfy hunger.[27] Thus, for many reasons, the feeding situation for children who fail to thrive may be emotionally unrewarding for child and caretakers and functionally insufficient to permit the child to obtain adequate nutrition for growth.

Maltreatment of the Child

Most children with failure to thrive do not experience physical abuse or intentional neglect.[5] However, it is important that clinicians recognize those children with failure to thrive who are suffering active maltreatment because the survival of these children is in jeopardy. Active withholding of food from children has been described, particularly in cases of so called "psychosocial dwarfism," and usually is associated with physical abuse.[86] A review of a number of studies suggests that approximately 10 per cent of children initially hospitalized for failure to thrive will sustain nonaccidental trauma.[17, 41, 48, 65, 107] Fatal outcomes have been noted by multiple investigators among children who suffer both failure to thrive and physical abuse.[83, 107] Among those who survive, the ensuing functional deficits are far more severe than those seen in children with failure to thrive who were not injured.[33, 40, 48] Therefore, when inflicted injury is identified in children with failure to thrive, out of home placement should be considered.

Implications for Psychosocial Treatment

The psychosocial factors contributing to failure to thrive are complex and vary widely from family to family, so that no single form of treatment is appropriate for all cases. Detailed and sensitive interviewing, usually extending over several contacts, is necessary to identify important stressors. Home visits enhance rapport and provide information not readily obtained in clinical settings. Formal evaluation of parents for potentially treatable psychiatric disorders, including major depression, psychosis, and substance abuse, may be helpful in selected cases.

Psychosocial interventions in failure to thrive must simultaneously address the material and interpersonal aspects of the child's environment. In cases in which poverty is a major cause of the child's failure to thrive, aggressive advocacy with public bureaucracies and private relief organizations is required to help families obtain needed services.[55] Less obvious is the optimal treatment of family dysfunction and interactive breakdown between parent and child. Extended hospitalization is counterproductive,[135] whereas brief placement in medically specialized foster homes with frequent visits by natural parents demonstrated positive effects in a small comparative study.[79] In addition, both classic behavioral modification treatment of feeding disorders[92] and nontraditional psychotherapy, involving extensive outreach, home visits, and treatment of parent and child together, have been found to exert a positive impact on parental competence and children's growth and development[52] in published case reports. A single controlled study in a low-income urban population found advocacy for concrete services as effective as parent–child or family therapy in promoting positive outcomes in children hospitalized under the age of 1 year for failure to thrive.[36] Further research in this area clearly is needed.

DEVELOPMENTAL FACTORS

The management of developmental issues in children who fail to thrive entails (1) recognition of the developmental risks associated with failure to thrive, (2) understanding the effects of malnutrition on the function and structure of the developing nervous system, and (3) advocating appropriate preventive and therapeutic interventions to minimize developmental morbidity (Table 4).

Evaluation of Developmental Impairment with Failure to Thrive

In infancy, many children with failure to thrive show developmental delays and abnormalities of posture and tone.[7, 20, 30, 48, 87, 118, 121, 125, 150] Clinical experience suggests that children presenting in the second year with failure to thrive that is

Table 4. *Developmental Management*

Malnutrition impairs brain structure and function.
Standardize developmental assessment.
Use center- or home-based developmental intervention.
Assess need for remedial education on school entry.

secondary to interactive feeding disorders are less likely to show developmental impairments than those presenting in infancy.[27]

During the preschool and school years, children hospitalized for failure to thrive in infancy continue to have depressed psychometric scores and high rates of school failure.[26, 41, 62, 77, 106, 135] Samples sometimes are biased by the fact that early investigators in this field required developmental or behavioral aberrations as a necessary criterion for diagnosis of nonorganic failure to thrive.[125, 150] In samples in which children are selected on the basis of anthropometric criteria alone, developmental deficits are less pervasive.[36, 37, 45] For example, in a study of children with failure to thrive who were identified in a primary care setting and never hospitalized, there were no significant differences in cognitive test scores compared to matched controls; both scored below standard norms.[101]

All children presenting with failure to thrive should undergo standardized developmental assessment when their acute medical condition has stabilized.[1, 17, 53, 122] The Denver Developmental Screening Test is insufficiently sensitive to the degree and types of deficit afflicting these children.[140] More extensive developmental evaluations, such as the Bayley Scales of Infant Development for infants under 30 months,[10] or the McCarthy Scales for older children, should be used.[98] Speech and language functions are often disproportionately delayed[105, 106, 121] and may warrant specific assessment. The qualitative aspects of a child's performance may be more revealing than simple psychometric scores. Children who fail to thrive typically show difficulty with sustained attention and do not engage well with the examiner or the test objects.

Because the neurodevelopmental derangements produced by concurrent malnutrition may be profound, clinicians should be cautious about diagnosing fixed neurologic disease such as hypotonic cerebral palsy or irreversible mental retardation at the time that the child is acutely malnourished. After their nutritional status has improved, children should be reassessed neurologically and developmentally to permit more accurate assessment of prognosis.

Mechanisms of Developmental Impairment in Failure to Thrive

The mechanisms mediating the relationship between failure to thrive and persistent developmental impairment are complex and cannot be ascribed to any single cause. On the one hand, hospitalization itself, as well as the socioenvironmental deprivation that often accompanies failure to thrive, may independently produce developmental deficits.[23, 37, 54] On the other hand, the functional and structural effects of malnutrition on the developing nervous system are known to impair cognition and behavior and to magnify the adverse effects of socioenvironmental deprivation on development.[4, 6, 9, 28, 32, 43, 54, 58–62]

At any age, undernutrition need not be severe or prolonged to produce behavioral changes that may have important implications for both parent–child interaction and the ability of the child to explore and master the inanimate environment. The amino acid composition of a single meal has been shown to influence the sleep behavior of human infants,[155] with obvious implications for parent–child interaction. In studies of infants and toddlers, iron deficiency, even without associated protein energy deficits, correlates with lowered scores on tests of mental and motor development, as well as with increased fearfulness, inatten-

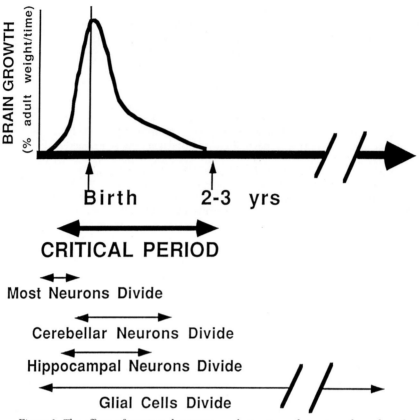

Figure 1. The effects of nutrient deprivation on brain size and structure depend on the timing, duration, and severity of malnutrition in relation to the development of the brain. See text for details.

tiveness, and decreased social responsiveness.[94, 95] These developmental deficits may persist after the iron deficiency has been treated.[94] Among children with IQs below the median, merely missing breakfast significantly increases errors on developmental scales.[116, 117] Protein-energy undernutrition reduces playful and exploratory activity, motivation and arousal, and increases apathy and irritability,[11, 28] even before anthropometric deficits occur. The physiologic mechanisms of these behavioral derangements are not fully understood but may be related to alterations in neurotransmitter synthesis and release.[6, 133]

While undernutrition produces functional alterations of behavior at any age, the brain is uniquely vulnerable to structural deficits during the critical period of rapid brain growth that extends from midgestation through the early preschool years (Fig. 1).[34, 35] The growing brain utilizes nutrients at very rapid rates, accounting for only 2 to 3 per cent of the child's body weight, but 60 per cent of the body's glucose utilization.[6, 151] During this critical period, the brain has biosynthetic abilities that do not persist into later life.[35] The germinal stem cell populations for neurons become inactive after early development, making it impossible to generate new neurons if substrate only becomes available after the critical period has passed.[133]

The effects of nutrient deprivation on brain size and structure depend on the timing, duration, and severity of malnutrition in relation to the development of the brain. When the brain is deprived of an optimal supply of nutrients, there are no discrete lesions. Rather, generalized morphologic distortion occurs, affecting those areas of the brain that were maturing at the time of nutrient deficit.[133] For example, in the cerebellum, which continues neurogenesis after birth, postnatal malnutrition leading to failure to thrive also could alter the number, location, and structure of all classes of cerebellar neurons.[133] As might be predicted from the critical period model, early undernutrition correlates with persistent fine- and gross-motor dysfunction, probably reflecting disordered cerebellar maturation.[4, 45, 58, 141]

In other areas of the brain, where most neuronal cells have differentiated during prenatal life, malnutrition in infancy reduces the formation of synapses and the branching of dendrites.[12, 32] Moreover, the nutritive and supporting glial cells of the brain, which are largely formed after birth, are reduced in number following undernutrition.[34] Reduced glial cells result in impairment of the myelinization necessary for normal nerve conduction.[151] Although glial cells, unlike neurons, are continually being replaced in the brain, early undernutrition may cause a large enough deficit that refeeding at a time after the critical period cannot fully restore glial numbers.[34, 133]

These structural alterations in brain size are reflected clinically in reduced head circumference.[141] If intensive nutritional resuscitation is undertaken while the brain is still in the critical period, catch-up growth in head circumference sometimes occurs. Occasionally, this growth is at such a rapid rate that there is widening of the cranial sutures without clinical signs of increased intercranial pressure.[110] In many cases, however, particularly if nutritional resuscitation is delayed or inadequate, deficits in head circumference are life long, although weight and length deficits may be largely restored.[4, 43, 59, 141]

Therapeutic Implications for Prevention and Treatment

Malnutrition during the critical period of brain growth should be identified promptly and treated vigorously to minimize central nervous system deficit. Nutritional resuscitation is a necessary but not sufficient mode of treatment. Data on children hospitalized for failure to thrive in the United States[26, 41, 63] and Australia,[105–107] and on malnourished children from the developing world[4, 28, 58–62, 67, 100, 102, 141] demonstrate clearly that medical care and nutritional resuscitation alone may restore physical growth but do not bring developmental functions into the normal range. Specific developmental interventions have been evaluated in only one small sample of nine infants with failure to thrive, in whom after 3 months of intervention there were trends toward improved vocal responding and mental and motor scores among the five infants who received intervention, compared to the four who did not.[121] In uncontrolled studies, investigators who offered families a variety of supportive interventions, such as visiting nurses, advocacy with social welfare agencies, and family therapy,[36, 37, 45] found improved developmental scores on followup 3 to 18 months after intervention. Long-term followup to school age has not been performed following such intervention.

Several studies from the developing world have shown encouraging results from prolonged developmental intervention offered in conjunction with acute nutritional and medical rehabilitation. Malnourished children who received focused and sustained center-[100, 102] or home-based[67] developmental intervention beginning before the age of 2 years and sustained for at least 3 years showed significantly better developmental scores at followup when compared to untreated malnourished children. Both groups continued to lag behind better nourished children of similar background, however.[67, 101, 102] Malnourished children from Korea who were adopted into privileged Western homes before the age of 2 years also showed high developmental functioning at school age.[91] These findings would suggest that the developmental concomitants of failure to thrive should be the subject of focused assessment and ongoing treatment from the time of diagnosis. Although deficits may not be fully reversible, they may be ameliorated; planning for long-term remedial education at school entry also may be necessary.

While nutritional interventions are insufficient to reverse developmental deficits that have already occurred, they serve an important preventive function. Several studies have suggested that high levels of nutritional supplementation offered to impoverished children in infancy and early childhood are correlated at school age with greater height and weight, improved scores on standard intelligence tests, and more optimal attentiveness and social behavior. These positive effects were noted when supplemented children were compared with unsupplemented siblings[74] or with age mates from the same village.[9] Thus, nutritional supplementation, such as that provided in the United States by the WIC program, may have an important role in the primary prevention of failure to thrive and developmental deficits among impoverished children.

CONCLUSIONS

Once growth failure has been ameliorated, developmental impairments and deficits in social–emotional function constitute the major long-term morbidity of malnutrition in early life among children diagnosed as having failure to thrive. Failure to thrive should thus be approached as a chronic condition, requiring long-term followup, with remissions and exacerbations expected. In handling such a multidimensional problem, the role of the pediatrician extends beyond the simple diagnosis and treatment of complicating medical conditions. Rather, the pediatrician must mobilize a team of health professionals. This team must assure that the child receives nutritional assessment and rehabilitation, has developmental impairments identified and treated, and receives psychosocial supports for the family. The ultimate goal of treatment is a thriving child in a thriving family.

ACKNOWLEDGMENT

This work was supported in part by the Failure to Thrive Consortium Grant from the Department of Public Health of the Commonwealth of Massachusetts (#33048106339A) (DF) and by grants from the National Institutes of Health (HE16727, CA26731), a Future Leader award from the International Life Sciences Institute-Nutrition Foundation, and the Competitive Research Grants Program of the United States Department of Agriculture (CRCR-1-2464) (SZ).

REFERENCES

1. Accardo PJ (ed): Failure to Thrive in Infancy and Early Childhood: A Multidisciplinary Team Approach. Baltimore, Maryland, University Park Press, 1982
2. Alderette P, deGraffenried DF: Nonorganic failure-to-thrive syndrome and the family system. Social Work: 207–210, 1986
3. Als H, Tronick E, Adamson L et al: Behavior of full-term but underweight infant. Develop Med Child Neurol 18:590–602, 1976
4. Ashem B, Jones M: Deleterious effects of chronic undernutrition on cognitive abilities. J Child Psychol Psychiatry 19:23–31, 1978
5. Ayoub CC, Milner JS: Failure to thrive: Parental indicators, types, and outcomes. Child Abuse and Neglect 9:491–499, 1985
6. Balazs R, Lewis PD, Patel A: Nutritional deficiencies and brain development. In Falkner F, Tanner JM (eds): Human Growth, Vol 3. New York, Plenum Press, 1979

7. Barbero G, Shaheen E: Environmental failure to thrive: A clinical view. J Pediatr 71:639–644, 1967
8. Barbour SD: Acquired immunodeficiency syndrome of childhood. Pediatr Clin North Am 34:247–268, 1987
9. Barrett D, Radke-Yarrow M, Klein RE: Chronic malnutrition and child behavior: Effects of early caloric supplementation on social and emotional functioning at school age. Dev Psychol 18:541–556, 1982
10. Bayley N: Bayley Scales of Infant Development Manual. New York, Psychological Corporation, 1969
11. Beaton GH: Energy in human nutrition: Perspectives and problems. Nutr Rev 41:325–340, 1982
12. Bedi KS, Thomas YM, Davies CA et al: Synapse-to-neuron ratios of frontal and cerebellar cortex of 30-day-old and adult rats undernourished during early postnatal life. J Comp Neurol 193:49–56, 1980
13. Berkowitz CD, Sklaren BC: Environmental failure to thrive: The need for intervention. Am Fam Physician 29:191–199, 1984
14. Berwick DM: Nonorganic failure-to-thrive. Pediatr Rev 1:265–270, 1980
15. Berwick DM, Levy JC, Kleinerman R: Failure to thrive: Diagnostic yield of hospitalization. Arch Dis Child 57:347–351, 1982
16. Bithoney WG: Elevated lead levels in children with nonorganic failure to thrive. Pediatrics 78:891–895, 1986
17. Bithoney WG, Rathbun JM: Failure to thrive. In Levine MD, Carey WB, Crocker AC, Gross RT (eds): Developmental-Behavioral Pediatrics. Philadelphia, W. B. Saunders, 1983
18. Brandt L: Growth dynamics of low birthweight infants with emphasis on the perinatal period. In Falkner F, Tanner J (eds): Human Growth, Neurobiology and Nutrition. New York, Plenum Press, 1979
19. Brown JL, Pizer HF: Living Hungry in America. New York, Macmillan, 1987
20. Bullard DM Jr, Glaser HH, Heagarty MC et al: Failure to thrive in the "neglected" child. Am J Orthopsychiatry 37:680–690, 1966
21. Casey PH: Failure to thrive: A reconceptualization. J Dev Behav Pediatr 4:63–66, 1983
22. Casey PH, Arnold WC: Compensatory growth in infants with severe failure to thrive. South Med J 78:1057–1060, 1985
23. Casey PH, Bradley R, Wortham B: Social and Nonsocial home environments of infants with nonorganic failure-to-thrive. Pediatrics 73:348–353, 1984
24. Casey PH, Wortham B, Nelson JY: Management of children with failure to thrive in a rural ambulatory setting. Clin Pediatr 23:325–330, 1984
25. Casey PH, Collie WR, Blakemore WM: Zinc nutrition in children who fail to thrive. In Drotar D (ed): New Directions in Failure to Thrive: Implications for Research and Practice. New York, Plenum Press, 1985
26. Chase HP, Martin HP: Undernutrition and child development. N Engl J Med 282:933–939, 1970
27. Chatoor I, Schaefer S, Dickson L et al: Nonorganic failure to thrive: A developmental perspective. Pediatr Ann 13:829–843, 1984
28. Chavez A, Martinez C: Consequences of insufficient nutrition on child character and behavior. In: Levitsky DA (ed): Malnutrition, Environment, and Behavior. New York, Cornell University Press, 1979
29. Children's Defense Fund: A Children's Defense Budget: FY 1988. Washington D.C., 1987
30. Coleman RW, Provence S: Environmental retardation (hospitalism) in infants living in families. Pediatrics 19:285–292, 1957
31. Cupoli JM, Hallock JA, Barness LA: Failure to thrive. In Gluck L (ed): Current Problems in Pediatrics. Chicago, Illinois, Year Book Medical, 1980
32. Davies CA, Katz HB: The comparative effects of early-life undernutrition and subsequent differential environments on the dendritic branching of pyramidal cells in rat visual cortex. J Comp Neurol 218:345–350, 1983
33. Dietrich KN, Starr RH Jr, Weisfeld GE: Infant maltreatment: caretaker-infant interaction and developmental consequences at different levels of parenting failure. Pediatrics 72:532–539, 1983
34. Dobbing J: Infant nutrition and later achievement. Nutr Rev 42:1–7, 1984

35. Dobbing J, Sands J: The quantitative growth and development of the human brain. Arch Dis Child 48:757–767, 1973
36. Drotar D, Malone C, Devost C et al.: Early preventive intervention in failure to thrive: Methods and early outcome. In Drotar D (ed): New Directions in Failure to Thrive: Implications for Research and Practice. New York, Plenum Press, 1985
37. Drotar D, Nowak M, Malone CA et al: Early psychological outcome in failure to thrive: Predictions from an interactional model. J Clin Child Psychol 14:105–111, 1985
38. Eid EE: A follow-up study of physical growth following failure to thrive with special reference to a critical period in the first year of life. Acta Pediatr Scand 60:39–48, 1971
39. Ellerstein NS, Ostrov BE: Growth patterns in children hospitalized because of caloric-deprivation failure to thrive. Am J Dis Child 139:164–166, 1985
40. Elmer E: A follow-up study of traumatized children. Pediatrics 59:273–279, 1977
41. Elmer E, Gregg GS, Ellison P: Late results of the "failure to thrive" syndrome. Clin Pediatr 8:584–589, 1969
42. English PC: Failure to thrive without organic reason. Pediatr Ann 7:83–97, 1978
43. Engsner V, Vahlquist B: Brain growth in children with protein energy malnutrition. In Bazier M (ed): Growth and Development of the Brain. New York, Raven Press, 1975
44. Evans SL, Reinhart JB, Succop RA: Failure to thrive: A study of 45 children and their families. J Am Acad Child Psychiatr 2:440–457, 1972
45. Field M: Follow-up developmental status of infants hospitalized for nonorganic failure to thrive. J Pediatr Psychol 9:241–256, 1984
46. Finnegan LP: Drugs and other substance abuse in pregnancy. In Stern C (ed): Drug Use in Pregnancy. Boston, Science Press, 1984
47. Fischhoff J, Whitten CF, Petit MG: A psychiatric study of mothers of infants with growth failure secondary to maternal deprivation. J Pediatr 79:209–215, 1971
48. Fitch MJ, Cadol RV, Goldson E et al: Cognitive development of abused and failure-to-thrive children. J Pediatr Psychol:32–37, Spring 1976
49. Food and Nutrition Board: Recommended Dietary Allowances. Washington, D.C., National Academy of Sciences, 1980
50. Fomon ST: Infant Nutrition. Philadelphia, WB Saunders, 1974
51. Fosson A, Wilson J: Family interactions surrounding feedings of infants with nonorganic failure to thrive. Clin Pediatr 26:518–523, 1987
52. Fraiberg S, Adelsen E, Shapiro V: Ghosts in the nursery. J Am Acad Child Psychiatr 14:387–422, 1975
53. Frank DA: Biologic risks in "nonorganic" failure to thrive: Diagnostic and therapeutic implications. In Drotar D (ed): New Directions in Failure to Thrive: Implications for Research and Practice. New York, Plenum Press, 1985
54. Frank DA: Malnutrition and child behavior: A view from the bedside. In Brozek J, Schurch B (eds): Malnutrition and Behavior: Critical Assessment of Key Issues. Lausanne, Switzerland, Nestle Foundation, 1984
55. Frank DA, Allen D, Brown JL: Primary prevention of failure to thrive: Social policy implications. In Drotar D (ed): New Directions in Failure to Thrive: Implications for Research and Practice. New York, Plenum Press, 1985
56 Gaensbauer TJ, Sands K: Distorted affective communications in abused/neglected infants and their potential impact on caretakers. J Am Acad Child Psychiatr 18:236–249, 1979
57. Gagan RJ, Cupoli JM, Watkins AH: The families of children who fail to thrive: Preliminary investigations of parental deprivation among organic and non-organic cases. Child Abuse and Neglect 8:93–103, 1984
58. Galler JR, Ramsey F, Solimano G: A followup study of the effects of early malnutrition on subsequent development. II. Fine motor skills in adolescence. Pediatr Res 19:524–527, 1985
59. Galler JR, Ramsey F, Solimano G et al: The influence of early malnutrition on subsequent behavioral development. I. Degree of impairment in intellectual performance. J Am Acad Child Psychiatry 22:8–15, 1983a
60. Galler JR, Ramsey F, Solimano G et al: The influence of early malnutrition on subsequent behavioral development. II. Classroom behavior. J Am Acad Child Psychiatry 22:16–22, 1983b
61. Galler JR, Ramsey F, Solimano G: The influence of early malnutrition on subsequent

behavioral development. III. Learning disabilities as a sequel to malnutrition. Pediatr Res 18:309–313, 1984

62. Galler JR, Ramsey F, Solimano G: The influence of early malnutrition on subsequent behavioral development. V. Child's behavior at home. J Am Acad Child Psychiatry 24:58–64, 1985

63. Glaser HH, Heagarty MC, Bullard DM Jr et al: Physical and psychological development of children with early failure to thrive. J Pediatr 73:690–698, 1980

64. Goldbloom RB: Failure to thrive. Pediatr Clin North Am 29:151–165, 1982

65. Goldson E, Cadol RV, Fitch MJ et al: Nonaccidental trauma and failure to thrive. Am J Dis Child 130:490–492, 1976

66. Gomez F, Galvan R, Frenk S et al: Mortality in second and third degree malnutrition. J Trop Pediatr 2:77–83, 1956

67. Grantham-McGregor S, Schofield W, Powell C: Development of severely malnourished children who receive psychosocial stimulation: Six-year follow-up. Pediatrics 79:247–254, 1987

68. Gupta MC, Urrutia JJ: Effect of periodic antiascaris and antigiardia treatment on nutritional status of preschool children. Am J Clin Nutr 36:79–86, 1982

69. Habicht JP, Yarbrough C, Martorell R et al: Height and weight standards for preschool children: How relevant are ethnic differences to growth potential? Lancet 1:611–614, 1974

70. Hannaway PJ: Failure to thrive: A study of 100 infants and children. Clin Pediatr 9:96–99, 1970

71. Hanson JW, Jones KL, Smith DW: Fetal alcohol syndrome. JAMA 235:1458–1460, 1976

72. Hanson JW, Smith DW: The fetal hydantoin syndrome. J Pediatr 87:285–290, 1975

73. Hayward I, Stein MT, Gibson MI: Nutritional rickets in San Diego. Am J Dis Child 141:1060–1062, 1987

74. Hicks LE, Langham RA, Takenaka J: Cognitive and health measures following early nutritional supplementation: A sibling study. Am J Public Health 72:1110–1118, 1982

75. Homer C, Ludwig S: Categorization of etiology of failure to thrive. Am J Dis Child 135:848–851, 1981

76. Hoorweg J, Stanfield J: The effect of protein energy malnutrition in early childhood on intellectual and motor abilities in later childhood and adolescence. Develop Med Child Neurol 18:330–350, 1976

77. Hufton IW, Oates RK: Nonorganic failure to thrive: A long-term follow-up. Pediatrics 59:73–76, 1977

78. Kappy MS: Regulation of growth in children with chronic illness: Therapeutic implications for the year 2000. Am J Dis Child 141:489–493, 1987

79. Karniski W, Van Buren L, Cupoli JM: A treatment program for failure to thrive: A cost/effectiveness analysis. Child Abuse and Neglect 10:471–478, 1986

80. Kerr MA, Bogue JL, Kerr DS: Psychosocial functioning of mothers of malnourished children. Pediatrics 62:778–784, 1978

81. Keys SA, Brozek J, Henschel A et al: The Biology of Human Starvation, Vol II. Minneapolis, Minnesota, University of Minnesota Press, 1950

82. Kielman A, McCord C: Weight-for-age as an index of risk of death in children. Lancet 1:1247–1250, 1978

83. Koel BS: Failure to thrive and fatal injury as a continuum. Am J Dis Child 188:565–567, 1969

84. Kotelchuck M: Non-organic failure to thrive: The status of interactional and environmental etiology theories. Adv Behav Pediatr 1, 1980

85. Koumjian LL, Marks R: Catching Up! Annual Report for Failure to Thrive Program in Massachusetts 1985. Massachusetts Department of Public Health, Division of Family Health Services, Statistics and Evaluation Unit, 1985

86. Krieger I: Food restriction as a form of child abuse in ten cases of psychological deprivation dwarfism. Clin Pediatr 13:127–133, 1974

87. Krieger I, Sargent DA: A postural sign in the sensory deprivation syndrome in infants. J Pediatr 70:332–339, 1967

88. Lansky SB, Stephenson L, Weller E et al: Failure to thrive during infancy in siblings of pediatric cancer patients. Am J Pediatr Hematol Oncol 4:361–366, 1982

89. Lattimer A: Testimony before house agricultural committee. Subcommittee on Nutrition, October 20, 1983

90. Leonard MF, Rhymes JP, Solnit AJ: Failure to thrive in infants: A family problem. Am J Dis Child 111:600–612, 1966
91. Lien NM, Meyer K, Winick M: Early malnutrition and "late" adoption: A study of their effects on the development of Korean orphans adopted into American families. Am J Clin Nutr 30:1734–1739, 1977
92. Linscheid TR, Rasnake LK: Behavioral approaches to the treatment of failure to thrive. In Drotar D (ed): New Directions in Failure to Thrive: Implications for Research and Practice. New York, Plenum Press, 1980
93. Listernick R, Cristoffel K, Pace J et al: Severe primary malnutrition in U.S. children. Am J Dis Child 139:1157–1160, 1985
94. Lozoff B, Brittenham GM, Wolf AW et al: Iron deficiency anemia and iron therapy effects on infant developmental test performance. Pediatrics 79:981–995, 1987
95. Lozoff B, Wolf A: Does abnormal behavior account for low Bayley scores in iron deficient infants? Pediatr Res 17:100A, 1983
96. MacLean WC, de Romana GL, Masse E et al: Nutritional management of chronic diarrhea and malnutrition: Primary reliance on oral feeding. J Pediatr 97:316–323, 1980
97. Mahaffey KR, Annest JL, Roberts J et al: National estimates of blood lead levels: United States 1976–1980: Associated with selected demographics and socioeconomic factors. N Engl J Med 307:573–579, 1982
98. McCarthy D: Manual for McCarthy Scales of Children's Abilities. New York, Psychological Corporation, 1972
99. McJunkin JE, Bithoney WG, McCormick MC: Errors in formula concentration in an outpatient population. J Pediatr 111:848–850, 1987
100. McKay H, Sinisterra L, McKay L et al: Improving cognitive ability in chronically deprived children. Science 200:270–277, 1978
101. Mitchell WG, Gorrell RW, Greenberg RA: Failure-to-Thrive: A study in a primary care setting: Epidemiology and follow-up. Pediatrics 65:971–976, 1980
102. Mora JO, Clement J, Christianson H et al: Nutritional supplement, early stimulation, and child development. In: Brozek J (ed): Behavioral Effects on Energy and Protein Deficits. Bethesda, Maryland, Department of Health, Education and Welfare, National Institutes of Health, 1979
103. Murray C, Glassman M: Nutrient requirements during growth and recovery from failure to thrive. In: Accardo PJ (ed): Failure to Thrive in Infancy and Early Childhood. Baltimore, Maryland, University Park Press, 1981
104. Newberger EH, Hampton RL, Marx TJ et al: Child abuse and pediatric social illness: An epidemiological analysis and ecological reformulation. Am J Orthopsychiatry 56:589–601, 1986
105. Oates RK, Peacock A, Forrest D: Development in Children Following Abuse and Nonorganic Failure to Thrive. Am J Dis Child 138:764–767, 1984
106. Oates RK, Peacock A, Forrest D: Long-term effects of nonorganic failure to thrive. Pediatrics 75:36–40, 1985
107. Oates RK, Yu JS: Children with non-organic failure to thrive: A community problem. Med J Aust 2:199–203, 1971
108. Oatis P, Bobo R, Herman D: Nutritional status in hospitalized children (effect of socioeconomic status). Pediatr Res 4:583, 1982
109. Patton RG, Gardner LI: Influence of family environment on growth: The syndrome of "maternal deprivation." Pediatrics 301:957–962, 1962
110. Pearl M, Finkelstein J, Berman MR: Temporary widening of cranial sutures during recovery from failure to thrive. Clin Pediatr 11:427–430, 1972
111. Peterson KE, Rathbun JM, Herrera MA: Growth rate analysis in failure to thrive treatment and research. In Drotar D (ed): New Directions in Failure to Thrive: Implications for Research and Practice. New York, Plenum Press, 1985
112. Peterson KE, Washington J, Rathbun JM: Team management of failure to thrive. J Am Diet Assoc 84:810–815, 1984
113. Pollitt E: Failure to thrive: Socioeconomic, dietary intake and mother-child interaction. Fed Proc 34:1593–1597, 1975
114. Pollit E, Eichler A: Behavioral disturbances among failure-to-thrive children. Am J Dis Child 130:24–29, 1976

115. Pollit E, Eichler AW, Chan C: Psychological development and behavior of mothers of failure-to-thrive children. Am J Orthopsychiatry 45:525–537, 1975
116. Pollitt E, Leibel R, Greenfield D: Brief fasting, stress, and cognition in children. Am J Clin Nutr 34:1526–1533, 1981
117. Pollitt E, Lewis NL, Garza C et al: Fasting and cognitive function. J Psychiatr Res 17:169–174, 1983
118. Powell F, Low J: Behavior in nonorganic failure to thrive. J Dev Behav Pediatr 4:26–33, 1983
119. Powell GF, Brasel JA, Raiti S et al: Emotional deprivation and growth retardation simulating idiopathic hypopituitarism. N Engl J Med 276:1277–1282, 1967
120. Pugliese MT, Weyman-Daum M, Moses N et al: Parental health beliefs as a cause of nonorganic failure to thrive. Pediatrics 80:175–182, 1987
121. Ramey CT: Nutritional response-contingent stimulation, and the maternal deprivation syndrome: Results of an early intervention program. Merill-Palmer Q 21:45–53, 1975
122. Rathbun JM, Peterson KE: Nutrition in failure to thrive. In: Grand RJ, Sutphen JL, Dietz WH Jr (eds): Pediatric Nutrition: Theory and Practice. Boston, Butterworth Publishers, 1987
123. Richardson SA: The long-range consequences of malnutrition in infancy: A study of children in Jamaica, West Indies. In: Wharton B (ed): Topics in Pediatrics 2: Nutrition in Childhood. Tunbridge Wells, Great Britain, Pitman Medical, Kent, 1980
124. Riley RL, Landwirth J, Kaplan SA: Failure to thrive: An analysis of 83 cases. California Medicine 108:32–38, 1968
125. Rosenn DW, Stein Loeb L, Bates Jura M: Differentiation of organic from nonorganic failure to thrive syndrome in infancy. Pediatrics 66:698–702, 1980
126. Rudolph AJ: Failure to thrive in the perinatal period. Acta Pediatr Scand 319:55–61, 1985
127. Sameroff A, Chandler MJ: Reproductive risk and the continuum of caretaking casualty. In: Horowitz PD (ed): Review of Child Development Research. Chicago, Illinois, University of Chicago Press, 1978
128. Schiffman R, Faber J, Eidelman AI: Obstructive hypertrophic adenoids and tonsils as a cause of infantile failure to thrive: Reversed by tonsillectomy and adenoidectomy. Int J Pediatr Otorhinolaryngol 9:183–187, 1985
129. Schwartz J, Angle C, Pitcher H: Relationship between childhood blood lead levels and stature. Pediatrics 77:281–288, 1986
130. Shaheen E, Alexander D, Truskowsky M et al: Failure to thrive: A retrospective profile. Clin Pediatr 7:255–261, 1986
131. Sheridan MD: The intelligence of 100 neglectful mothers. Br Med J 91–93, Jan 1956
132. Sherrod KB, O'Connor S, Vietze PM et al.: Child health and maltreatment. Child Develop 55:1174–1183, 1984
133. Shoemaker WJ, Bloom FE: Effect of undernutrition on brain morphology. In Wurtman JJ, Wurtman RJ (eds): Nutrition and the Brain, Vol 2. New York, Raven Press, 1979
134. Sills RH: Failure to thrive. Am J Dis Child 132:967–969, 1978
135. Singer L: Long-term hospitalization of failure-to-thrive infants: Developmental outcome at three years. Child Abuse and Neglect 10:479–486, 1986
136. Skuse DH: Non-organic failure to thrive. Arch Dis Child 60:173–178, 1985
137. Smeeding T: Is the safety net still intact? In Bowden DL (ed): The social contract revisited: Aims and Outcomes of President Reagan's Social Welfare Policy. Washington, D.C., The Urban Institute Press, 1984
138. Solomons NW: Assessment of nutritional status: Functional indicators of pediatric nutriture. Pediatr Clin North Am 32:319–334, 1985
139. Spitz R: Hospitalism, an inquiry into the psychiatric conditions of early childhood. The Psychoanalytic Study of the Child 1:53–74, 1945
140. Sterner RA, Green JA, Funk SG: Preschool Denver developmental screening test as a predictor of later school problems. J Pediatr 107:615–621
141. Stoch M, Smythe P, Moodie A et al: Psychosocial outcome and CT findings after gross undernourishment during infancy: A 20-year developmental study. Dev Med Child Neurol 24:419–436, 1982
142. Suskind RM: Malnutrition and the immune response. In: Suskind RM (ed): Textbook of Pediatric Nutrition. New York, Raven Press, 1981

143. Togut MR, Allen JE, Lelchuck L: A psychological exploration of the nonorganic failure-to-thrive syndrome. Dev Med Child Neurol 11:601–607, 1969
144. Trowbridge FL: Prevalence of growth stunting and obesity: pediatric nutrition surveillance system. MMWR 32:55, 23–26ss, 1984
145. Vietze P, O'Connor S, Sandler H et al: Newborn behavior and interactional characteristics of non-organic failure to thrive infants. In Martin I, Field P, Goldberg S et al (eds): High-risk Infants and Children: Adult and Peer Interactions. New York, Academic Press, 1980
146. Villar J, Smeriglio V, Martorell R et al: Heterogenous growth and mental development in intrauterine growth-retarded infants during the first three years of life. Pediatrics 74:783–791, 1984
147. Viteri F: Primary protein-calorie malnutrition. In Suskind RM (ed): Textbook of Pediatric Nutrition. New York, Raven Press, 1981
148. Waterlow JC: Classification and definition of protein-calorie malnutrition. Br Med J 3:566–569, 1972
149. White JL, Malcolm R, Roper K et al: Psychosocial and developmental factors in failure to thrive: One- to three-year follow-up. J Dev Behav Pediatr 2:112–114, 1981
150. Whitten CF, Pettit MG, Fischhoff J: Evidence that growth failure from maternal deprivation is secondary to undereating. JAMA 209:1675–1682, 1969
151. Winick M, Morgan BLG: Nutrition and brain development. In: Walker WA, Watkins JB (eds): Nutrition in Pediatrics. Boston: Little, Brown & Co, 1985
152. Woolston JL: Eating disorders in infancy and early childhood. J Am Acad Child Psychiatr 22:114–121, 1983
153. World Health Organization: A Growth Chart for Use in Maternal and Child Health Care. Geneva, Switzerland, World Health Organization, 1978
154. World Health Organization: Measuring Changes in Nutritional Status. Geneva, Switzerland, World Health Organization, 1983
155. Yogman MW, Zeisel SH: Diet and sleep patterns in newborn infants. N Engl J Med 309:1147–1149, 1983
156. Zmora E, Gorodicher R, Bar-Ziv J: Multiple nutritional deficiencies in infants from a strict vegetarian community. Am J Dis Child 133:141–144, 1979

Failure to Thrive Program
FGH-3
Boston City Hospital
818 Harrison Avenue
Boston, Massachusetts 02118

Premature Graduates of the Newborn Intensive Care Unit: A Guide to Followup

Howard Bauchner, MD,* Elizabeth Brown, MD,†
and Joy Peskin, MD‡

Over the past two decades there has been a marked increase in the survival of low birth weight infants (LBW; ≤2500 gm) both in this country and abroad.[10, 52] This is true for both very low birth weight infants (VLBW, ≤1500 gm) and moderately low birth weight infants (MLBW, 1501–2500 gm). Of the 3.7 million live births annually in the United States, approximately 250,000 (6.8 per cent) are LBW and 41,000 (1.1 per cent) VLBW.[10, 14]

Caring for the LBW infant is difficult. Primary care providers need to be aware of the many medical, developmental, psychological, and neurological issues that are relevant to these infants and their families. This article will review the growth, health, and development of LBW infants. Particular attention will be paid to the special problems of the premature infant, including: routine immunization, the natural history of developmental and neurological functioning, bronchopulmonary dysplasia/chronic lung disease, complications of intraventicular hemmorrage, risk of cerebral palsy, apnea, and retinopathy of prematurity. A general review regarding screening the premature infant for developmental delay as well as some of the newer techniques for assessing the developmental capabilities of LBW infants are also included.

SURVIVAL OF PREMATURE INFANTS

Over the past decade survival among LBW and VLBW infants has improved. Although many of the recent studies include infants with different birthweights and with varying degrees of medical complications, their results are consistent (Table

*Assistant Professor of Pediatrics and Public Health, Boston University School of Medicine; Boston City Hospital, Division of Developmental and Behavioral Pediatrics, Boston, Massachusetts

†Associate Professor of Pediatrics, Boston University School of Medicine; Director, Division of Neonatology, Boston City Hospital, Boston, Massachusetts

‡Fellow, Division of Developmental and Behavioral Pediatrics, Boston University School of Medicine; Boston City Hospital, Boston, Massachusetts

Table 1. *Newborn Survival*

BIRTHWEIGHT (GM)	SURVIVAL (%)
600–700	<25
701–800	50
801–900	65
901–1000	85
1001–1250	90
1251–1500	95

1).[11, 25, 34, 36, 56, 65, 71, 81, 83, 101–103, 107, 112, 128, 133] For infants with birth weights greater than 750 gm, survival is likely (>50 per cent) and for infants with birth weights greater than 1000 gm it is probable (>90 per cent). With current methods of high-risk pregnancy identification and neonatal intensive care in perinatal referral centers, fewer than 5 per cent of moderately premature infants with birth weights greater than 1500 gm will die. With the emphasis shifted from issues of survival to the complications seen as part of survival, most pediatricians will be caring for an increasing number of infants born prematurely.

GROWTH AND ROUTINE HEALTH CARE MAINTENANCE

Growth of preterm appropriate-for-gestational-age (AGA) infants has been extensively studied and reviewed by Brandt.[19] Preterm AGA infants, when plotted by postconceptional (corrected age) rather than chronologic age, follow the same growth curve as AGA term infants. Corrected age is postnatal age less the number of weeks the child was premature. Acceptable weight gain should be just under 1 oz per day until 6 months of age, length increases about 1 cm per week until term, 0.75 cm per week from term to 3 months, and 0.5 cm per week from 3 to 6 months.[4] Head circumference increases about 0.5 cm per week until 3 months and 0.25 cm per week until 6 months of age.[4] Initially following birth head circumference increases before weight and length.[74] The difference between corrected and chronologic age loses significance after 1.5 years for head circumference, 2 years for weight, and 3.5 years for height.

Infants who are both small for gestational age (SGA) and preterm follow one of two patterns for growth. The difference in these patterns for head circumference has clinical implications. Usually, catch-up growth of head circumference occurs primarily in the first 8 months of life.[5] SGA preterm infants whose head circumference is within normal range for corrected age by 8 months have comparable neurodevelopmental outcomes to AGA preterm infants. On the other hand, SGA preterm infants who do not exhibit this early catch-up growth are at much higher risk for both developmental delay and neurologic handicap.[5, 53]

Although preterm infants have a variety of reasons for relative immunodeficiency, they have a normal response to immunization. An investigation by Bernbaum and others demonstrated that if the timing of the immunization is based on *postnatal* rather than postconceptional age, preterm infants mount a competent immunologic response.[13] Therefore, the American Academy of Pediatrics has recommended that preterm infants be immunized in the same standard schedule used for term infants. The same contraindications for pertussis vaccination apply: (1) previous severe reaction to DPT, (2) a poorly controlled seizure disorder, and (3) emerging or progressive neurologic disease.

Table 2. *Continuity of Developmental Status from Age 1 to 3 Years*

	3-YEAR STATUS		
1-YEAR STATUS	*Normal (%)*	*Suspect (%)*	*Abnormal (%)*
Normal (N = 69)	84	12	4
Suspect (N = 17)	29	29	42
Abnormal (N = 8)	25	0	75

DEVELOPMENTAL AND NEUROLOGIC OUTCOME AND ASSESSMENT

Developmental Outcome

Summarizing the developmental outcomes for these groups of infants is difficult due to the methodologic differences among the reports. Many of the studies include no control groups and there is wide variability in both the developmental tests used to assess the infants and the definitions of "normal." Perinatal risk factors for poor developmental outcome include not only birth weight, but also transport circumstances, gestational age, use and length of mechanical ventilation, asphyxia, intraventricular hemorrhage, and infection. Although a large number of reports are encouraging with respect to intelligence quotient (IQ), longer and more sophisticated followup reveals that a substantial number of these infants develop more subtle problems, such as learning disabilities, particularly visual–motor integration problems. In general, however, for surviving infants with birth weights less than 1000 gm approximately 50 per cent will demonstrate "normal" cognitive (developmental quotient ≥85) and motor development at 2 years of age. For those infants whose birthweights are between 1000 and 1500 gm, 75 per cent can be expected to be "normal" at 2 years of age, and for infants weighing more than 1500 gm, approximately 90 per cent will be normal.[25, 65, 71, 102–104, 107, 133]

Recent followup studies have addressed the stability of an infant's developmental and neurologic status over time, an important concern for pediatricians who monitor the development of premature infants. In other words, do infants classified as normal early in life remain normal? Ross and others reported on the developmental status of 94 VLBW infants (mean birth weight 1173 gm) followed until 3 to 4 years of age.[102] At 1 year, 73 per cent of the infants were considered to have a normal developmental index (Bayley Scales of Infant Development ≥ 85), 18 per cent a suspect score (Bayley score 71–84), and 9 per cent an abnormal score (Bayley score <70). At 3 years of age, of those infants classified as normal at 1 year, 84 per cent still had a normal score, 12 per cent were considered suspect, and 4 per cent had an abnormal score (Table 2). Of those infants in the suspect group at 1 year, 29 per cent were considered normal, 29 per cent suspect, and 42 per cent abnormal at 3 years. For the eight infants who were considered abnormal at a year, 25 per cent were considered normal at 3 years and 75 per cent still abnormal. Overall, of those infants classified as normal or abnormal at 1 year (77 of 94), 83 per cent remained in the same category at 3 years. This study demonstrates the general continuity in developmental level for those infants considered normal or abnormal at 1 year of age.

Although there is stability in general developmental scores during the preschool years, recent studies have suggested that LBW infants develop more subtle problems as they enter school. For example, in a study of 42 infants (mean birth weight = 1247 gm) followed until 7 years of age, despite normal IQ scores and age-appropriate reading skills, 10 of 22 infants had visual–motor integration problems.[128] For the infants who were abnormal or suspect at 7 years of age with regard to their developmental level, 13 of 17 demonstrated poor visual motor skills, and 11 were reading below the 50th percentile. With regard to school placement, 8 of the 42 infants were in special education classes and 21 were receiving some form of supplemental services (speech and language, remedial mathematics). In another study, 46 VLBW infants (mean birth weight = 1216 gm) with normal intelligence and no neurologic abnormalities at 5 years of age were matched to a control group of children who were full term and in the same kindergarten or preschool class.[65] The VLBW infants did significantly less well on tests of spatial relations and visual–motor integration. In conclusion, longer followup of these infants often reveals the development of subtle learning problems and school dysfunction, despite normal IQ scores. Premature infants with normal development, but who are having difficulty in school, should be evaluated for the presence of a specific learning disability.

When speaking with parents about their premature infant, pediatricians need to be aware of a number of additional issues. First, pediatricians can aid parents in dealing with their grief. Few parents anticipate that their infant may be premature and are unprepared for the medical and psychological consequences. Parents may deny problems, become angry with the pediatrician or other professionals, and feel isolated from friends. Second, the studies reporting on long-term followup are concerned with the performance of large groups of children. All of these studies report relatively wide variation in the performance of children classified in any group. Hence, for any individual child, it is difficult to predict precisely how they will perform. Parents often have a difficult time dealing with the uncertainty that exists about prognosis. Third, developmental problems may arise at virtually any time. It is important for pediatricians to monitor these children regularly and refer them for further evaluation and early intervention when the infants demonstrate delay after correcting for prematurity or when parents feel the need for another professional opinion. Finally, prematurity is a major contributor to the "vulnerable child syndrome." Frequently parents describe these infants as "difficult." It is important for pediatricians to give parents a hopeful view of their child and explore their feelings about the child with them.

Neurologic Outcome

The neurologic followup of LBW infants includes evaluation for possible visual and auditory deficits and for the presence of hydrocephalus and cerebral palsy. This section will be confined to a discussion of cerebral palsy, since the other medical conditions will be discussed in the following section.

Although most LBW infants will not develop cerebral palsy, prematurity is still an important risk factor.[45, 87] In the Collaborative Perinatal Project of the National Institute of Neurological and Communicative Disorders and Stroke, 189 (0.4 per cent) of 45,559 children, followed to the age of 7 years, developed cerebral palsy.[82] Twenty-one per cent of the children who developed cerebral palsy had gestational ages less than 32 weeks (approximate birth weights = 1500 gm). However of the 1503 children in this study with gestational ages $\leq$ 32 weeks only 2.7 per cent developed cerebral palsy. In a number of recent studies, the incidence of cerebral palsy in infants weighing less than 1500 gm was approximately 15 per cent.[67, 71, 104, 107, 133] These studies, taken as a whole, suggest that although prematurity is a risk factor for cerebral palsy, most LBW infants will not develop cerebral palsy and that most infants who do develop cerebral palsy are not premature. Moreover, unlike the situation with full-term infants with cerebral palsy, premature infants with cerebral palsy will not be at an appreciably higher risk for mental retardation as are full-term infants.

The stability of neurologic classification is also important. In the same study reviewed in the section on developmental outcome, the authors also examined the stability of the diagnosis of cerebral palsy over time.[102] At 1 year of age, 77 per cent

Table 3. *Continuity of Cerebral Palsy Classification from Age 1 to 3 Years*

	3-YEAR STATUS		
1-YEAR STATUS	Normal (%)	Suspect (%)	Abnormal (%)
Normal (N = 72)	97	3	0
Mild CP (N = 7)	86	14	0
Moderate/severe CP (N = 15)	13	13	73

of the infants (72 of 94) did not manifest cerebral palsy, while 7 per cent had mild cerebral palsy and 16 per cent had moderate to severe cerebral palsy. At 3 years of age, only 3 per cent of the infants classified as normal at 1 year were diagnosed with cerebral palsy (Table 3). For those infants with mild cerebral palsy at 1 year, 86 per cent had no cerebral palsy at 3 years and 14 per cent continued to have mild cerebral palsy. For the moderate to severe group at 1 year, 73 per cent still had moderate to severe cerebral palsy at 3 years, and 13 per cent showed either no cerebral palsy or mild cerebral palsy. Thus, most infants who show no signs of cerebral palsy at 1 year continued to have a normal neurologic examination. Most infants who are suspect or have mild cerebral palsy at 1 year will improve with age. The prognosis is worse for those infants with a definitive diagnosis of severe or moderate cerebral palsy at 1 year. Most of these infants will continue to demonstrate signs of cerebral palsy as they get older.

Contribution of the Environment to Developmental Outcome

Understanding the process of development can aid the pediatrician in assessing the development of premature infants. Currently, single risk factors, such as prematurity, are felt to be insufficient in determining the developmental outcome of these infants.[9, 27, 38, 108] Current theory suggests that children interact with their environment, with the behaviors of each being modified by the other. Both the child and caretaker adapt and change as a result of their interactions. To predict outcome, the "biologic risk" of prematurity and quality of the environment need to be assessed.

Numerous studies have confirmed the importance of the environment as a major factor in the developmental outcome of premature infants. Escalona studied 86 LBW infants and found an appreciable decline in cognitive development associated with low socioeconomic status.[37] The 21 infants in the lowest quartile of socioeconomic status manifested a decline in IQ scores from 96 to 80 between 7 and 45 months of age. In marked contrast, the 25 infants in the highest quartile of socioeconomic status showed no such decline. Escalona concluded that infants born at biologic risk from prematurity, and environmental risk, from low SES groups, are at "double hazard" for poor developmental outcomes.[38]

In another study, Beckwith and Parmelee reported that 15 LBW infants reared in a more responsive caregiving environment had higher intelligence scores at the age of 5 years than a group of 34 LBW infants who were raised in a less responsive caregiving environment.[7] The caregiving environment was assessed when the infant was 1, 8, and 24 months of age, from naturalistic home observations. These investigators concluded that, "It is likely that single risk factors are insufficient in determining outcome for most infants."

In a related study of 215 full-term 4-year-old children, in which 10 risk factors were assessed, Sameroff and others reported that the variability in verbal IQ scores was directly related to the number of risk factors each infant accumulated.[108] The risk factors were maternal mental health, anxiety, interactive behaviors, level of education, parental perspectives, occupation of head of household, minority group status, family social support, family size, and stressful life events. Regardless of socioeconomic status, infants with four or more risk factors had IQ scores that were 15 points less than infants with zero to one risk factors. Although this investigation involved full-term infants, it is likely that similar risk factors are even more important when assessing premature infants due to the biovulnerability associated with premature birth.

In summary, the caretaking environment has a profound impact on the premature infant's long term development. An infant's resilience to biologic insults can be ameliorated by a supportive and stimulating environment, or exacerbated by a nonoptimal environment.

Developmental Assessment

Assessing the development of premature infants in an office setting is difficult. Most pediatricians do not have the time nor are trained to performed detailed assessments. However, there are screening tools that pediatricians can use that will facilitate following these infants.

The Denver Developmental Screening Test (DDST) is the most popular screening tool that pediatricians use to assess young infants.[36] Unfortunately, there have been few reports discussing its efficacy in evaluating the LBW infant. Because it is a familiar tool to pediatricians, however, it can be used as a framework to observe infants' skills. When using the DDST, as is the case with any assessment tool for premature infants, the age of the infant should be corrected for the extent of prematurity, until the infant reaches 1 year of age.[119]

How should the DDST be used? A recent report by Sciarillo and others suggested that DDST did not identify a significant number of 62 LBW infants who received suspect or abnormal evaluations on more sophisticated neurodevelopmental assessment.[111] However, the screeners' clinical impression, which was based on observations made during the administration of the DDST, did identify infants with abnormal development. The screener's clinical judgment appropriately identified seven of the eight infants who received low scores on the Bayley. Some younger infants were inappropriately labeled as abnormal. However, since the goal of screening is to identify the majority of children with a poor outcome (high sensitivity) prior to further diagnostic evaluation, the process of administering the DDST and formulating a clinical impression is a useful screening procedure. In conclusion, the results of this study suggest that the DDST may not accurately identify those infants who do poorly on more extensive evaluation, but it does provide a framework for systematically observing premature infants and formulating an overall clinical impression. The clinical impression derived from performing the DDST is particularly accurate with infants who are older than 1 year.

A child should be referred for further developmental evaluation based on a clinical impression of developmental problems and an understanding of environmental factors that may facilitate or impede development. A number of assessment tools have been designed to aid the pediatrician in assessing the quality of the home environment (Home Observation for Measurement of the Environment—HOME and Home Screening Questionnaire—HSQ), social supports (Maternal Social Support Index—MSSI), and life stresses (Life Event Scale).[27] These questionnaires are self-administered and can be completed while a parent and child are waiting to be seen. Although these tests can be a useful adjunct in following the families of premature infants, since pediatricians are aware of a family's resources and strengths these structured tools may not be necessary.

Neurologic Assessment

Assessing LBW infants for the presence or absence of cerebral palsy is another important task for the pediatrician. Although cerebral palsy is defined as a fixed motor deficit, it is often difficult to make a definitive diagnosis early in life because of its changing clinical picture. After 1 year of age, as discussed above, infants who are normal or have moderate to severe cerebral palsy demonstrate general stability with regard to their neurologic status. Recently Graziani and others described the relationship between neonatal ultrasound and cerebral palsy.[50] In a cohort of 139 infants followed for 5 years, a diagnosis of cerebral palsy was made in 15 children. The gestational ages, birth weight, Apgar scores, and need for mechanical ventilation were similar for infants with and without cerebral palsy. The results of cerebral ultrasound were quite helpful in distinguishing the two groups. All 15 infants who developed cerebral palsy had specific abnormal ultrasound images (grade III or IV intracranial hemorrhage with periventricular cysts, porencephaly, or hydrocephalus) and only 3 of 124 infants who did not develop cerebral palsy had the same specific abnormal ultrasound images. Because most LBW infants are routinely evaluated by cranial ultrasound, pediatricians can use this information as a marker of risk for the development of cerebral palsy.

During the first year of life, a delay in the achievement of motor milestones can be a sign of cerebral palsy. Poor muscle tone, hypertonia, hypotonia, increased deep tendon reflexes, and persistence of primitive reflexes are of concern. Although many LBW infants will demonstrate increased lower extremity tone and increased truncal tone during the first year of life, "transient dystonia of prematurity," the persistence of these findings beyond 1 year should alert the pediatrician to the possibility of cerebral palsy. Geogieff and others recently reported that 62 per cent of 34 VLBW infants had increased lower extremity tone at 6 months' (corrected age), but that the incidence declined to 9 per cent by 18 months' corrected age.[48] A referral for complete evaluation is appropriate when there is the presence of poor motor development, persistence of increased tone, hyper-reflexia, or asymmetric abnormalities in tone or reflexes. Because the treatment of cerebral palsy is complex and has been extensively reviewed elsewhere, it will not be discussed here.[123] However, pediatricians are cautioned not to label LBW infants as having cerebral palsy unless there is a reasonably certain diagnosis due to transient neurologic abnormalities.

Early Intervention

After identifying infants who are doing poorly because of either biologic or environmental risks, pediatricians need to consider if early intervention would be appropriate. Over the past decade, there have been a number of reviews that have highlighted both the risks and benefits of early infant intervention. The authors of these reviews make the following points:[28, 51, 86, 98, 101, 105, 118, 120]

1. The identification of infants who will do poorly is complicated and must include assessment of the infant, parent, and environment.

2. Early intervention programs are efficacious, particularly for those infants in whom biologic risk is coupled with environmental risk.

3. Initial gains in IQ scores may be transient, but other benefits, such as less need for special educational services and repetition of grades in school, are evident in long-term followup studies.

4. Structured curriculum, extensive parental involvement, family counseling and support services, and interventions involving the parent and child together are important factors in those programs demonstrating the most effectiveness.

5. Frequently early intervention preschool special education programs need to be followed by further special education efforts once the child reaches elementary school.

6. Earlier referral seems to be more efficacious than later referral.

Pediatricians should be careful not to refer every LBW infant to early intervention programs because there are potential adverse risks. First, these programs involve a commitment of time and energy on behalf of the parents. Second, most LBW infants will do relatively well without any intervention. There are no data suggesting that all premature infants should be referred to early intervention programs. Referral should be reserved for those children who demonstrate delay in the first year of life and those with environmental risk factors.

When a referral is made to a program, a pediatrician can be helpful by being familiar with the intake process, the specific types of services offered, and the format of the intervention. The pediatrician should communicate with the staff about the infant's medical problems and in turn receive information about the infant's developmental progress. This information then can be used in the ongoing discussions with the family.

NEW TECHNIQUES OF DEVELOPMENTAL ASSESSMENT

Previously, premature infants were assessed while in the newborn intensive care unit (NICU) using clinically derived scales. These scales attempted to link prognosis to prenatal and perinatal events.[32, 126] Measures such as the Optimality Scale and the Obstetric, Postnatal, and Pediatric Complications Scales assigned scores to various medical risk factors present in the perinatal period in an attempt to predict outcome.[49, 114] However, the prognostic capabilities of these scales were poor. Initially, Apgar scores also were thought to have potential in predicting future outcome.[31] However, as recently summarized by the Committee on the Fetus and Newborn, low Apgar scores at 1 and 5 minutes alone are "not evident of sufficient hypoxia to result in neurologic damage." In addition, over the years, the Apgar score has not been found to reliably predict the development of the premature infant.[115] More recently, two new tests, acoustical analysis of cry and the Fagan Test of Infant Intelligence (FTIT), have been developed to identify premature infants who will have developmental problems.

For years it has been noted that there is an association between unusual cry features and neurologic damage or dysfunction. For example, high-pitched cries have been associated with infants with "cri du chat" syndrome or meningitis.[134] Recently, new computerized models of acoustic analysis have been developed permitting the rapid analysis of cries.[69] Cry features are affected by the stability of laryngeal coordination and vocal tract mobility, both of which are a reflection of neurologic maturity. In a study by Lester, the cries of 18 premature and 13 term infants were analyzed using a computer-based signaling system developed by Golub.[69] A significant correlation was found between certain characteristics of cry and developmental outcome as measured by the Bayley at 18 months and the McCarthy General Cognitive Index at 5 years of age.

Fagan and co-workers have recently developed another screening device to assess cognitive development.[39-41] The FTIT is a test that determines differences in recognition memory during infancy, measuring an infant's developing ability to perceive and to retain information. An infant is presented with two pictures, a novel one and a familiar one. The more developmentally advanced infant should choose the novel picture over the familiar one, since early novelty preferences reflect underlying memory and cognitive development. The predictive validity of the FTIT is good. Infants were tested between 3 and 7 months of age and then again at the age of 3 years. The FTIT had a predictive validity of 88 per cent in detecting developmental delay (IQ <70) and 91 per cent in predicting normality.[39]

Acoustic analysis of cry and the FTIT have been developed in an attempt to identify which premature infants will do poorly. However, both of these tools remain investigational at the moment. Additional data are needed before we can fully assess the value of these tests.

THE ENVIRONMENT OF THE NICU

The environment of the NICU has been viewed as both overstimulating and depriving. With increasing survival among VLBW infants and hence longer hospital stays (average length of stay for infants with birth weights less than 1000 gm is 60 days), our attention has been refocused on the physiologic and developmental effects of the environment. The goal of health care includes creating an appropriate environment for further growth and development.

During the 1960s and early 1970s there was a strong movement to increase the amount of stimulation in the seemingly deprived NICU environment. Multiple interventions were studied, measuring various outcomes. Some of the prevailing philosophies emphasized the importance of mimicking the *in utero* environment, whereas others attempted to create for the infant an environment similar to that of the home environment of full-term infants.[42, 70] Interventions included rocking, stroking, oscillating waterbeds, heartbeat recordings, and cycled lighting.[42, 58] Unfortunately, these early studies did not include assessments of the specific environmental deficiencies within the NICU. When studied, some areas of the NICU were found to be overstimulating, while other areas were found to be deficient. There are high levels of illumination with no day–night variation. Ambient noise levels are high due to radios, equipment, monitors, adult speech, and isolettes.[72] In contrast to elevated noise levels, speech directed toward the infant is miniscule, occurring only 5 per cent of the time.[42] Along with the high levels of stimulation in these areas, there is no rhythmicity or consistency in the infants' environment. There is little vestibular-kinesthetic stimulation, and gentle touching is infrequent.[6] This is true both while the infant is acutely ill, when it may be necessary, as well as when the infant is stable, when benefit from appropriate stimulation exists. More recent studies attempt to address some of these deficiencies.

Field and others studied the effects of giving pacifiers to VLBW infants with respiratory disease during all nasogastric feedings.[43] Sucking is a normal activity of newborns and of the *in utero* fetus and may help the premature infant attain some degree of control over his or her state of organization. Infants given the pacifiers during feeds had significantly greater weight gain and fewer hospitalized days as compared to control infants. They also had fewer medical problems and were quicker to make the transition to breast- or bottle-feeding. Growth parameters were still significantly better for the study subjects at 1 year of age.[42, 43]

Another area investigated by Field and others is tactile-kinesthetic supplementary stimulation.[44] They theorized that premature infants may be similar to maternally deprived babies and need tactile-kinesthetic stimulation that replicates maternal touching behaviors that normal newborns receive. Twenty premature infants were compared to twenty control infants of similar gestational age (<36 weeks), birth weight (<1500 gm), and medical risks. Stimulation was given for 15 minutes at the beginning of 3 consecutive hours for 10 weekdays after the morning feed. The intervention group demonstrated significantly greater weight gain, increased motor activity, more alertness, and better performance on the Brazelton Neonatal Assessment Scale than did the control group.

A recent report by Als and others described an attempt to provide stimulation in a consistent and time-appropriate manner.[1] The group studied eight experimental and eight control infants with birth weights less than 1250 gm, gestational ages less than 28 weeks, and mechanical ventilation for more than 24 of the first 48 hours of life. The infants who received the intervention were observed prior to treatment so that a more individualized program could be developed in conjunction with the primary nurses. Examples of these interventions include: avoidance of proximity to faucets and sinks; reduction in telephone and radio noise level, lighting, and traffic; and the opportunity to suck during and between feedings. Overall these interventions created for the infant a calmer, more contained world with increased sensitivity toward the infant's alertness, space, and position, and his or her need for rest and sleep. This emphasis on stress reduction and increase of self-regulatory competence decreased the number of days on the respirator and need for supplemental oxygen, and improved feeding transition to oral nutrition.[1]

In summary, recent data suggest that supplemental stimulation in the NICU is not an "all or none" phenomenon. Rather, more adaptive individualized interventions that emphasize stress reduction and self-regulatory skills are necessary. This approach will create for the premature infant a more optimal environment for growth and development. Pediatricians should try to ensure that, particularly when a premature infant is well, the infant receives appropriate supplemental stimulation.

LONG-TERM MEDICAL COMPLICATIONS

Premature infants have increased risks both in terms of morbidity and mortality in the first year of life. Followup care of these children requires more than "routine" health surveillance. LBW infants have twice the risk of rehospitalization during the first year of life, whereas VLBW infants have 4.5 times the increased risk. As with term infants, factors associated with rehospitalization include congenital anomalies, developmental delay, and low socioeconomic status.[78] The degree of risk is greatly increased in infants with discharge diagnoses in three categories: chronic lung disease, intraventricular hemorrhage, and retinopathy of prematurity. In addition, all premature infants are at increased risk for hearing loss, apnea, and perhaps sudden infant death syndrome (SIDS).

Chronic Lung Disease

Bronchopulmonary dysplasia (BPD) is the major chronic lung disease. It is seen in 6 to 24 per cent of premature infants who require mechanical ventilation with increased oxygen concentration. Other factors associated with BPD include pulmonary immaturity, patent ductus arteriosus, excess intravenous fluid administration, and postnatal ventilator management.[20, 21, 33, 76, 80, 84, 100] New therapies such as vitamin A supplementation to reduce epithelial injury and high-frequency ventilation to decrease exposure to barotrauma are currently under study.

Although the definition of BPD has been controversial, the definition of O'Brodovich and Mellins has been well accepted. They define BPD as an acute lung injury in the first 2 weeks of life, persisting beyond 1 month, associated with the clinical findings of respiratory distress, cyanosis in room air, and chest radiograph findings of cystic or hyperinflated areas.[85] The lung pathology involves impaired ciliary function with accumulation of secretions in terminal and respiratory bronchioles; ulceration and necrosis of bronchiolar membranes, and widespread fibrosis.[18] The clinical symptoms and pulmonary function test abnormalities include chronic secretions with episodes of coughing and vomiting, a tendency to wheeze with respiratory infections, reactive airway disease, and chronic hypoxemia. The combination of hypoxemia and increased pulmonary vascular resistance places these infants at risk for development of cor pulmonale.

Management of infants with chronic lung disease after discharge from the NICU is directed toward maintenance of adequate growth, minimizing hypoxemia, decreasing airway hyper-reactivity if present, and avoiding lower respiratory tract infections. Infants with BPD have an increased caloric requirement due to both an increased oxygen consumption and increased work of breathing.[131] Methods for increasing caloric intake while maintaining fluid restriction include concentration of formula to 24 to 30 calories per ounce by addition of caloric supplements (medium-chain triglycerides, polycose) and use of diuretics. Early in the course of BPD, despite several potential serious complications, diuretic therapy can decrease airway resistance and increase lung compliance, both beneficial effects.[26, 59, 62–64, 92, 121, 127] However, the chronic use of diuretics is more controversial since no long-term studies are available and potential effects on pulmonary function and growth are unknown.

For infants with BDP, increased oxygen must be provided to prevent hypoxic vasoconstriction of the pulmonary vascular bed and to decrease the work of breathing. This will allow utilization of calories for growth. Oxygen should be administered continuously. Tent or hood oxygen is inappropriate as oxygen levels fluctuate with movement of the infant in and out of the apparatus. The best way to ensure that oxygen concentrations are constant is to use a nasal canula or nasal trough method. Oxygen flow should be adjusted to keep the arterial po_2 greater than 50 mm Hg. Oxygen levels below 50 mm Hg result in pulmonary vasocontriction and is associated with risk of cor pulmonale. Weaning from oxygen should be attempted only when both po_2 is greater than 50 mm Hg and an adequate rate of growth has been established. Too early weaning from oxygen may result in diminished growth and therefore slower recovery. Ultimately, improvement in lung function depends on increased lung size and hence adequate growth.

Lower respiratory tract infections are a major risk for both mortality and rehospitalization in infants with chronic lung disease. As many as 30 to 80 per cent of infants will develop either bronchiolitis or pneumonia in the first year of life.[22, 73, 109, 129] Although exposure to viral illness cannot be eliminated, care should be taken with BPD infants to minimize the risks. Elective admissions to hospital should not be done in the winter months during respiratory syncytial virus season; office visits should be scheduled in such a way that the infant goes directly to an examining room and does not wait in a area with sick toddlers. If day care is an absolute necessity, placement should be sought in a setting where the infant will not be exposed to toddlers. If an infant with BPD does develop lower respiratory tract disease, early aggressive management with bronchodilators may be indicated. In addition, since these infants can develop respiratory failure quickly when ill, they need to be carefully monitored.

Other complications seen in infants with BPD include tracheal stenosis (8 per cent of infants), upper airway obstruction secondary to subglottic cysts, hoarseness due to partial or complete vocal cord paralysis, and wheezing. When an infant with BPD presents with hoarseness or stridor, particularly in the absence of infection, full evaluation by an ear, nose, and throat specialist is indicated. Although wheezing with respiratory infection is common in infants with BPD, about 10 per cent of such infants will wheeze in the absense of infection.

There is growing evidence that infants with bronchopulmonary dysplasia do not recover completely.[24, 125] Studies in late childhood have indicated a high incidence of obstructive airway disease and ventilation/perfusion imbalance.[132] Long-term studies have shown persistent bronchial hyper-reactivity.[15, 121] Treatment with bronchodilators may be beneficial and should be tried in infants with persistant wheezing.[64]

Some infants with BPD have developmental delay. Most often this delay is related to delayed gross motor skills secondary to hypotonia. Because of the marked influence of motor delay on the overall assessment of developmental skills in the first year of life, care must be taken not to extrapolate early test results to anticipate later cognitive functioning of these infants.

The stress placed on the family of the BPD infant is considerable. Disturbed family relationships between parents and among siblings are common. All available services to help families with chronically ill children should be used, including visiting nursing, homemaking, early intervention, social services, respite care, and

Table 4. *Classification of Intraventricular Hemorrhage*

Grade I:	Subependymal hemorrhage without ventricular or parenchymal extension
Grade II:	Intraventricular hemorrhage without ventricular dilatation
Grade III:	Intraventricular hemorrhage with ventricular dilatation
Grade IV:	Intraventricular hemorrhage with parenchymal brain hemorrhage

parent groups. Attention to the medical needs of the child without providing for the needs of the entire family is incomplete care.

Posthemorrhagic Neurologic Complications

In nonasphyxiated preterm infants, the major cause of long-term neurologic disability is related to complications of intraventricular hemorrhage (IVH). IVH may occur in as many as 30 to 40 per cent of infants less that 1500 gm birth weight with a mortality rate as high as 28 per cent.[50] The hemorrhage usually occurs during the first 3 days of life and originates in the subependymal germinal matrix area. Risk factors include birth asphyxia, respiratory distress syndrome, acidosis, hypoxia, apnea, hypotension, infusion of hypertonic solutions (e.g., bicarbonate), seizures, and a requirement for ventilatory support.[66]

The major immediate complication of IVH is hydrocephalus, which occurs with increased frequency with increasing severity of hemorrhage. Most infants with blood filling more than 50 per cent of the ventricular space will develop hydrocephalus. Ventriculomegaly after IVH is common and occurs in at least 50 per cent of all infants with hemorrhage. Ventricular dilatation usually precedes an increase in head circumference, and all infants with IVH should have frequent ultrasounds in the weeks after an IVH to assess this complication. Of infants with posthemorrhagic hydrocephalus, half will have rapid progression and require immediate intervention. The other half may have a period of what Volpe calls "normal pressure" hydrocephalus, in which the infant has ventriculomegaly but with stable or slowly increasing ventricular size. About half of these infants will need a surgical drainage of their CSF.[54] The need for surgical intervention may be delayed between a few months and a year after the hemorrhage.

The long-term outcome for infants with hydrocephalus has not been reported for any large group of patients. Available information suggests that the overall outcome for this group is poor, particularly if the birth weight is less that 1000 gm. Infants with IVH but without hydrocephalus have a much better prognosis. Factors important in predicting outcome include the degree of the hemorrhage, the hemorrhagic destruction of both germinal matrix and periventricular white matter, intracranial hypertension and impaired cerebral perfusion, and the development of posthemorrhagic hydrocephalus.[130]

The long-term complications of IVH include neuromotor handicap and developmental delay. There is some relationship between severity of hemorrhage and outcome in so far as hemorrhage size predicts local cerebral ischemic damage. Papile and others reported that 60 per cent of infants with grade III or IV hemorrhage had major neuromotor handicap or developmental delay, neither of which was seen in infants with less severe bleeding.[88] (See Table 4 for grading system.) Scott and co-workers reported more subtle findings that appear at age 2 to 3 years.[113] At 24 months of age the DQ of infants with low-grade hemorrhage was significantly lower than that of matched controls without IVH, although almost all infants were still in the low normal or normal DQ range. When hydrocephalus complicates IVH, the long-term prognosis is worsened. Chaplin and colleagues reported that only 5 of 22 such infants had an IQ greater than 90, and of those 5, 2 had major neurologic handicap.[29]

Table 5. *Classification of Retinopathy of Prematurity*

Zone I:	From optic disk to twice the distance from the disk to center of the macula
Zone II:	From edge of Zone I to the nasal ora serrata and to an area near the temporal anatomic equator
Zone III:	Residual crescent of retina anterior to Zone II (This is the zone last vascularized in the eye of the infant and most frequently involved with ROP.)

There is considerable controversy as to whether IVH per se is responsible for the poor outcome or factors responsible for the hemorrhage are the real culprits. Schub and co-workers in Atlanta compared 33 infants with IVH to 30 infants without IVH but with matching Apgar scores, birth weight, and gestational age.[110] There were no differences in neuromotor outcome or development between the two groups.

Followup on infants with IVH should include careful assessment of head circumference and neurodevelopmental function throughout early childhood. Increased head circumference or clinical signs associated with increased intracranial pressure require repeated cranial ultrasound or computer tomographic (CT) studies until ventricular size has been stable for several months. Late progression to hydrocephalus severe enough to require a ventral–peritoneal shunt procedure has been reported as late as 2 years of age. Infants with evidence of any neuromotor abnormality should be carefully followed and enrolled in appropriate programs such as physical therapy, occupational therapy, and early intervention.

Retinopathy of Prematurity

The epidemic of retrolental fibroplasia (RLF) described in the early 1950s was clearly related to administration of increased concentration of oxygen with elevated pO_2. In recent years the term *retinopathy of prematurity* (ROP) has been adapted.

ROP can only occur if the retina is not vascularized. The extent of retinal vascularization is inversely related to gestational age. Younger premature infants have less peripheral vascularization. The association between elevated pO_2 and ROP is thought to result from hyperoxic vasoconstriction in the most immature part of the retina (usually the temporal area) followed by hypoxic injury to the devascularized retina after hyperoxia ends. Neovascularization then proceeds and the changes occur as outlined in Table 5.[2]

Even with careful oxygen monitoring, ROP still occurs in infants in whom no hyperoxia can be demonstrated. Other causes associated with ROP besides hyperoxia and prematurity include hypercapnia, hypoxia, intraventricular hemorrhage, seizures, apnea, and exchange transfusion with adult blood, which may alter oxygen delivery to the tissues.[23, 97, 99, 106, 117]

A new international classification (Table 6) has resulted in more uniform diagnostic categorization of the lesion and has enabled investigators to conduct multicenter trials of new pharmacologic and surgical therapies for the disorder.[47] With consistent definitions of the lesion, the epidemiology of ROP has become clearer. Phelps documented a ROP incidence of 2.2 per cent in infants weighing 1000 to 1500 gm at birth.[93] There is a marked increase in incidence in infants less than 1000 gm birth weight. Merritt and Kraybill reported that 59.5 per cent of infants weighing less than 1000 gm at birth developed ROP, compared to 13.9 per cent of infants weighing 1001 to 1399 and 6 per cent of infants weighing 1400 to 1799 gm.[79] Only 1 per cent of preterm infants weighing more than 1799 gm at birth developed ROP. Whereas the authors demonstrated an overall incidence of ROP of 20 per cent in their population, only 1.8 per cent had severe disease and were

Table 6. *Stages of Retinopathy of Prematurity*

Stage I:	Demarcation line—This white line separates the avascular retina from vascularized retina. There is abnormal branching of vessels that lead to the demarcation line.
Stage II:	Ridge—Although the demarcation line does not extend anterior out of the plane of the retina, as the disease progresses, this area develops as tufts of new vessels appear.
Stage III:	Extraretinal fibrovascular proliferation—These are located posterior to the ridge or into the vitreous.
Stage IV:	Retinal detachment

Plus disease (+): When posterior veins are enlarged or arterioles are tortuous, a "+" is added to the ROP stage designation.

blind. The early changes of ROP regress spontaneously in about 90 per cent of cases.

Several new therapies for ROP have been tried in recent years. Hittner and co-workers reported a decreased incidence of severe ROP but no overall decrease in incidence of ROP in infants treated with parenteral vitamin E, an antioxidant, from the first day of life.[57] Other studies have either reported no benefit or have raised concern about possible toxicity. Routine use of vitamin E for the purpose of ROP prevention is not yet indicated based on currently available data.[94, 95]

Two surgical interventions have been attempted. Cryotherapy has been used based on the hypothesis that destroying spindle cells ultimately may decrease vascular proliferation and thus prevent progression of the disease. Repair of retinal detachment also has been attempted but unless done early has not been very effective in restoring useful vision. Both therapies currently are under study in nationwide trials and should be thought of as experimental, pending further data.

All infants at risk should be examined at 4 to 6 weeks of age by an ophthalmologist. Infants who remain on oxygen therapy should be examined again several weeks after oxygen has been discontinued. Infants with vascular proliferative changes should be examined every 3 to 6 months until the changes resolve or until cicatricial changes (scarring) have been identified. Infants with cicatricial changes require lifelong followup. Mild scarring often results in myopic changes, most often correctable with lenses. Many myopic infants present with secondary strabismus, and surgical repair is the most common surgical procedure in the first year of life in preterm infants. More severe scarring is associated with retinal detachment. Secondary glaucoma has been reported in infants with severe cicatricial changes.[96]

Hearing Screening in Preterm Infants

Very low birth weight is one of the seven risk criteria for identifying children who should be screened for hearing impairment (other risk factors include: (1) a family history of deafness, (2) congenital perinatal infection, (3) anatomic malformation involving the head or neck, (4) hyperbilirubinemia, (5) bacterial meningitis, and (6) severe asphyxia).[61] High-risk infants have two to five times the risk of moderate to profound hearing loss compared to infants without risk factors. The incidence of hearing loss in infants without any risk factors is about 1 per cent. Preterm infants should be screened by 3 to 6 months of age. Multiple methods are available, including emittance audiometry (not useful at <3 months of age); Crib-o-Gram, which measures an infant's gross body movements in response to an intense sound stimulus; auditory response cradle, which is similar to a Crib-o-Gram; and auditory brain stem response audiometry, which is helpful in identifying children with less serious hearing loss.[12, 46]

Diagnosis of hearing loss should be established early (<6 months of age) and services for the hearing impaired provided. Hearing is closely linked to speech development, and early intervention is important.

Apnea of Prematurity

Apnea of prematurity (AP) is a diagnosis of exclusion, made when preterm infants have a respiratory pause greater than 20 seconds associated with cyanosis and bradycardia. Other causes, such as anemia, patent ductus arteriosus, hypoxia, airway obstruction, seizures, and sepsis, must be ruled out. AP has been thought to be a maturational delay in development of the respiratory control system and usually resolves as the preterm infant reaches term dates.[75] Infants who do not resolve their apnea by the time of discharge may be treated at home with methylxanthines (theophylline or caffeine). If apnea is well controlled on pharmacologic therapy, the drug should be continued until 2 to 3 months post-term dates and then discontinued while the infant is on an apnea monitor. If no further apneic episodes occur it can then be discontinued. If apneic episodes recur then methylxanthines should be restarted and the infant retested at 6 months. Theophylline blood levels need to be tested frequently and maintained in the therapeutic range (6–16 μg per ml) since the infants' growth rates accelerate rapidly. Doses needed to provide a stable blood level vary widely but usually approximate 6.5 mg per kg per day divided into four doses.

Infants whose AP is not well controlled on methylxanthine treatment should be considered candidates for home apnea monitoring. The monitoring should be done through an organized program with a coordinated multidisciplinary team approach.

Although graduates of NICUs have an increased risk of SIDS in comparison to normal infants, apnea of prematurity does not pose an additional risk. A normal pneumogram should not be interpreted to mean a low risk for SIDS in this population.[17, 122]

CONCLUSION

Over the next decade pediatricians will care for an increasing number of premature graduates of the NICU. Their care is complicated because many have complex medical problems, delayed development, and concerned and anxious parents. It is important for pediatricians to see these infants regularly, assiduously monitoring their growth, health, and development. Problems need to be identified early so appropriate services can be provided. Although many specialists may be involved with the low birth weight infant, it is the pediatrician who knows the family best and can integrate the subspecialty medical information, provide guidance for the parents, and offer emotional support.

ACKNOWLEDGMENT

Support was provided by an Academic Training Program Grant in Behavioral Pediatrics, funded by the Bureau of Health Care Delivery and Assistance, Maternal and Child Health Branch (#MCJ-009094). We would also like to thank Barry Zuckerman, MD, and Steven Parker, MD, for their guidance and thoughtful critique of the article.

REFERENCES

1. Als H, Lawhon G, Brown E, et al: Individualized behavioral and environmental care for the very low birth weight preterm infant at high risk for bronchopulmonary dysplasia:

Neonatal intensive care unit and developmental outcome. Pediatrics 78:1123–1132, 1986

2. Ashton N: The pathogenesis of retrolental fibroplasia. Ophthalmology 86:1695, 1979
3. Avery M, Tooley W, Keller J et al: Is chronic lung disease in low birth weight infants preventable? A survey of eight centers. Pediatrics 79:26–30, 1987
4. Babson S: Growth of low birth weight infants. J Pediatr 77:11–18, 1970
5. Babson S, Henderson N: Fetal undergrowth: Relation of head growth to later intellectual performance. Pediatrics 53:890–894, 1974
6. Barnard K, Bee H: The impact of temporally patterned stimulation on the development of preterm infants. Child Dev 54:1157–1167, 1983
7. Beckwith L, Parmelee A: EEG patterns of preterm infants, home environment, and later IQ. Child Dev 57:777–789, 1986
8. Beckwith L, Cohen S, Kopp et al: Caregiver-infant interaction and early cognitive development in preterm infants. Child Development 47:579–587, 1976
9. Bee H, Barnard K, Eyres S, Gray C et al: Prediction of IQ and language skill from perinatal status, child performance, family characteristics, and mother-infant interaction. Child Dev 53:1134–1156, 1982
10. Behrman R: Preventing low birth weight: A pediatric perspective. J Pediatr 107:842–854, 1985
11. Bennett F, Robinson N, Sells C: Growth and development of infants weighing less than 800 grams at birth. Pediatrics 71:319–323, 1983
12. Bennet M, Wade H: Computerized hearing test for neonates. Hear Aid J 10:52, 1981
13. Bernbaum J, Daft A, Anolik R et al: Response of preterm infants to diphtheria-tetanus-pertussis immunizations. J Pediatr 107:184–188, 1985
14. Bernbaum J, Hoffman-Williamson M: Following the NICU graduate. Contemp Pediatr 3:22–37, 1986
15. Bertrand J, Riley S, Popkin J et al: The long-term pulmonary sequelae of prematurity: The role of familial airway hyperreactivity and the respiratory distress syndrome. N Engl J Med 312:742, 1985
16. Besharov D, Hartle T: Head start: Making a popular program work. Pediatrics 79:440–445, 1987
17. Black L, David R, Broullette R et al: Effects of birth weight and ethnicity on incidence of sudden death syndrome. J Pediatr 108:209, 1986
18. Bonikos S, Bensch K, Northway W et al: Bronchopulmonary dysplasia: The pulmonary pathologic sequel of necrotizing bronchiolitis and pulmonary fibrosis. Hum Pathol 7:643, 1976
19. Brandt I: Growth dynamics of low-birth weight infants with emphasis on the perinatal period. In Falkner F, Tanner JM (eds): Human Growth, Vol 2. Postnatal Growth. New York, Plenum Press, 1978, pp 557–617
20. Brown E: Increased risk of bronchopulmonary dysplasia in infants with patent ductus arteriosus. J Pediatr 95:865, 1979
21. Brown E, Stark A, Sosenki I et al: Bronchopulmonary dysplasia: Possible relationship to pulmonary edema. J Pediatr 92:982, 1978
22. Brown E: Long-term sequelae of preterm birth (in press)
23. Brown D, Milley R, Ripepi U et al: Retinopathy of prematurity: Risk factors in a five-year cohort of critically ill premature neonates. Am J Dis Child 141:141–154, 1987
24. Bryan M, Hardie M, Reilly B et al: Pulmonary function studies during the first year of life in infants recovering from the respiratory distress syndrome. Pediatrics 52:169, 1973
25. Buckwald S, Zorn W, Egan E: Mortality and follow-up data for neonates weighing 500 to 800 g at birth. Am J Dis Child 138:779–782, 1984
26. Callahan J, Haller J, Cacciarell A et al: Cholelithiasis in infants: Association with total parenteral nutrition and furosemide. Radiology 143:437, 1982
27. Casey P, Bradley R, Caldwell B et al: Developmental intervention: A pediatric clinical review. Pediatr Clin North Am 33:899–923, 1986
28. Chamberlin R: Developmental assessment and early intervention programs for young children: Lessons learned from longitudinal research. Pediatr Rev 8:237–247, 1987
29. Chaplin E, Goldstein G, Myerberg J et al: Posthemorrhagic hydrocephalus in the preterm infant. Pediatrics 65:901, 1980

30. Cohen S, Parmelee A: Prediction of five-year Stanford-Binet scores in preterm infants. Child Dev 54:1242–1253, 1983
31. Drage J, Kennedy C, Berendes H et al: The Apgar score as an index of infant morbidity. Dev Med Child Neurol 8:141, 1966
32. Dubowitz L, Dubowitz V, Palmer P et al: Correlation of neurologic assessment in the preterm newborn infant with outcome at one year. Pediatrics 105:452–457, 1984
33. Edwards D, Wayne M, Northway W: Twelve years experience with bronchopulmonary dysplasia. Pediatrics 59:839, 1977
34. Eilers B, Desai N, Wilson M et al: Classroom performance and social factors of children with birth weights of 1,250 grams or less: Follow-up at 5 to 8 years of age. Pediatrics 77:203–208, 1986
35. Epstein M: Personal communication, November 11, 1987
36. Elliman A, Bryan E, Elliman A et al: Denver developmental screening test and preterm infants. Arch Dis Child 60:20–24, 1985
37. Escalona S: Babies at double hazard: Early development of infants at biologic and social risk. Pediatrics 70:670–676, 1982
38. Escalona S: Social and other environmental influences on the cognitive and personality development of low birthweight infants. Am J Ment Defic 88:508–512, 1984
39. Fagan J, Singer L, Montie J et al: Selective screening device for the early detection of normal or delayed cognitive development in infants at risk for later mental retardation. Pediatrics 78:1021–1026, 1986
40. Fagan J, Singer L: Infant recognition memory as a measure of intelligence. In Lipsett LP (ed): Advances in Infancy Research. Norwood, New Jersey, Ablex 2, 1983, pp 31–78
41. Fagan J, Singer L, Montie M: An experimental selective screening device for the early detection of intellectual deficit in at-risk infants. In Frankenburg W, Emde R, Sullivan J (eds): Early Identification of Children at Risk: An International Perspective. New York, Plenum Press, 1985, pp 257–266
42. Field T: Interventions for premature infants. J Pediatr 109:183–191, 1986
43. Field T, Ignatoff E, Stringer S et al: Nonnutritive sucking during tube feedings: Effects on preterm neonates in an ICU. Pediatrics 70:381, 1982
44. Field T, Schanberg S, Scafidi F et al: Effects of tactile/kinesthetic stimulation on preterm neonates. Pediatrics 77:654, 1986
45. Freeman J: National Institutes of Health report on causes of mental retardation and cerebral palsy. Pediatrics 76:457–459, 1985
46. Galambos R, Hicks G, Wilson M: The auditory brain stem response reliably predicts hearing loss on graduates of tertiary intensive care nursery. Ear Hear 5:254, 1984
47. Garner A: An international classification of retinopathy of prematurity. Pediatrics 74:127–133, 1984
48. Geogieff M, Bernbaum J, Hoffman-Williamson M, Daft A: Abnormal truncal muscle tone as a useful early marker for developmental delay in low birth weight infants. Pediatrics 77:659–663, 1986
49. Gorski P, Lewkowicz D, Huntington L: Advances in neonatal and infant behavioral assessment: Toward a comprehensive evaluation of early patterns of development. Develop Behav Ped 8:1, 1987
50. Graziani L, Pasto M, Stanley C et al: Neonatal neurosonographic correlates of cerebral palsy in preterm infants. Pediatrics 78:88–95, 1986
51. Green M, Ferry P, Russman B et al: Early intervention programs: Where do pediatricians fit in? Contemp Pediatr: 92–118, March, 1987
52. Hack M, Fanaroff A, Merkatz I: The low-birth weight infant—evolution of a changing outlook. N Engl J Med 301:1162–1165, 1979
53. Hack M, Breslau N: Very low birth weight infants: Effects of brain growth during infancy on intelligence quotient at 3 years of age. Pediatrics 77:196–202, 1986
54. Hill A, Volpe J: Normal pressure hydrocephalus in the newborn. Pediatrics 68:623, 1981
55. Hill A, Wolpe J: Seizures, hypoxic-ischemic brain injury, and intraventricular hemorrhage in the newborn. Ann Neurol 10:109, 1981
56. Hirata T, Epcar J, Walsh A et al: Survival and outcome of infants 501 to 750 gm: A six-year experience. J Pediatr 102:741–748, 1983
57. Hittner H, Godio L, Speer M et al: Retrolental fibroplasia: Further clinical evidence

and ultrastructural support for efficacy of vitamin E in the preterm infant. Pediatrics 71:423, 1983

58. Holmes T, Reich N, Pasternak J: The development of the infant born at risk. Hillsdale, NJ, 1984, p 216
59. Hufnagle K, Kahn S, Penn D et al: Renal calcifications. Pediatrics 70:360, 1982
60. Hunt J: Predicting intellectual disorders in childhood for high-risk preterm infants. In Freidman S, Sigman M (eds): Preterm Birth and Psychological Development. New York, Academic Press, pp 329–351, 1981
61. Joint Committee on Infant Hearing Position Statement. Ear Hear 4:3, 1983
62. Kao L, Warburton D, Sargent C et al: Furosemide acutely decreases airway resistance in chronic bronchopulmonary dysplasia. J Pediatr 103:624, 1983
63. Kao L, Durand D, Phillips B et al: Oral theophylline and diuretics improve pulmonary mechanics in infants with bronchopulmonary dysplasia. J Pediatr 111:439–444, 1987
64. Kao L, Warburton D, Platzker A et al: Effect of isoproterenol inhalation on airway resistance in chronic bronchopulmonary dysplasia. Pediatrics 73:509–514, 1984
65. Klein N, Hack M, Gallagher J et al: Preschool performance of children with normal intelligence who were very low-birth-weight infants. Pediatrics 75:531–537, 1985
66. Kosmetatos N, Dinter J, Williams M et al: Intracranial hemorrhage in the premature: Its predictive features and outcome. Am J Dis Child 134:855, 1980
67. Largo R, Molinari L, Weber M et al: Early development of locomotion: Significance of prematurity, cerebral palsy and sex. Dev Med Child Neurol 27:183–191, 1985
68. Leib S, Benfield D, Guidabaldi J: Effects of early intervention and stimulation on the preterm infant. Pediatrics 66:83–90, 1980
69. Lester B: Developmental outcome prediction from acoustic cry analysis in term and preterm infants. Pediatrics 80:529, 1987
70. Linn P, Horowitz F, Fox H: Stimulation in the NICU: Is more necessarily better? Clin Perinatol 12:407–423, 1985
71. Lloyd B: Outcome of very-low-birthweight babies from Wolverhampton. Lancet: 739–741, 1984
72. Long J, Philip A, Lucey J: Noise and hypoxemia in the intensive care nursery. Pediatrics 65:143–145, 1980
73. Markestad T, Fitzhardinge P: Growth and development in children recovering from bronchopulmonary dysplasia. J Pediatr 98:597, 1981
74. Marks K, Marsels M, Moore E et al: Head growth in sick premature infants in a longitudinal study. J Pediatr 94:282–285, 1979
75. Martin R, Miller M, Waldemar A: Pathogenesis of apnea in preterm infants. J Pediatr 109:733–741, 1986
76. McCarthy K, Bhogal M, Nardi M et al: Pathogenic factors in bronchopulmonary dysplasia. Pediatr Res 18:483, 1984
77. McCormick M, Shapiro B, Starfield B: Factors associated with maternal opinion of infant development—clues to the vulnerable child? Pediatrics 69:537–543, 1982
78. McCormick M, Shapiro S, Starfield B: Rehospitalization in the first year of life for high-risk survivors. Pediatrics 66:991–999, 1980
79. Merritt J, Kraybill E: Retrolental fibroplasia: A five-year experience in a tertiary perinatal center. Ann Ophthalmol 18:65–67, 1986
80. Merritt T, Cochrane C: Elastase and alpha-1-protease inhibitor activity in tracheal aspirates during respiratory distress syndrome. J Clin Invest 72:656, 1983
81. Michelsson K, Lindahl E, Parre M et al: Nine-year follow-up of infants weighing 1500 g or less at birth. Acta Paediatr Scand 73:835–841, 1984
82. Nelson K, Ellenberg J: Antecedents of cerebral palsy. N Engl J Med 315:81–86, 1986
83. Nickel R, Bennet F, Lamson F: School performance of children with birth weights of 1,000 g or less. Am J Dis Child 136:105–110, 1982
84. Nickerson B, Taussig L: Family history of asthma in infants with bronchopulmonary dysplasia. Pediatrics 65:1140, 1980
85. O'Brodovich H, Mellins R: Bronchopulmonary dysplasia. Am Rev Respir Dis 132:694, 1985
86. Palfrey J, Walker D, Sullivan M et al: Targeted early childhood programming. Am J Dis 141:55–59, 1987
87. Paneth N: Birth and the origins of cerebral palsy. N Engl J Med 315:124–126, 1986

88. Papile L, Munsick G, Weaver N et al: Cerebral intraventricular hemorrhage in infants less than 1500 grams: Developmental outcome at one year. Pediatr Res 13:528, 1979
89. Parmelee A: Sensory stimulation in the nursery: How much and when? Develop Behav Ped 6:242–243, 1985
90. Parmelee A, Wenner W, Akiyama Y et al: Sleep states in premature infants. Dev Med Child Neurol 9:70–77, 1967
91. Patz A: Current concepts of the effect of oxygen on the developing retina. Curr Eye Res 3:159, 1984
92. Perlman J, Moore V, Siegel M et al: Is chlorides depletion an important contributing cause of death in infants with bronchopulmonary dysplasia? Pediatrics 77:212–216, 1986
93. Phelps D: Retinopathy of prematurity: An estimate of vision loss in the United States—1979. Pediatrics 67:924, 1981
94. Phelps D: Vitamin E and retrolental fibroplasia in 1982. Pediatrics 70:420, 1982
95. Phelps D, Rosenbaum A, Isenberg S et al: Tocopherol efficacy and safety for preventing retinopathy of prematurity: A randomized, controlled, double-masked trial. Pediatrics 79:489–500, 1987
96. Pollard Z: Secondary angle-closure glaucoma in cicatricicial retrolental fibroplasia. Am J Ophthalmol 89:651–653, 1980
97. Procianoy R, Garcia-Prats J, Hittner H et al: An association between retinopathy of prematurity and intraventricular hemorrhage in very low birth weight infants. Acta Paediatr Scand 70:473–477, 1981
98. Provence S: On the efficacy of early intervention programs. 6:363–366, 1985
99. Purohit D, Ellison R, Zierler S et al: Risk factors for retrolental fibroplasia: Experience with 3025 premature infants. Pediatrics 76:339–344, 1985
100. Reynolds E, Taghizadek A: Improved prognosis of infants mechanically ventilated for hyaline membrane disease. Arch Dis Child 49:505, 1974
101. Ross G: Home intervention for premature infants of low-income families. Am J Orthopsychiatry 54:263–270, 1984
102. Ross G, Lipper E, Auld P: Consistency and change in the development of premature infants weighing less than 1,501 grams at birth. Pediatrics 76:885–891, 1985
103. Ross G, Lipper E, Auld P: Early predictors of neurodevelopmental outcome of very low-birthweight infants at three years. Dev Med Child Neurol 28:171–179, 1986
104. Ross G, Lipper E, Auld P: Physical growth and developmental outcome in very low birth weight premature infants at 3 years of age. J Pediatr: 284–286, 1985
105. Russman B: Early intervention for the biologically handicapped infant and young child: Is it of value? Pediatr Rev 5:51–55, 1983
106. Sacks L, Shaffer D, Anday E et al: Retrolental fibroplasia and blood transfusion in very low birth weight infants. Pediatrics 68:770–774, 1981
107. Saigal S, Rosenbaum P, Stoskopf B et al: Outcome in infants 501 to 1000 gm birth weight delivered to residents of the McMaster health region. J Pediatr 105:969–976, 1984
108. Sameroff A, Seifer R, Barocas R et al: Intelligence Quotient scores of 4-year-old children: Social-environmental risk factors. Pediatrics 79:343–350, 1987
109. Sauve R, Singhai N: Long-term morbidity of infants with BPD. Pediatrics 76:725, 1985
110. Schub H, Ahmann P, Dykes F et al: Prospective, long-term follow up of prematures with subependymal/intraventricular hemorrhage. Pediatr Res 15:711, 1981
111. Sciarillo W, Brown M, Robinson N et al: Effectiveness of the Denver developmental screening test with biologically vulnerable infants. Develop Behav Pediatr 7:77–83, 1986
112. Scott D: Premature infants in later childhood: Some recent follow-up results. Semin Perinatol 11:191–199, 1987
113. Scott D, Ment L, Warshaw J: Follow up of very low birthweight infants: Late developmental sequelae in GMH/IVH survivors. Pediatr Res 15:341, 1982
114. Sell E, Gainew J, Gluckman C et al: Early identification of learning problems in neonatal intensive care graduates. Am J Dis Child: 139, 1985
115. Sell E: Outcome of very low birth/weight infants. Clin Perinatol 13:2, 1986
116. Shenai J, Kennedy K, Chytil F et al: Clinical trial of vitamin A supplementation in infants susceptible to bronchopulmonary dysplasia. J Pediatr 111:269–277, 1987
117. Shohat M, Reisner S, Krikler R et al: Retinopathy of prematurity: Incidence and risk factors. Pediatrics 72:159–163, 1983

118. Shonkoff J, Hauser-Cram P: Early intervention for disabled infants and their families—a quantitive analysis. Pediatrics (in press)
119. Siegel L: Correction for prematurity and its consequences for the assessment of the very low birth weight infant. Child Dev 54:1176–1188, 1983
120. Simeonsson R, Cooper D, Scheiner A: A review and analysis of the effectiveness of early intervention programs. Pediatrics 69:635–640, 1982
121. Smyth J, Tabachnik E, Duncan W et al: Pulmonary function and bronchial hyperactivity in long-term survivors of bronchopulmonary dysplasia. Pediatrics 68:336, 1981
122. Southall D, Richards J, Rhoden K et al: Prolonged apnea and cardiac arrhythmias in infants discharged from neonatal intensive care units. Failure to predict an increased risk for sudden infant death syndrome. Pediatrics 70:844, 1982
123. Taft L: Cerebral palsy. Pediatr Rev 6:35–45, 1984
124. Taft H, Roin J: Effect of furosemide administration on calcium excretion. Br Med J 1:437, 1971
125. Tepper R, Morgan W, Cota K et al: Expiratory flow limitation in infants with bronchopulmonary dysplasia. J Pediatr 109:1040–1046, 1986
126. Tronick E, Scanlon K, Scanlon J: A comparative analysis of the validity of several approaches to the scoring of the behavior of the preterm infant. Infant Behav Dev 8:395–411, 1985
127. Venkataraman B, Han B, Tsang R et al: Secondary hyperparathyroidism and bone disease in infants receiving long-term furosemide therapy. Am J Dis Child 137:1157, 1983
128. Vohr B, Garcia Coll C: Neurodevelopmental and school performance of very low-birth-weight infants: A seven-year longitudinal study. Pediatrics 76:345–350, 1985
129. Vohr B, Bell E, Oh W: Infants with bronchopulmonary dysplasia: Growth pattern and neurologic and developmental outcome. Am J Dis Child 136:443, 1982
130. Volpe J: Evaluation of neonatal periventricular–intraventricular hemorrhage. Am J Dis Child 134:1023, 1980
131. Weinstein M, Oh W: Oxygen consumption in infants with bronchopulmonary dysplasia. J Pediatr 99:959, 1981
132. Wheeler W, Castile R, Brown E et al: Pulmonary function in survivors of prematurity. Am Rev Respir Dis 129:218, 1984
133. Yu V, Loke H, Bajuk B et al: Prognosis for infants born at 23 to 28 weeks' gestation. Br Med J 293:1202–1204, 1986
134. Zeskind P: Production and spectral analysis of neonatal crying and its relation to other biobehavioral systems in the infant at risk. In Field, Sostek (eds): Infants Born at Risk: Physiological, Perceptual and Cognitive Processes. New York, Grune & Stratton, 1983

HOB 2
Boston City Hospital
818 Harrison Avenue
Boston, Massachusetts 02118

0031-3955/88 $0.00 + .20

Double Jeopardy: The Impact of Poverty on Early Child Development

Steven Parker, MD, * *Steven Greer, MD,* †
and Barry Zuckerman, MD ‡

It is clear that poverty places children at risk for a variety of adverse behavioral and developmental outcomes; it is less clear why this is so. Children growing up in similarly impoverished environments commonly have very different outcomes. Even within the same family, one child may fail while another excels. The risk factors associated with poverty frequently, but not invariably, lead to untoward outcomes for children. In this article we shall discuss the mechanisms by which poverty impacts on early developmental functioning and suggest interventions to ameliorate these effects.

Children living in poverty experience double jeopardy. First, they are exposed more frequently to such risks as medical illnesses, family stress, inadequate social support, and parental depression. Secondly, they experience more serious consequences from these risks than do children from higher socioeconomic status. It is the synergistic double jeopardy of increased exposure to and greater sequelae from environmental risks that predisposes children living in poverty to adverse developmental outcomes.

It is important to acknowledge an important limitation of the literature in this area: an inordinate emphasis is placed on the intelligence quotient (IQ) as an outcome measure. IQ tests are easily quantified and widely used. However, there are many other aspects of early childhood functioning of equal importance. Outcomes such as a child's sense of mastery, self-esteem, motivation to learn, and joy in life are rarely addressed. Consequently, the complexity and richness of childhood functioning are notably absent from most studies. The available data provide a very limited understanding of the impact of poverty on child development and, if anything, underestimate its true cost.

POVERTY AND CHILD DEVELOPMENT: A TRANSACTIONAL MODEL

Early theories of child development implied that negative developmental outcomes could result from a single risk factor, such as an early insult to the central

---

*Assistant Professor of Pediatrics, Boston University School of Medicine; Director, Developmental Assessment Clinic, Boston City Hospital, Boston, Massachusetts

†Instructor in Pediatrics, Boston University School of Medicine; Fellow in Developmental and Behavioral Pediatrics, Boston City Hospital, Boston, Massachusetts

‡Professor of Pediatrics, Boston University School of Medicine; Director, Division of Developmental and Behavioral Pediatrics, Boston City Hospital, Boston, Massachusetts

nervous system. This approach is called the *main effect* model and implies a linear cause-and-effect relationship between risk and outcome. It was best articulated and gained wide acceptance after a retrospective study by Pasaminick and Knobloch,[55] in which they hypothesized a "continuum of reproductive causality" to describe the relationship between perinatal factors (e.g., perinatal asphyxia, low birthweight, delivery complications) and poor outcomes (e.g., cerebral palsy, epilepsy, mental retardation, or learning disorders).

With such a model in mind, researchers in the 1970s were confronted with a curious fact: the best predictor of long-term developmental outcomes for infants born at risk was parental socioeconomic status (SES), rather than the type or degree of neonatal illness. For example, in a landmark followup study of 26,760 infants enrolled in the National Collaborative Perinatal Project, SES and maternal education were the factors most predictive of children's intellectual performance at 4 years.[13] This finding was unexpected to the researchers, who included 158 biomedical and only 11 sociobehavioral independent variables in their analysis.

Perhaps the most elegant and sustained longitudinal study of developmental outcomes for children has been conducted by Werner.[90] Her group has reported data at 18 years on 88 per cent of all 698 children born in 1955 on the island of Kauai, Hawaii. A significant interaction between the quality of the caretaking environment and the amount of perinatal stress has been apparent at each stage of followup. For example, 2-year-old children from high SES who had experienced perinatal complications had mean IQ scores 5 to 7 points lower than children from the same social class with no perinatal problems. In contrast, 2 year olds from low SES with perinatal complications had IQs 19 to 37 points less than their unstressed counterparts.[91]

Werner found that children from high SES with the most severe perinatal complications had mean IQ scores similar to children with no perinatal complications from poor homes. The children with the most significant delays had experienced severe perinatal complications and grew up in the poorest homes. By 18 years of age, ten times as many children with poor behavioral or developmental outcomes lived in poverty than had been exposed to significant perinatal stress. Other studies[6, 49] have since confirmed that poverty places children at greater developmental risk from perinatal insults.

In a recent study of 215 full-term children, Sameroff et al.[67] demonstrated the cumulative nature of social risk factors in predicting IQ at 4 years. These risk factors included: maternal mental health problems, maternal anxiety, impaired mother–child interactions, low maternal education, negative parental attitudes and values, unemployment, minority group status, inadequate social support, large family size, and stressful life events. Although these risk factors tended to cluster in poor families, a cumulative deleterious effect was evident regardless of SES. In the highest SES group, for example, the mean IQ of 4 year olds with zero to one risk factor was 120, compared to a mean IQ of 100 for children exposed to four or more risk factors. The lowest SES group demonstrated a similar trend, with a mean IQ of 113 associated with zero to one risk factor and a mean IQ of 91 with 4 or more risk factors.

These data demonstrate that SES is a marker for potential psychosocial risk factors that may lead to developmental and behavioral morbidity.[64] These factors additively or synergistically interact with the child's inherent strengths and vulnerabilities to shape outcomes. This viewpoint was articulated by Sameroff and Chandler in 1975 and called a *transactional* model of child development.[65] It evolved out of the studies that demonstrated developmental outcomes to be largely unexplainable solely by the presence or degree of a biologic insult such as perinatal asphyxia,[21] neurologic insults,[50] abnormal neonatal neurologic examination,[53] and prematurity,[25, 39] unless these insults were of the most severe variety with clear organic sequelae. In this model of development, outcomes can only be understood by considering the transaction between the *content* of the child's behaviors and the *context* in which they are manifested.

The transactional model addresses the dynamic interplay between the environment and the child. Characteristics of the child (e.g., genetic endowment, temperament, health) shape his or her responses to the environment. These interactions, in turn, transform environmental responsivity. Just as the child is shaped by his environment, so is the environment actively modified by the child. The child brings a host of attributes to the transaction. Three that have been particularly well studied are genetic endowment, temperamental style, and health status. These characteristics in part determine how the child will respond to the environment.

The environment likewise brings specific attributes to the transactions with the child. (In referring to environmental characteristics, the term *low SES* will be used interchangeably with *poverty*, although there are many other ways to define SES.) In a low SES environment, more risk factors for adverse developmental and behavioral outcomes are likely to be present. The most pertinent of these include increased stress, diminished social support, and maternal depression. These risk factors, in turn, exert their influence on the child through the quality of the home environment and the parent–child interactions, to name two of the most widely studied mechanisms.

As an example of a transactional view of child development, consider a child born at 34 weeks' gestation to a single mother living in poverty who received minimal prenatal care. Following a 3-week hospitalization, the infant was mildly hypotonic and had difficulty maintaining an alert state. The mother felt overwhelmed, depressed, and bereft of emotional support. The child's passivity engendered maternal feelings of inadequacy that resulted in a deepening of her depression. Positive interactions with her child were rare. The child did not look to the environment for stimulation and rarely vocalized. This further heightened the mother's feelings of inadequacy and depression. By 2 years the child was clearly delayed in his language and cognitive development.

What is the etiology of this child's developmental delays? Is it biologic vulnerability secondary to prematurity? Maternal depression? Temperamental passivity? Inadequate environmental stimulation? Insufficient social support? A transactional analysis considers all of these factors as operating together to shape this outcome. Each factor modifies and potentiates the other. Together they weave a complex pattern that cannot be understood by examining the thread of only a single risk.

While adding considerable complexity to the determinants of child outcomes, such a model also suggests practical strategies for intervention. Changes in any aspect of the ecology of the child's world (e.g., maternal depression) can create positive transformations in another (e.g., environmental stimulation). Although characteristics of the child and the environment are discussed separately in this article, these distinctions are arbitrary and for purposes of clarity only.

CHILD CHARACTERISTICS

Genetic Endowment

An analysis of the interaction between the child and her environment must begin with an understanding of the child's role in that transaction. No variable has been demonstrated to be a more powerful predictor of cognitive outcomes than the child's genetic endowment.

The most compelling data concerning the heritability of intelligence derives from comparisons of identical twins raised together or apart.[10] In one study the correlation for cognitive development at age 36 years for monozygotic twins raised apart was 0.58, compared to 0.66 for identical twins raised together. In comparison, a summary of 11 studies found the average IQ correlation for adoptive siblings from different biologic parents to be 0.30.[10] Although studies of adopted children demonstrate IQ scores about 6 to 10 points higher than their biologic parents due to the enriched environment of the adoptive home, their IQs are still more closely correlated to the biological than the adoptive parents.[71] Thus, individuals with similar genotypes raised apart are far more alike in intellectual functioning than are individuals with disparate genotypes raised in similar environments.

Estimates of the contribution of genotype to the variance of IQs range from 40 to 60 per cent.[56] This means that genotypes account for one half of the observed differences in IQs between individuals. Such data do not support strict nativists who believe genes are destiny, nor strict environmentalists who believe in the limitless potential for intellectual achievement in every person. Intelligence is malleable, but only within the limits circumscribed by a child's genotype.

Scarr and McCartney have proposed a transactional resolution to this nature/nurture controversy.[70] They believe that the child's genetic endowment drives development by determining early responsivity to the environment. These genotypically determined responses not only shape the interaction with the environment but also influence the kind of experiences sought by the child. This active influence of the child's genotype explains the variability of outcomes for children raised in similar environments and the startling similarities in personalities and intelligence of identical twins reared apart. Poverty's risk factors may be attenuated by a resilient constitution or accentuated by a child who requires more environmental stimulation to achieve his or her true potential.

Temperament

Every infant is born with a distinct temperamental style. The importance of temperament in the developmental process was first highlighted by the pioneering work of Thomas and Chess.[78] They describe temperament as the "how" of behavior, as compared to motivations (the "why" of behavior) and abilities (the "what" of behavior). Nine temperamental dimensions are identified in their model: activity level, regularity of biologic functions, approach/avoidance tendencies, adaptability, responsivity to stimuli, intensity of reactions, quality of mood, distractibility, and persistence.

Thomas and Chess followed a cohort of 133 middle-class children from birth to young adulthood to relate early temperamental characteristics to long-term outcomes. Forty per cent of their sample were described as having an "easy" temperament, characterized by a predominantly positive mood, high adaptability to change, and a positive approach to unfamiliar stimuli. Children with irregular biologic functions, withdrawal from novel stimuli, and intense expressions of mood were characterized as "difficult" and constituted 10 per cent of the sample. A third group, labeled the "slow-to-warm-up child," constituted 15 per cent of the sample. The remainder of the children did not fall into any category.

Children with difficult temperaments were more likely to have behavioral problems in the first 5 years of life.[79] By early adulthood, however, this relationship was not seen. In analyzing the development of each child, Thomas and Chess found the nature of the interaction between the child's temperament *and* the environment to be the best predictor of long-term outcomes. They rated this interaction by its "goodness of fit." If the environmental expectations were compatible with the child's style, healthy development occurred. When the environment made inappropriate demands on the child, especially in relation to his innate temperament, a poor fit resulted, which left that child vulnerable to behavioral dysfunction in young adulthood.

Temperamental characteristics have not been directly associated with SES.[44] However, an easy disposition may moderate the impact of stress on a child.[41] In the Kauai Longitudinal Study, for example, temperamental traits considered rewarding to caretakers, such as social responsiveness and a normal activity level, were associated with fewer learning and behavioral problems at age 10 years.[90] Children who are more adaptable, less intense, and more responsive are less likely to manifest behavioral problems when stressed.[4] Additionally, children with a positive mood, high regularity, and high adaptability are less likely to be the target of parental hostility, criticism, and irritability.[63] Difficult temperaments are associated with a higher incidence of physical abuse when other family stresses are also present.[83] A child with a difficult temperament is a source of added stress, especially to parents who already feel overwhelmed and unsupported.

Biologic Insults

Children born into poverty are at greater risk for a host of biologic insults that can affect outcomes. The data support both a higher prevalence and greater sequelae of illnesses for poor children.[27] In the prenatal period, for example, low SES increases the risk of contracting a cytomegalovirus (CMV) infection.[2] Infants infected with CMV from poor families have lower IQ scores and 2.7 times more school failure than do matched controls.[36] In contrast, these outcomes were not seen for infected infants of middle or upper class backgrounds. Poverty exposes children to double jeopardy from CMV infections: more exposure and greater developmental morbidity.

There are numerous other examples of increased biologic risks for children in poverty that are detailed in this volume. Prenatal insults to the developing nervous system from maternal drug use, malnutrition, intrauterine infections, or other medical illnesses are more common. The incidence of low birthweight is two to three times higher and developmental morbidity greater in low SES groups.[49] Poor children are also far more likely to experience lead poisoning, failure to thrive, otitis media, and other infectious diseases. In reviewing the effects of biologic insults on child development, Shonkoff[73] concludes that children in poverty "carry a disproportionate burden of biologic vulnerability that is largely related to the increased health risks of poverty. . . . Their developmental outcomes will be determined by a highly complex series of transactions among a great number of biological and environmental facilitators and constraints." In the next section some of these environmental constraints will be discussed.

ENVIRONMENTAL RISKS

Stress

The concept of stress was introduced by Hans Selye[72] in 1950 to explain a number of physiologic disorders caused by hypersecretion of the adrenal gland. The psychogenic causes of stress have since been catalogued,[25] but there is still no consensus as to its definition. Most recently, Garmezy and Rutter[33] have defined stress as a stimulus "requiring a change in adaptation (strain), mental state (distress), and bodily reaction or response."

People living in poverty experience stress more frequently and more chronically than do middle and upper class families. For example, Roghmann et al.[61] examined the rates of stressful life events in different social classes. The incidence of major stressors (e.g., housing problems, financial shortfalls, death of a relative or friend, school difficulties) was two to four times greater for mothers with incomes of less than $6000 (in 1969) than for those with more financial resources. Stress appears to be especially high for poor women with children under 6 years of age.[15]

In addition to a higher frequency of stressful events, there is evidence that stress begets stress. For example, inadequate financial resources greatly exacerbate the problems experienced by children and parents in divorced families.[20] Equivalent levels of stress also engender more clinical depression among women from lower SES.[15] Chronic stress, in the form of unemployment, lack of material goods, and so forth is also more prevalent in poor families and far more likely to have negative consequences than acutely stressful events.[8]

Stress is associated with adverse consequences for parents and, directly or indirectly, for children. Children from highly stressed environments are at increased risk for a variety of developmental and behavioral problems, including poorer performance on developmental tests at 8 months,[30] lower IQ scores and impaired language development at 4 years,[7] and poorer emotional adjustment and increased school problems at school age.[69] This last relationship is strongest for children in low SES/high-stress families and much less apparent for children in high SES/high-stress families. These findings suggest that the psychological and material resources associated with higher social class buffer families from the vicissitudes of stress.

Increased stress interferes with the mother's ability to respond appropriately to her infant. It has been associated with impaired bonding behaviors between mothers and their premature infants[35] and less positive interactions at 4 months.[23] Toddlers in families exposed to high stress appear to be less secure in their attachment to their mothers regardless of social class.[80] There is also less consistency of attachment behaviors over time by these infants.[82] It is well established that insecure attachments are associated with an increased risk for subsequent behavioral and emotional problems.[42] The data suggest that stress causes negative outcomes by inhibiting positive interactions and the attachment between parent and child.

Inadequate Social Support

Social support is defined as "the availability of meaningful and enduring relationships that provide nurturance, security and a sense of interpersonal commitment."[74] The benefits of social support fall into three categories: material supports (e.g., day care, nutritional supplements, availability of emergency help), emotional supports (e.g., friendships, counseling), and information/referral services (e.g., community resource availability, child-rearing techniques). Social support may derive from formal networks (e.g., health care providers, educational services, or peer groups) or informal networks (e.g., family, friends, or the media).[81]

Families living in poverty are at greater risk for experiencing inadequate social support. The most common problem mentioned by poor families living in hotel rooms, for example, is the lack of emotional support.[18] Pascoe et al.[54] demonstrated an association between low SES and low social support. Single parents are especially susceptible to social isolation.[85] Since the absence of social support is particularly damaging to families under stress,[23, 48, 74] their children are again placed in double jeopardy. For example, low levels of social support are associated with decreased cognitive abilities at 8 months,[30] more behavior problems among 5 to 8 year olds,[69] lower IQ and receptive language skills at 4 years,[7] and a higher incidence of child abuse.[38]

Social support exerts its influence on childrens' development by direct and indirect means.[17] Indirect effects occur by providing parents with access to emotional support, material assistance, external monitoring of their child rearing practices, and positive role models. These are especially important for infants and young children, who frequently have little contact with anyone other than their primary caretakers. The direct benefits of providing the child with cognitive and social stimulation, emotional support, positive role models, and a widened social network may play a larger role, especially when they are lacking in the child's home environment.

Adequate social support has been associated with enhanced parental functioning. Mothers with high social support appear to be more satisfied with their lives in general[23] and feel more positively about their maternal role.[1] Additionally, the protective role of social support in reducing the incidence of maternal depression,[51] anxiety,[46] and other psychiatric problems[15] has been well established.

More positive parent-child interactions are seen in families with helpful support networks. Mothers who feel supported, for example, use less punishment and are more responsive to their 8-month-old infants[30] and are more actively involved with their infants in general.[81] They continue to exhibit more optimal interactions with their children at 2 to 4 years.[85] This improvement in mother–child interactions helps to explain the positive relationship found between social support and secure attachment behaviors of toddlers who had been irritable infants.[24]

In addition to enhancing parent-child interactions, the presence of adequate social support is associated with a more stimulating and appropriate home environment for the child. Pascoe et al.[54] demonstrated that, regardless of stress levels, mothers who reported more social support provided more stimulation to their 3-year-old infants. Strong associations also were seen between social support and a more organized physical environment, the provision of appropriate play materials, and a wider range of available stimulation for the child. Numerous studies have shown the quality of the home environment to be one of the most powerful predictors of developmental outcomes for children.[11] By enabling stressed parents to fashion a more stimulating and responsive environment, social support can improve outcomes for children.

Maternal Depression

Depression is defined as a mood characterized by sadness, helplessness, gloom, loss of interest, emotional emptiness, and a feeling of "flatness."[95] Inadequate financial resources,[43, 52] lower educational attainment,[84] recent immigrant status,[92] race,[26] dissatisfaction with housing,[47] stressful life events,[22] and inadequate social support[16] can all contribute to an increased incidence of depression. With these risk factors in mind, it is not surprising that numerous studies report an association between low SES and depression.[3, 66] Brown et al.,[15] for example, described the prevalence of depression in a London borough as 5 per cent for middle class women and 25 per cent for lower class women.

Mothers of young children are at much higher risk for becoming depressed. The prevalence of depression in such circumstances has been estimated from 12 per cent (when strict diagnostic criteria are used)[12] to 52 per cent (when self-reported symptoms are used).[47] The younger the mother at the time of her first child[45] and the greater the number of young children,[16] the greater the risk for depression. Low SES mothers of young children are therefore the most vulnerable for depression and, in conjunction with poor social support and increased stress, may experience the most severe consequences.

Maternal depression has been linked to adverse health outcomes for their children such as lower birthweights,[93] more accidents,[14] failure to thrive,[57] complaints of headaches and stomachs,[96] and more surgical procedures.[87] Maternal depression also is associated with a number of negative behavioral and developmental outcomes for children, such as sleep problems,[60, 97] depression,[5] attention deficit disorder,[87] socially isolating behaviors at school age,[86] and withdrawn and defiant behaviors during adolescence.[87]

A number of studies have examined the mechanisms underlying these associations. Three-month-old infants will respond negatively when their mothers simulate a depressed mood.[19] Depressed mothers have been shown to display less spontaneity, more unhappy affect, fewer vocalizations, and diminished physical contact with their 4 month olds.[68] These infants already manifest fewer vocalizations and happy expressions toward their mothers.[29] By the toddler stage, maternal depression is associated with infants demonstrating anxious and avoidant behaviors toward their mothers following a brief separation.[58, 77] The level of negative child outcomes engendered by maternal depression appears to vary with the degree to which depressive symptoms are evidenced in the parent–child interaction.

Maternal depression, like stress and diminished social support, places children living in poverty at double jeopardy for poor outcomes. These risk factors are highly intercorrelated and their effects are synergistic. Stress is exacerbated by a lack of support. Depression inhibits seeking adequate supports. The cycle becomes self-perpetuating because stress causes more depression, which elicits less support, which causes more stress. Ultimately, through the parent–child relationship and the quality of the home environment, these risks are passed on to the child.

PROTECTIVE MECHANISMS: STRESS-RESISTANT CHILDREN

We have discussed the world of children living in poverty as filled with potential risk factors that through their transactions with the child, lead to negative outcomes. However, as Garmezy noted over 15 years ago:

> In the study of high risk and vulnerable children, we have come across another group of children whose prognosis could be viewed as unfavorable on the basis of familial or ecological factors, but who upset our prediction tables and in childhood bear the visible indices that are the hallmarks of competence: good peer relations, academic achievement, commitment to education and to purposive life goals, early and successful work histories. . . . Were we to study the forces that move such children to survival and to adaptation, the long range benefits to our society might be far more significant than our many efforts to construct models of primary prevention designed to curtail the incidence of vulnerability.[31]

Some view the issue of vulnerability versus resiliency as more semantic than real. Rather than designating "risk factors," one can as easily call their opposite "protective factors." If low social support is a risk factor, then high social support must be a protective factor. However, protective mechanisms are more than merely the absence of risk factors. The process by which resiliency occurs appears to be qualitatively different than that of vulnerability.[63] For example, a shy personality protects against delinquency, but an outgoing personality does not predispose one to antisocial behaviors. Focusing only on vulnerabilities prevents an understanding of how protective mechanisms shield children from risk.

A constructive approach is to identify the factors that promote successful adaptation in children. In the past decade, efforts to understand "invulnerable" children have begun. Garmezy has proposed three categories of protective factors:[32] (1) the personality characteristics of the child; (2) a supportive, stable, and cohesive family unit; and (3) external support systems that enhance coping and project positive values.

Recently, investigators have looked to the child's self-concept as a key determinant of successful outcomes.[63] It is suggested that children with positive feelings of self-esteem, mastery, and control can more easily negotiate stressful experiences. These children elicit more positive experiences from their environment. They show initiative in task accomplishment and relationship formation. Even in stressed families, the presence of one good relationship with a parent reduces psychiatric risk for children.[62] For older children, the presence of a close, enduring relationship with an external support figure (e.g., schoolteacher) may likewise serve a protective function. A child with a positive self-concept seeks, establishes, and maintains the kind of supportive relationships and experiences that promote successful outcomes. These successes enhance the child's self-esteem and sense of mastery, which leads to further positive experiences and relationships. The cycle of success can be as self-perpetuating as that of failure. One goal of social support and therapeutic interventions must be to establish environments and relationships for the child that promote a positive self-concept.

IMPLICATIONS FOR INTERVENTION

The developmental costs of poverty for children are excessively high. Approximately two thirds of all children who test as mildly retarded have grown up in poverty.[73] The cost to society can be measured in terms of school dropout, unemployment, delinquency, unwanted pregnancies, and the intergenerational perpetuation of failure. Successful interventions require both the amelioration of risk factors and the enhancement of protective mechanisms.

The care of adolescent mothers and their infants is an example of the necessity of such an approach. It is known that the adolescent mother's nutritional status plays an important role in the increased incidence of low birthweight among their infants.[98] The child's subsequent developmental and social functioning will be related to birthweight, as well as social support from the maternal grandmother,[99] the level of involvement of the baby's father, and the mother's mental health status.[94] Optimal interventions for adolescent mothers should address all of these factors by providing ongoing nutritional, emotional, and psychological support for mother and child.

The most ambitious and comprehensive intervention of this type has recently begun in Chicago. This program, called the Beethoven Project, is providing pregnant women living in poverty and their children with nutritional, medical, educational, and social support from the prenatal period through the first 5 years of the child's life. It is an exciting effort that addresses child health and the ecology of family functioning in an early, continuous, and comprehensive fashion. If it proves successful and cost effective, it will serve as a model program in the future.

Transactional theory implies that even partial interventions may benefit other areas of functioning. For example, improving the health status of children can lessen their vulnerability to a disorganized home environment. Interventions also have benefits beyond their intended scope. The first studies of the Head Start programs, founded in the 1960s, revealed only short-term gains in IQ scores. More creative researchers then looked at other areas of functioning and discovered marked long-term benefits in such areas as diminished special education services and less grade retention.[40] Subsequent studies have demonstrated that early intervention services decrease juvenile delinquency, teenage pregnancy, and unemployment during young adulthood.[9] These studies have lead the House Select Committee on Children, Youth, and Families to estimate that every $1.00 spent on preschool education saves at least $4.75 in later educational and social costs.[37]

Early intervention is effective for children at biologic[76] or environmental risk.[59] Current research is examining the necessary and sufficient interventions to achieve long-term benefits. Until this question is resolved, current wisdom dictates that interventions start early, be comprehensive, and continue for as long as possible.

The first level of intervention must address basic needs for children and their parents living in poverty. Such interventions are best accomplished by public health measures such as the provision of material support (e.g., food, shelter, and money) and accessible medical care. The emphasis on improved prenatal care for women at risk, for example, has reduced the incidence of low birth weight deliveries and saved $3.38 in medical costs for every $1.00 invested.[37] The developmental benefits of these interventions, although more difficult to quantify, may be even more impressive.

Pediatricians are comfortable with assessment and intervention for medical risks. However, the prevention of developmental and behavioral morbidity secondary to poverty requires a broader focus. During a health care visit the family's material resources for nutrition, housing, and other finances should be addressed. The clinician can evaluate the child's temperamental characteristics and the "goodness of fit" with the environment. The earlier a mismatch is identified, the more successful can be the interventions.

The clinician should also attend to potential social risks for the child in the environment. Is there significant family stress? Do the parents appear depressed and overwhelmed? What is the level of social support available for the family? What is the quality of the parent–child interaction seen in the office? What sort of home environment awaits the child after the visit? Any or all of these questions can be addressed in the medical setting. The answers will determine the appropriate interventions. For one family, social support in the form of a visiting nurse may be helpful. For another, advocacy for adequate housing is necessary. A third may require a comprehensive early intervention program to provide the child with adequate stimulation and emotional nurturance.

Finally, the clinician should try to identify these risks to developmental and behavioral outcomes as early as possible. Developmental screening tests alone, however, poorly predict long-term problems unless the context of the child's environment also is considered. Using such an approach at Boston City Hospital, early childhood educators have been integrated into medical settings such as the failure to thrive, lead poisoning, adolescent mother, and neurology clinics, as well as the inpatient wards. The goal has been to identify children in need of services to prevent developmental morbidity. The assessment includes not only developmental testing but an evaluation of the child's learning style, self-esteem, sense of mastery, the parent–child interaction, "goodness of fit," and health and social risk factors. Using this approach, 23 per cent of the first 853 children were judged to be in need of new or additional services. Health care settings provide the earliest and best opportunity to intervene with children at risk. The challenge for us all is to recognize risk early and draw on available resources to eliminate the double jeopardy for children living in poverty.

ACKNOWLEDGMENT

Support was provided by Academic Training Program in Behavioral Pediatrics funded by Bureau of Health Care Delivery and Assistance, Maternal and Child Health Branch (Grant #MCJ-009094), the Boston Foundation, and the Jessie B. Cox Charitable Trust. We thank Ms. Margaret Stanhope and Ms. Jeanne McCarthy for their help in preparing the manuscript for this article. Bill Harris's tireless efforts and commitment to improve the health and well-being of children living in poverty has been a special source of support and inspiration.

REFERENCES

1. Abernathy V: Social network and response to the maternal role. Intl J Soc Family 3:86–92, 1973
2. Alford C: Prenatal infections and psychosocial development in children born into low socioeconomic settings. In Mittler P (ed): Research in Mental Retardation. Baltimore, University Park Press, 1977, pp 251–259
3. Aneshensel C, Clark V, Fredrichs R: Race, ethnicity and depression: A confirmation analysis. J Personality Soc Psych 44:385–398, 1983

4. Bates J: Temperament in infancy. In Osofsky J (ed): Handbook of Infant Development. New York, John Wiley and Sons, 1987
5. Beardslee W, Keller M, Klerman G: Children of parents with affective disorders. Int J Fam Psychiatry 6(3):283–299, 1985
6. Beckwith L, Parmelee A: EEG patterns of preterm infants, home environment, and later IQ. Child Dev 57:777–789, 1986
7. Bee H, Hammond M, Etres S et al: The impact of parental life changes of the early development of children. Res Nurs Health 9:65–74, 1986
8. Belle D: The social network as a source of both stress and support to low income mothers. Presented at the Society for Research in Child Development, 1981
9. Berrueta-Clement J, Schweinhart L, Barnett W et al: Changed Lives: The Effects of the Perry Preschool Project on Youths Through Age 19. Ypsilanti, Michigan, High Scope Educational Research Foundation, 1986
10. Bouchard T, McGue M: Familial studies of intelligence: A review. Science 212:1055–1059, 1981
11. Bradley R, Caldwell B: Pediatric usefulness of home assessment. Adv Behav Pediatr 2:61–80, 1981
12. Bromet E, Solomon Z, Dunn L et al: Affective disorders in mothers of young children. Br J Psychiatry 140:30–36, 1982
13. Broman S, Nichols R, Kennedy W: Preschool IQ: Prenatal and Early Developmental Correlates. Hillsdale, New Jersey, Laurence Erlbaum, 1975
14. Brown G, Davidson S: Social class: Psychiatric disorder of mothers and accidents to children. Lancet 1:378, 1978
15. Brown G, Bhrolchain M, Harris T: Social class and psychiatric disturbance among women in an urban population. Soc 9:225–254, 1975
16. Brown G, Harris T: The Social Origins of Depression. London, Tavistock Publications, 1978
17. Cochran J, Brassard J: Child development and personal social networks. Child Dev 50:601–616, 1979
18. Cohen C, Adler A: Assessing the role of social network interventions with an inner city population. Am J Orthopsychiatry 56:278–288, 1986
19. Cohn J, Tronick E: Three-month-old infants' reaction to simulated maternal depression. Child Dev 54:185–193, 1983
20. Colletta N: Divorced mothers at two income levels: Stress, support and child rearing practices. Dissert Abstr Intl 38(12-B):6114, 1978
21. Corah N, Anthony E, Painter P et al: Effects of perinatal anoxia after seven years. Psychol Mongr 79:3, 1965
22. Costello C: Social factors associated with depression: A retrospective community study. Psychol Med 12:329–339, 1982
23. Crnic K, Greenberg M, Ragozin A et al: Effects of stress and social support on mothers and premature and full term infants. Child Dev 54:209–219, 1983
24. Crockenberg S: Infant irritability, mother responsiveness, and social support influences on the security of infant-mother attachment. Child Dev 52:857–865, 1981
25. Drillien C: A longitudinal study of the growth and development of prematurely and maturely born children: Mental Development at 2–5 years. Arch Dis Child 36:233, 1961
26. Eaton W, Kessler L: Rates of symptoms of depression in a national sample. Am J Epidemiol 114:528–538, 1981
27. Egbuonu L, Starfield B: Child health and social status. Pediatrics 69:550–557, 1982
28. Escalona S: Babies at double hazard: Early development of infants at biologic and social risk. Pediatrics 70:343–350, 1982
29. Field T: Early interactions between infants and their postpartum depressed mothers. Infant Behav Dev 7:517–522, 1984
30. Garcia-Coll C, Vohr B, Hoffman J et al: Maternal and environmental factors affecting developmental outcome of infants of adolescent mothers. Dev Behav Pediatr 7:230–236, 1986
31. Garmezy N: Vulnerability research and the issue of primary intervention. Am J Orthopsychiatry 41:101–116, 1971
32. Garmezy N: Stress, competence and development: Continuities in the study of schizo-

phrenic adults, children vulnerable to psychopathology, and the search for the stress-resistant child. Am J Orthopsychiatry 57:159–174, 1987

33. Garmezy N, Rutter M: Stress, Coping and Development in Children. New York, McGraw Hill, 1983
34. Ghodsian M, Zajicek E, Wolkind S: A longitudinal study of maternal depression and child behavior problems. J Child Psychol Psychiatr 25:91–109, 1984
35. Grossman P: Prematurity, poverty related stress, and the mother–infant relationship. Dissert Abstr Intl 40(4-B):1954, 1979
36. Hanshaw J, Scheiner A, Moxley A et al: School failure and deafness after silent congenital cytomegalovirus infection. N Engl J Med 295:468–470, 1976
37. House Select Committee on Children, Youth, and Families: Yearly Report, 1986
38. Hunter F, Kilstrom N: Breaking the cycle in abusing families. Am J Psychiatry 136:1320–1322, 1979
39. Illsley R: Early prediction of perinatal risk. Proc Royal Soc Med 59:181–184, 1966
40. Lazar I, Darlington A: Lasting effects after preschool. Monogr Soc Res Child Dev 47 (2 and 3):1982
41. Lerner R, East P: The role of temperament in stress, coping and socioemotional functioning in early development. Infant Ment Health J 5:148–159, 1984
42. Main M, Kaplan K, Cassidy J: Security in infancy, childhood and adulthood. Monogr Soc Res Child Dev 50:66–104, 1985
43. Makosky V: Sources of stress: Events or conditions? In Belle D (ed): Lives in Stress: Women and Depression. Beverly Hills, Sage Publications, 1982, pp 35–53
44. Maziade M, Boudreault M, Thivierge J et al: Infant temperament: SES and gender differences and reliability of measurement in a large Quebec sample. Merrill-Palmer Q 30:213–226, 1984
45. McGee R, Williams S, Kaskani J: Prevalence of self-reported depressive symptoms and associated social factors of mothers in Donedin. Br J Psychiatry 143:473–479, 1983
46. Miller P, Ingham J: Friends, confidants and symptoms. Soc Psychiatry 11:51, 1976
47. Moss P, Plewis I: Mental distress of preschool children in inner London. Psychol Med 7:614–652, 1977
48. Mueller D: Social networks: A promising direction for research on the relationship of the social environment to psychiatric disorder. Soc Sci Med 40:147–161, 1980
49. National Center for Health Statistics: Factors associated with low birthweight: 1976. Pub.# 80–1915. Washington, D.C., U.S. Dept. of Health and Human Services, 1980
50. Niswander K, Gordon M (eds): The Collaborative Perinatal Study of the National Institute of Neurologic Diseases and Stroke. Philadelphia, W.B. Saunders, 1972
51. Nuckolls K, Cassel J, Kaplan B: Psychosocial assets, life crisis and the prognosis of pregnancy. Am J Epidemiol 95:431–441, 1972
52. Orr S, James S: Maternal depression in an urban pediatric practice: Implications for health care delivery. Am J Public Health 74:363–365, 1984
53. Parmelee A, Michaelis R: Neurologic Examination of the Newborn. In Hellmuth J (ed): Exceptional Infants: Studies in Abnormalities. New York, Brunner/Mazel, 1971
54. Pascoe J, Loda F, Jeffries V, Earp J: The association between mothers' social support and provision of stimulation to their children. J Dev Behav Pediatr 2:15–19, 1981
55. Pasaminick B, Knobloch H: Retrospective studies on the epidemiology of reproductive casuality: Old and new. Merrill-Palmer Q 12:7–26, 1966
56. Plomin R: Behavioral genetics and intervention. In Gallagher J, Ramey C (eds): The Malleability of Children. Baltimore, Brookes, 1987, pp 15–24
57. Pollitt E, Eichler A, Chan C: Psychosocial development and behavior of mothers in failure to thrive syndrome. Am J Orthopsychiatry 45:525, 1975
58. Radke-Yarrow M, Cummings E, Kuczynski L, et al: Patterns of attachment in two- and three-year-olds in normal families and families with parental depression. Child Dev 56:884–893, 1985
59. Ramey C, Campbell F: Preventive education for high-risk children: Cognitive consequences of the Carolina Abecedarian Project. Am J Ment Defic 88:515–523, 1984
60. Richman N: A community survey of characteristics of one- to two-year-olds with sleep disruptions. J Am Acad Child Psychiatry 20:281–291, 1981
61. Roghmann K, Hecht P, Haggerty R: Coping with stress. In Haggerty R, Roghmann K, Pless I (eds): Child Health and the Community. New York, John Wiley and Sons, 1975, pp 54–66

62. Rutter M: Early sources of security and competence. In Bruner J, Garten A (eds): Human Growth and Development. London, Oxford University Press, 1978
63. Rutter M: Psychosocial resilience and protective mechanisms. Am J Orthopsychiatry 57:316–331, 1987
64. Sameroff A: Environmental context of child development. J Pediatr 109:192–199, 1986
65. Sameroff A, Chandler M: Reproductive risk and the continuum of caretaking casualty. In Horowitz F, Hetherington M, Scarr–Salanatek S et al (eds): Review of Child Development Research. Chicago, University of Chicago Press, 1975, pp 187–244
66. Sameroff A, Seifer R: Familial risk and child competence. Child Dev 54:1254–1268, 1983
67. Sameroff A, Seifer R, Barocas et al: Intelligence quotient scores of 4-year-old children: Social environmental risk factors. Pediatrics 79:343–350, 1987
68. Sameroff A, Seifer R, Zax M: Early development of children at risk for emotional disorders. Monogr Soc Res Child Dev 47:1–71, 1982
69. Sandler W, Block M: Life stresses and maladjustment of poor children. Am J Commun Psychol 8:41–52, 1980
70. Scarr S, McCartney K: How people make their own environments: A theory of genotype–environmental effects. Child Dev 54:424–435, 1983
71. Scarr S, Weinberg R: The influence of "family background" on intellectual attainment. Am Soc Rev 43:674–692, 1987
72. Selye H: The physiology and pathology of stress. Montreal, Acta, 1950
73. Shonkoff J: Biologic and social factors contributing to mild mental retardation. In Heller K, Holtzman W, Messiuk S (eds): Placing Children in Special Education: A Strategy for Equity. Washington, National Academy Press, 1982
75. Shonkoff J: Social support and vulnerability to stress: A pediatric perspective. Pediatr Ann 14:550–554, 1985
76. Shonkoff J, Hauser-Cram P: Early intervention for disabled infants and their families: A quantitative analysis. Pediatrics 80:650–658, 1987
77. Spieker S: Patterns of very insecure attachment found in samples of high-risk infants and toddlers. Top Early Child Spec Educ 6:37–53, 1986
78. Thomas A, Chess S: Temperament and Development. New York, Brunner/Mazel, 1977
79. Thomas A, Chess S: Genesis and evolution of behavioral disorders from infancy to early adult life. Am J Psychiatry 141:1–9, 1984
80. Thompson R: Stability of infant–mother attachment and its relationship to changing life circumstances in an unselected middle class sample. Child Dev 53:144–148, 1982
81. Unger D, Powell D: Supporting families under stress: The role of social networks. Fam Relat 29:566–574, 1980
82. Vaughn B, Egeland B, Sroufe L et al: Individual differences in infant–mother attachment at 12 and 18 months: Stability and change in families under stress. Child Dev 50:971–975, 1979
83. Vietze P, Falsey S, Sandler H et al: Transactional approach to prediction of child maltreatment. Inf Ment Health J 1:248–261, 1980
84. Warren L, McEachern C: Psychosocial correlates of depressive symptomology in adult women. J Abnorm Psychol 92:151–160, 1983
85. Weinraub M, Wolf B: Effects of stress and social supports on mother–infant interactions in single and two parent families. Child Dev 54:1297–1311, 1983
86. Weintraub S, Neale J, Liebert D: Teachers' ratings of children vulnerable to psychopathology. Am J Orthopsychiatry 45:839–849, 1975
87. Weissman M, John K, Merikangas K et al: Depressed parents and their children: General health, social and psychiatric problems. Am J Dis Child 140:801–809, 1986
88. Weissman M, Prusoff B, Gammon G et al: Psychopathology in the children (age 6–18) of depressed and normal parents. J Am Acad Child Psychiatry 23:78–84, 1986
89. Weissman M, Siegal R: The depressed woman and her rebellious adolescent. Social Casework 53:563–570, 1972
90. Werner E, Smith R: Kauai's Children Come of Age. Honolulu, Hawaii, University of Hawaii Press, 1977
91. Werner E, Simonian K, Bierman J, et al: Cumulative effect of perinatal complications and deprived social environment on physical, intellectual, and social development of preschool children. Pediatrics 39:480–505, 1967
92. Williams H, Carmichael A: Depression of mothers in a multiethnic urban industrial municipality. J Child Psychol Psychiatr 26:277–288, 1985

93. Wolkind S: Prenatal emotional stress: Effects on the fetus. In Wolkind S, Zajicek E (eds): Pregnancy: A Psychological and Social Study. Orlando, Florida, Grune Stratton, 1981, pp 177–193

94. Zuckerman B, Amaro H, Beardslee W: Mental health of adolescent mothers: The implications for depression and drug use. Dev Behav Pediatr 8:111–116, 1987

95. Zuckerman B, Beardslee W: Maternal depression: A concern for pediatricians. Pediatrics 79:110–117, 1987

96. Zuckerman B, Stevenson J, Bailey V: Stomachaches and headaches in a community of sample of preschool children. Pediatrics 79:677–682, 1987

97. Zuckerman B, Stevenson J, Bailey V: Sleep problems in early childhood: Continuities, predictive factors, and behavioral correlates. Pediatrics 80:664–671, 1987

98. Zuckerman B, Hingson R, Alpert J et al: Neonatal outcome: Is adolescent pregnancy a risk factor? Pediatrics 71:489–495, 1983

99. Zuckerman B, Walker D, Frank D et al: Adolescent pregnancy: Biobehavioral determinants of outcome. J Pediatr 105:857–862, 1984

Division of Developmental and Behavioral Pediatrics
Department of Pediatrics
Boston City Hospital
Boston, Massachusetts 02118

Foster Care

Edward L. Schor, MD*

Our society has always been faced with the problem of providing care for children without living parents or whose parents are unable or unwilling to care for them. In preindustrial America there was incentive for taking such children into a family because they could be expected to materially contribute to the welfare of the family. Seen as important resources and necessary to the economy, dependent children were apprenticed or "bound out" to other families until the age of majority. This provided the child with some sense of permanency while he or she was expected to pay his or her own way. It also led to abuses of child labor. As the country developed, childhood became a more protected life stage, in which expectations of children to contribute materially were limited. The late 1800s also were characterized by immigration from both outside and within the country or region. Industrialization created a dispersion of extended families and isolated individuals from established systems of social support. These circumstances contribute to family dysfunction and in the extreme case the inability of more parents to parent their children adequately. As a consequence, society responded by developing institutions for the care of children, foundling homes and orphanages.[10] The minority of children were truly orphans, and most came from homes that were unable to care adequately for them.

At the 1909 White House Conference on Children, the principles of supporting families so that they could continue caring for their children, or alternatively, placing children in foster families to be cared for until their biologic families were able to resume care, were adopted.[10] This recommendation was formalized in law when in 1935, Congress enacted Title IV-A, Aid to Dependent Children, as a component of the Social Security Act. The objective of this Title was to provide financial assistance to widows and widowers to avoid the breakup of families from economic hardship. The title was subsequently amended to include assistance to the parent and certain specified relatives and the name was changed to its current one, Aid to Families with Dependent Children (AFDC). The program has changed considerably since its inception, especially in the decade from 1967 to 1976 when the number of supported children increased from 3.6 to 8.1 million. The upward trend was accompanied by a marked decrease in children who were paternal orphans to a rapid increase in children with living fathers absent from the home. Despite programs to support the family, the number of children in need of substitute parenting increased. In 1961, Title IV-A was amended to provide Federal matching

*Clinical Associate Professor, Department of Pediatrics, Stanford University School of Medicine; Program Officer, The Henry J. Kaiser Family Foundation, Menlo Park, California

payments to States for AFDC eligible children who might be removed from their home and placed in foster care.[5c] This change has resulted in the foster care system increasingly serving poor, minority, single-parent, and female-headed households.[5c]

For the greater part of the history of child welfare in the United States, there has been little evidence of central, governmental planning based on a general social concern for the well-being of children. The patchwork planning represented within the Social Security Act and the AFDC program has been continuously subject to political influence, placing child welfare policy within a highly partisan process. Major public child welfare legislation and regulation largely reflect political ideology about families, children, and the proper role of government. Family policy formulated by the government is often viewed as an invasion of family autonomy, an intrusion into private, moral decisions.[24] This is reflected in the reluctance of the courts to interfere with the "natural family," so that it is difficult for children to be freed for adoption. In addition, few services are made available for the family to address problems that lead to inadequate child care in the home, in part for fear of rewarding welfare dependency.

Over the past decade the circumstances that lead to a need for foster care for children (e.g., poverty, lack of social supports, parental physical and mental illness, and substance abuse), coupled with limited institutional resources that effectively screen out the more manageable cases for foster care placement has skewed the foster child population toward greater need for therapeutic and rehabilitative services. Since 1983 the foster care population nationally has been growing in absolute size and contains a higher proportion of older and special-needs children.[5h] Foster children today have more serious physical and emotional health problems than they did in the past. Sexually assaulted children make up an increasing proportion of children in foster care. Infants with AIDS whose parents are themselves usually drug abusers and have contracted AIDS are requiring foster care. Because they are difficult to place, children with AIDS are frequently boarded in hospitals and special units.

In the past the health care needs of children in foster care did not differ remarkably from those of other children. Today the number of children in care and the nature and severity of their health problems has required that special, organized systems of care be developed for them. During the past decade some progress has been made in this regard.

DEFINITION AND EPIDEMIOLOGY

Foster Care and Its Goals

Placement of a child in foster care is intended to be a planned, temporary service to strengthen families and to enhance the quality of life for children. During the placement families are to receive the social support and counsel they require to be reunited. During the period of placement, communities, through their social service agencies, assume the responsibility for ensuring that the children's physical and emotional health and educational needs are met. In theory, if, after study and investigation reuniting the child with the family is not deemed possible or is considered not to be in the best interests of the child, parental rights are to be terminated and the child is to be placed with an adoptive family. For some children neither reunion nor adoption is feasible, and they remain impermanently with a foster family or in another setting until they reach the age of majority, or in the case of children with AIDS, until they die.

Children in Foster Care

The total children in foster care increased from 272,000 in 1972 to 502,000 in 1977 and decreased to 243,000 by the end of 1982.[5c] However, in 1983 the downward trend halted and the number of children entering foster care began rising. This trend was not uniform and showed regional variation. The increase seems to be due to more children entering foster care rather than fewer children leaving.[5c]

There are approximately equal numbers of males and females in foster care. The mean age of children in care increased from 9.6 in 1977 to 10.1 in 1982; the median age remained unchanged. About 40 per cent of children in care are minority, with proportionately more black children than their ratio in the population than one would expect. About one fourth of the foster care population is handicapped.[5a]

The Foster Care System

Three-quarters of the children in foster care are there because of child maltreatment (48 per cent) or the absence or condition of the parent (26 per cent).[5d] In 1984, of all children in substitute care, 68 per cent were in foster family care, 10 per cent were in institutions, 9 per cent were in group homes, 7 per cent were in their own home, and 6 per cent were in other or unknown settings.[5h]

Most children entering foster care return to their biologic families within the first year. In 1983, children left the system for the following reasons: reunification with parents or relatives (55 per cent), adoption (11 per cent), emancipation or reaching the age of majority (9 per cent), transfer to another agency (3 per cent), ran away (3 per cent), and other reasons (19 per cent).[5f] However, about 25 per cent of children remain in care 2 years after initial placement, and they are likely to remain in care for many years thereafter. More than one third of the white children, and greater than one half the black children have been in care for more than 2 years.[14, 27] Slightly over one half of the children experience only one placement setting while in care; over one-fourth experience three or more placement settings.[5a]

Twenty per cent of foster children reenter foster care within 1 year of discharge. The reentry of a child into the foster care system may be due to (1) a system failure for not preparing the child and family adequately for reunification; (2) a failed effort despite the best efforts of the agency, the family, and others involved in the process; (3) added stress, such as unemployment, housing crisis, lack of child care, and so forth.[5f]

The amount of time children spend in foster care is critical to their development. The longer the child remains in continuous care the more likely that strong attachments will develop with foster parents, especially if involvement of the biologic parents decreases. The younger child, having a different sense of time, is likely to quickly come to relate to the foster parents as psychological parents.[19]

Concerns about the length of time in care were central to changes in federal policy leading to the enactment of the Adoption Assistance and Child Welfare Act of 1980, P.L. 96–272. The act specifically attempts to reduce the duration of care. This was influenced, in part, by the results of a 1977 survey of children in foster care that revealed that more than 100,000 children had been in care for 6 or more years.[48] The new legislation mandated that child welfare agencies develop care plans for children in foster care that provide for a sense of permanency in their lives. External citizen and judicial review processes were instituted to ensure that permanency planning occurred. Consequently, there has been a large decline in the duration of care. In 1961, 38 per cent of children were in care for 5 years or more; in 1984 this had decreased to 18 per cent. Similarly, the mean duration of placement decreased from 46 to 22 months.[5g]

The increase in child maltreatment reporting has had a substantial impact on the foster care system. It has altered the types of services that need to be provided by child welfare agencies, the likelihood of reunion of the family, and the emotional status of the children entering care.

Specialized foster homes have been developed to address a variety of health problems of children in care. Some of these homes are designed to care for children with emotional disturbances. Others have foster parents trained to provide specialized "nursing" care to chronically ill children. Recently, efforts have been made to alleviate the boarding of infants with AIDS in hospital settings by developing AIDS-specialized foster family homes.[21]

While the number of children entering care and the severity of their physical, emotional, developmental, and social problems are increasing, agencies are having increasing difficulty recruiting and retaining qualified foster parents. This is particularly true in larger urban areas. Persons willing to serve as foster parents generally take on this responsibility to fulfill a sense of social responsibility, altruism, personal need, or religious conviction. The rate of payment from child welfare agencies to foster families barely covers essential child care costs and in no way can be construed as remuneration for professional parenting services. The average monthly rate in 1985 was $255.95. The standard rate includes the basic monthly rate plus, where applicable, special clothing allowances and personal and incidental allowances. It does not include additional payments for special needs children or any other extraordinary payments.[5h] Given the increasing age of children in care and the increasing prevalence of special needs children, the inadequacy of these rates becomes progressively problematic. Parents of specialized foster homes receive a substantially higher rate.

The child welfare system is plagued with problems that impede the provision of appropriate services to children and families.[36] Administration of child welfare agencies is hampered by inadequate budgets, insufficient and poorly trained personnel, and a plethora of paperwork and legal mandates. Between 1958 and 1977 the proportion of professionally trained graduate social workers employed by child welfare agencies decreased from 51 to 9 per cent.[5g] Turnover of personnel is exceedingly high and often prevents coherent planning and continuity of services.

RISK FACTORS FOR FOSTER CARE PLACEMENT

The risks for entering foster care should be examined not only as emanating from the unique problems of individual families, but also as reflections of larger social patterns and problems. Therefore one must look beyond the increasing rate of physical and sexual child abuse, and to the social context in which this occurs. During the past decade there has been a retreat from the commitments of the 1960s to the families and children burdened by poverty and racism. There has been a significant increase in poverty in America.[11, 35] Children now constitute the largest segment of the population who live in poverty.[4] More than 40 per cent of black children and almost 40 per cent of Hispanic children are poor. Benefits that affect children have been cut extensively. Programs that administer food stamps, Medicaid, AFDC, school lunch, and day care have been severely affected.[34] Regardless of race, a child in a female-headed family is five times more likely to be poor than a child in a male-headed or two-parent family.[4] In 1983, 70 per cent of children who lived in households headed by minority females were poor.[34] Children from AFDC families are about four times more likely to enter foster care than are other children; therefore, coming from a poor, single-parent household greatly increases the risk of a child entering foster care.[5i]

In addition to poverty, risk factors for foster care include migration within the country, immigration, teenage parenthood, single parents, lack of social support, alcoholism and substance abuse, AIDS, homelessness, and mental illness. These of course are not independent factors but interact to magnify the risk to children in families experiencing such circumstances.

Within the foster care system itself, social factors have been found to be important. For example, the time children spend in care, once placed, differs according to ethnic group. Overall, though more white children are in care (58 per cent) than other racial groups, in large urban areas more minorities are in care. Minority status leads to increased risk of placement. Although black children compose a smaller than expected proportion of the population, they are at greater risk for being identified in need of foster care; conversely, when they are in greater numbers than expected, they are less likely to be in care. The length of stay in foster care is significantly influenced by the proportion of families with children who are in poverty in a community. Thus, time in care is partially predictable by social and economic factors.[28]

HEALTH PROBLEMS OF FOSTER CHILDREN

Studies of the foster child population have consistently shown higher than expected rates of chronic health problems.[20, 25, 29, 44] These problems include a wide variety of chronic medical disorders and dental needs, and increasingly include prenatal exposure to drugs and congenital infections, including acquired immune deficiency syndrome. Chronic health problems are exceedingly common, affecting 40 to 76 per cent of these children.[20, 26, 29, 44] Foster children have been found to be over-represented in pediatric specialty clinics, especially those caring for neuromuscular, pulmonary, and visual disorders, and myelomeningocele and cystic fibrosis.[6]

Physical health problems are almost uniformly encountered. In one prospective study of 149 children entering foster care because of abuse or neglect, it was found that only 13 per cent of the children had entirely normal physical examinations. Thirty-four per cent had potentially serious medical problems requiring one or more subspecialty consultations.[26] Problems with physical growth are frequently encountered.[7, 25, 29, 44] Although no longitudinal studies have been done on foster children to investigate the incidence of growth retardation, the presumption is that these children's short stature reflects nonorganic failure to thrive. This has implications not only in terms of the care of these children prior to placement but portends poorly for their subsequent cognitive development.[7] In addition to abnormalities in growth, decreased visual and auditory acuity and dental problems are frequent.[26, 29, 44] Preventive health care services are less likely to have been provided,[29, 44] and documentation of such services is difficult to obtain.

Children in foster care appear to have an elevated rate of developmental delays and educational problems.[29, 41, 44] This may, in part, reflect their impoverished origins and emotional deprivation experienced while with their own family.[9] They have been found to have cognitive and academic function at the low end of the average range. These functional levels are similar to the levels of low SES and minority children living with their own families.[14, 16]

The most frequently identified health problems of children in foster care are mental health disorders. Prevalence data on serious emotional problems among foster children range from 35 to 95 per cent.[17, 22, 26, 31, 32, 44, 50] The circumstances that lead to children's placement in foster care, especially their experiences with abuse and neglect, render them at risk for psychological disorders.[18, 49]

Most excess health problems of children in foster care can be related to prenatal factors and preplacement social circumstances. Most foster children come from homes in which poverty and lack of education can adversely influence dietary habits and health behaviors and can limit access to regular health care. Their mothers are less likely to have obtained adequate prenatal care. The children may not have received regular health care supervision and preventive services. Medical care of acute health care problems may have been delayed and predispose to chronicity. They may have experienced poorly coordinated care for identified health problems.

Removal from the family home, though intended as a therapeutic intervention, may contribute to the child's poor health. Ongoing health care may be interrupted, especially because information about present and past health problems is inconsistently obtained and transmitted by child welfare workers.[26, 30] In addition, the removal itself may lead to abandonment of the child by his biologic parents, leaving the child vulnerable to lifelong feelings of loss, rejection, and diminished self-worth.[13, 40] Unfortunately, once in foster care many of their health problems persist and, in fact, may be compounded after placement.[29, 44, 53] Foster children ordinarily do not have available to them an organized system of health care that is able to address their health problems effectively. In addition, it also has been suggested that the impermanence of foster care, including the lack of long-term planning and placement in multiple foster homes, contributes to lifelong problems in establishing emotional intimacy, and to the high rate of mental health disorders and delinquent behavior.[17, 19, 40, 42, 44]

INTERFACE BETWEEN SYSTEMS OF SOCIAL SERVICE AND HEALTH CARE

Problems

The foster care system has been accused of substituting societal for parental neglect.[1] Child abuse within foster homes is not uncommon. Child welfare agencies have been sued successfully for harming children under their care through inadequately selecting, licensing, training, and supervising foster parents, failing to match foster children with suitable homes, overcrowding foster homes, failing to provide adequate medical, psychological and educational services, and assigning excessive caseloads to child care workers.[33]

The Adoption Assistance and Child Welfare Act of 1980, P.L. 96–272, initiated important changes in the system of foster care, some of which had indirect effects on the health of children in care. The major thrust of this law was to encourage permanency planning for children in foster care. Through its implementation there has been a decrease in the number of children in foster care, and the duration of placement has been reduced.[5b] The Act also provided federal funds to facilitate the adoption of otherwise hard to place children by providing matching funding to cover postadoption maintenance costs and medical or other special services that the comprehensive care of a child might require.[5e]

While addressing the important issue of permanency planning and providing additional funds for health care services that could facilitate adoption, P.L. 96–272 did not address the lack of a regulated and organized approach, which is the fundamental problem in the system of health care available to children in foster care. In addition, child welfare agencies generally give low priority to health care, are not well educated about child health and development, and are administratively unable to monitor services and quality.

Children entering foster care often do so during a crisis that includes their abrupt removal from their family home. Initial health care is sought either to gather evidence regarding possible abuse and sexual assault, or to screen for the presence of contagious diseases to protect members of the foster parents' household. Although a comprehensive health assessment should follow placement, this happens inconsistently, rarely follows a uniform plan, and infrequently includes screening for mental health problems.[23, 54] Ordinarily, foster parents are given little direction from the child welfare agency as to where and when to obtain health care services for a child in their care.[23, 43] Since most children in foster care have their health care paid for by a state-operated Medicaid program, foster parents are dependent upon those physicians willing to accept this source and level of reimbursement.[54] The number of such physicians is apparently decreasing.[37] The eligibility procedures for Medicaid programs are cumbersome and can prevent obtaining timely care at placement of the child. In many states the scope, frequency, and quality of services, especially for mental health problems, are unduly restricted by the Medicaid programs.

Given the lack of an organized system of standards and policies relating to child health care it is not surprising that health care is fragmented. In the absence of ascribed priority to health matters, caseworkers, burdened by excessive caseloads and an uneven background in child development and child health, neglect attending to health care issues except the most obvious physical and emotional disabilities.[2, 23, 43] Thus, past medical information, such as information about prior medical care, mental health evaluations, or immunization status, is usually not available to the foster parents or to physicians caring for foster children.[23, 26, 29]

The types of health problems presented by foster children require time-consuming, coordinated, comprehensive, and continuous care from competent and conscientious health care providers. However, the lack of direction and oversight and the poor record keeping by child welfare agencies, the potentially temporary and transient nature of foster care placement, and the poor level and restrictions on payment for health care services militate against foster children receiving the quality of care they deserve and require. Compounding the problem, health care providers usually are not familiar with the foster care system, including the relationship among the agency staff, foster and biologic parents and the children, the special needs of the children, and the resources that are available.[23]

Models of Care

There have been some successful efforts to improve the health care provided to children in foster care. The acceptance of Medicaid eligible children into prepaid, capitated systems of health care delivery offers a ready-made, organized system of comprehensive care. This model has been applied successfully in Baltimore, Maryland, where for over a decade the Chesapeake Health Plan, a staff model health maintenance organization, has offered care for the city's children in foster care.[47] In New York City, the Children's Aid Society has offered primary health care services on site at the agency to the majority of children under its supervision. Other efforts to develop centralized sources of comprehensive care, some mandated by the courts, are underway across the country.[33] In other locales, child welfare agencies are attempting to identify preferred providers, pediatricians who are both willing and able to provide the quality of health services that children in care require. All of these approaches must guarantee to the child welfare agency that high quality health care is being provided.

The retention of a portable, abbreviated health care record by the foster parent has long been advocated by child health providers.[1] The Commonwealth of Massachusetts has adopted such a medical passport, and has linked its use with a computerized system to track medical services provided to children in care. There is federal legislation pending that would require that a health record be a part of every social service case record.

In 1988, the Child Welfare League of America, in consultation with the American Academy of Pediatrics, issued standards for the health care of children in foster care. This document, based on a consensus paper developed by a panel of experts in the field of child welfare and health, addresses problems at every level of the delivery of health services to children in care, and will serve as the basis for the development of local systems of health care, professional education, and administrative responsibility.[46] Additional recommendations specific to the clinical role of pediatricians are also available.[2, 3, 45]

RECOMMENDATIONS

Primary Prevention

Since foster care is an institutional response to family dysfunction rooted in pervasive social problems, it is likely to continue to be needed as long as those problems remain. The litany of risk factors that predispose to foster care placement are major problems that programs addressing poverty, malnutrition, teenage pregnancy, drug abuse, unemployment, and educational inequality must resolve. Meanwhile, family preservation efforts that seek to keep children from troubled families out of dependent care by assisting the families to remain intact, and that address the problems that are leading to dysfunction should be encouraged.[3, 39] Over 30 states have developed State trust funds for children, with special concern for child abuse. These funds are typically financed through taxes on birth certificates and marriage licenses and offer additional sources of funding for family support programs.[38]

Secondary Prevention

Once a child has been remanded to the child welfare system it is imperative that comprehensive health care be provided so that existing physical, emotional, developmental, and educational problems can be recognized and treated appropriately. Centralized systems of care seem superior in this regard.[44, 50] Case management should be used to ensure comprehensiveness and continuity of care. Although it does not include adequate provisions for the identification and treatment of mental health disorders, the Early Periodic Screening Diagnosis and Treatment Program, available to all children who qualify for Title XIX funding, should be used to facilitate access to pediatric care.

Child welfare agencies must improve their internal system of monitoring the health care of children for whom they are responsible, and for ensuring that the care that is being provided meets accepted levels of quality. This will entail adoption of new or revised policies, procedures and standards, simplified record keeping, automated, computerized information systems, the use of consultation from child health professionals, and training of agency staff and foster parents.

Tertiary Prevention

Given the very high prevalence of chronic physical and emotional problems among children in foster care, extensive efforts should be undertaken to limit the debilitating effects of these disorders. Unfortunately, the system of foster care primarily is designed to transport, adjudicate, and provide placement services for children and not to serve their long-term medical, developmental and emotional needs.[23] Health care services for children in foster care must include ready access to the variety of medical specialists, subspecialists, and other professionals needed to address their needs. Care plans devised by child welfare agencies should be made in conjunction with health care professionals to ensure that appropriate and comprehensive medical care plans are included.

Specialized foster homes should be developed to provide a therapeutic environment for children with chronic medical and emotional disorders. When provided with sufficient professional backup support, these can be successful placements for psychiatrically disturbed and medically fragile children and adolescents, and may be useful additions to the range of treatments available.[15, 55] Foster parents can also be guided to work with the biologic parents, to nurture and support them, so that they will be able to reestablish primary responsibility for parenting their child.

One important intervention is to move children out of foster care and back to their biologic families or into adoptive homes. Although permanency planning has great potential, there is a need to improve the process, especially the provision of community services to the biologic family so as to facilitate return of the child.[51] Sadly, biologic parents of foster children rarely are offered services designed to build on their strengths to enable them to restore their homes as viable abodes for their children.[12]

FUTURE NEEDS

Demonstration Projects

There are a large number of initiatives that can be undertaken that have the potential to improve the circumstances and health of children in foster care. First, the several models of providing health care services to children in care need further testing. This can be accomplished through a combination of reorganization of child welfare agencies' procedures for obtaining and monitoring health care services, and creative use of existing health care funding mechanisms. The latter include the use of Medicaid waivers, capitated health care, and capturing other sources of Federal funding such as increasing claims for matching funds through Title IV-B, IV-E, and V of the Social Security Act.[39, 54] Availability of Medicaid funds should be expanded to cover health care services for some period following the return of a child to his biologic family or upon emancipation.

Increased effort and resources should be directed toward family preservation efforts. For example, this could be facilitated by providing Medicaid waivers to pay for in-home services needed by at-risk families, and using Medicaid for counseling and therapy services to eligible families.[39]

Accountability of Social Service System

Child welfare agencies have only rarely been held accountable for the quality of health care provided to children under their supervision.[33] With the publication of standards for the health care of children in foster care by the Child Welfare League of America, agencies will have clearer guidelines for the parameters of their responsibility. Child advocates including health professionals, children's rights attorneys, and the judiciary will have an easier time ascertaining whether appropriate efforts are being undertaken on behalf of the health of children in care.

Training

Without exception, all those involved in the health care of dependent children are in need of additional training. Child welfare professionals need to know more about the health care system, child health problems, and child development. Foster parents need similar training and should be offered child specific education when caring for a child with a unique, complex, or difficult to manage health problem. Judges and attorneys should have a better grounding in basic principles of child development and parent–child relationships.[19] Health care professionals must become more familiar with the organization, goals, and operation of the foster care system, and with the special health care needs of children in care.

Biologic Parents

Biologic parents are too often either neglected by the foster care system or are purposefully excluded from the ongoing lives and care of their children. If reconstitution of the family is indeed a goal of foster care, then the parents should play an active and ongoing role. They can be the source of otherwise unavailable information about the child, and ascribing importance to their contribution to the child's care while in placement can enhance the likelihood of a return home. Continuing contact has also been shown to have a beneficial effect on the child's mental health status.[52] Biologic parents remain central to the emotional lives of children in care, even when the possibility of reunion has been excluded. Therefore, the presence of biologic parents should be acknowledged, and they should play as active a role during their child's placement as is warranted and possible.

Specialized Care by Foster Parents

Foster parents are valued for the shelter they provide children in care but are not routinely offered the training and incentive to play an active role in the child's and biologic family's treatment and rehabilitation. There have been a number of successful initiatives using foster care to meet the special needs of some children, particularly those with chronic medical and emotional problems. Foster parents can not only provide care for the child but can assume responsibility for teaching the biologic parents the skills necessary to provide that care themselves.[15, 55] Efforts should be made to increase the availability of therapeutic foster homes, employing the foster family as members of a therapeutic team. Specialized foster parent training should be made available, and board rates should reflect the service and expertise that is then offered.

Foster Children with AIDS

Children with AIDS will constitute a small but growing proportion of the foster child population for the foreseeable future. Their care presents complex social, ethical, legal, educational, physical, and emotional health issues, which the foster care system is presently ill prepared to address. The needs of these children, and the consequences of public assumption of responsibility for their care, will require careful monitoring and ongoing study and definition.[8, 21]

REFERENCES

1. American Academy of Pediatrics, Committee on Adoption and Dependent Care: The needs of the child in foster family care. Pediatrics 59:465, 1977
2. American Academy of Pediatrics, Committee on Early Childhood, Adoption, and Dependent Care: Health care of foster children. Pediatrics 79(4):644–646, 1987
3. Chadwick DL: Dependency as a therapeutic process. California Pediatrician Summer:29–32, 1985
4. Child Poverty Rate Stays High: CDF Reports 9(4):1–8, 1987
5. Child Welfare Research Notes, Administration for Children, Youth and Families, HDS, DHHS:
5a. #1: Characteristics of Children in Foster Care, December 1983
5b. #4: Impact of P.L. 96–272, Section 427 Protections, March 1984
5c. #8: Gershenson CP: The twenty year trend of federally assisted foster care, July 1984
5d. #11: Gershenson CP: 1983 Trend of children in foster care, April 1985
5e. #12: Maza PL: Trends in adoption assistance, July 1985
5f. #14: Gershenson CP: An assessment of children re-entering foster care, January 1986
5g. #16: Gershenson CP: A re-examination of the duration of foster care for children served by public agencies, December 1986
5h. #17: Collins RC: Foster care rates: Trends and implications, May 1987
5i. #18: Gershenson CP. Title IV-E federally assisted children in foster care, May 1987
6. Dalby JT, Fox SL, Haslam RHA: Adoption and foster care rates in pediatric disorders. Develop Behav Pediatr 3:61–64, 1982

7. Dowdney L, Skuse D, Heptinstall E et al: Growth retardation and developmental delay amongst inner-city children. J Child Psychol Psychiatr 28:529–541, 1987
8. Education and foster care of children infected with human T-lymphotropic virus type III/ lymphadenopathy-associated virus. MMWR 34(34):517–521, 1985
9. Eisenberg L: The sins of the fathers: Urban decay and social pathology. Am J Orthopsychiatry 32:5–17, 1962
10. English PC: Pediatrics and the unwanted child in history: Foundling homes, disease, and the origins of foster care in New York City, 1860 to 1920. Pediatrics 73(5):699–711, 1984
11. Families in Poverty: Changes in the "Safety Net." Washington D.C., U.S. Government Printing Office, 1984
12. Fanshel D: The exit of children from foster care: An interim research report. Child Welfare 50:65–81, 1971
13. Fanshel D: Decision-making under uncertainty: Foster care for abused or neglected children? Am J Public Health 71(7):685–686, 1981
14. Fanshel D, Shinn EG: Children in Foster Care: A Longitudinal Investigation. New York, Columbia University Press, 1978
15. Foster PH, Whitworth JM: Medical foster care. Children Today 15(4):12–16, 1986
16. Fox M, Arcuri K: Cognitive and academic functioning in foster children. Child Welfare 59(8):491–496, 1980
17. Frank G: Treatment needs of children in foster care. Am J Orthopsychiatry 50(2):256–263, 1980
18. Friedrich WN, Einbender AJ: The abused child: A psychological review. J Clin Child Psychol 12:244–256, 1983
19. Goldstein J, Freud A, Solnit A: Beyond the best interests of the child. New York, Macmillan, 1976
20. Gruber AR: Children in Foster Care. New York, Human Sciences Press, 1978, pp 180–183
21. Gurdin P, Anderson GR: Quality care for ill children: AIDS-specialized foster family homes. Child Welfare 56(4):291–302, 1987
22. Halfon N, Klee L: Health care for foster children in California. Report prepared for the David and Lucile Packard Foundation, January 15, 1986
23. Halfon N, Klee L: Health services for California's foster children: Current practices and policy recommendations. Pediatrics 80(2):183–191, 1987
24. Hartley EK: Government leadership to protect children from foster care "drift." Child Abuse and Neglect 8:337–342, 1984
25. Hochstasdt NJ, Jaudes PK: The MAPS Project—Medical and Psychosocial Screening: A Survey of the Medical and Psychosocial Needs of Children Entering the Care of the Department of Children and Family Services. Chicago, Illinois, La Rabida Children's Hospital and Research Center, December, 1984
26. Hochstadt NJ, Jaudes PK, Zimo KA et al: The medical and psychosocial needs of children entering foster care. Child Abuse and Neglect 11:53–62, 1987
27. Jenkins S: Duration of foster care: Some relevant antecedent variables. Child Welfare 46:450–455, 1967
28. Jenkins S, Diamond B: Ethnicity and foster care: Census data as predictors of placement variables. Am J Orthopsychiatry 55(2):267–276, 1985
29. Kavaler F, Swire MR: Foster Child Health Care. Lexington, Massachusetts, Lexington Books, DC Heath & Col, 1983
30. Klee L, Halfon N: Communicating health information in the California foster care system: Problems and recommendations. Children and Youth Services Review 9:171–185, 1987
31. McIntyre A, Keesler TY: Psychological disorders among foster children. J Clin Child Psychol 15(4):297–303, 1986
32. Moffatt ME, Peddie M, Stulginskas J et al: Health care delivery to foster children: A study. Health Soc Work 10:129–137, 1985
33. Mushlin MB, Levitt L, Anderson L: Court-ordered foster family care reform: A case study. Child Welfare 65(2):141–154, 1986
34. Newberger CM, Melnicoe LH, Newberger EH: The American family in crisis: implications for children. Current Problems in Pediatrics 16(12):669–739, 1986
35. O'Hare WP: Poverty in America: trends and new patterns. Population Bull 40:1, 1985

36. Oreskes M, Daley S, Rimer S: A system overloaded: The foster-care crisis. New York Times, Sunday, March 15, 1987, p 1
37. Perloff JD: Trends in pediatrician participation in state Medicaid programs: state report for California, Working Paper 11-A. Elk Grove Village, Illinois, American Academy of Pediatrics, January 1985
38. Poertner J: The Kansas Family and Children Trust Fund: Five years later. Child Welfare 66:3–12, 1987
39. Preserving Families in Crisis: Financial and Political Options. Washington D.C., The Center for the Study of Social Policy, May 1986
40. Rest ER, Watson KW: Growing up in foster care. Child Welfare 63(4):291–306, 1984
41. Rowe J, Lambert L: Children who wait: A study of children needing substitute families. London, Assoc of British Adoption Agencies, 1973, pp 50–51
42. Runyan DK, Gould CL: Foster care for child maltreatment: Impact on delinquent behavior. Pediatrics 75(3):562–568, 1985
43. Schor E: Health supervision of foster children. Child Welfare 60:313–319, 1981
44. Schor EL: The foster care system and health status of foster children. Pediatrics 69:521–528, 1982
45. Schor E: Pediatric care of foster children. In Dershewitz R (ed): Ambulatory Pediatric Care. Philadelphia, JB Lippincott, 1988
46. Schor E, Aptekar R, Scannell T: The Health Care of Children In and Out of Home Care. A White Paper. Washington, D.C., Child Welfare League of America, 1988
47. Schor E, Neff JM, LaAsmar JL: The Chesapeake Health Plan: An HMO model for foster children. Child Welfare 63:431–440, 1984
48. Shyne AW, Schroeder AG: National study of social services to children and their families: Overview. Bulletin 017–091–0025–8. Washington, D.C., U.S. Government Printing Office, 1978
49. Stricklin AB, Austad CS: Perceptions of neglected children and negligent parents about causes for removal from parental homes. Psycholog Rep 51:1103–1108, 1982
50. Swire MR, Kavaler F: Health services for foster children: Factors associated with health care costs. J Health Politics Policy Law 3:251–263, 1978
51. Turner J: Reuniting children in foster care with their biological parents. Social Work 29:501–505, 1984
52. Vasaly SM: Foster care in five states: A synthesis and analysis of studies from Arizona, California, Iowa, Massachusetts, and Vermont, publication (OHD) 76–300–157. Washington, D.C., U.S. Department of Health, Education, and Welfare, 1974
53. White R, Benedict M: Health status and utilization patterns of children in foster care. Final Report: DHHS, OHDS, ACYF (90-pd-86509), 1985
54. White RB, Benedict MI, Jaffe SM: Foster child health care supervision policy. Child Welfare 66(5):387–398, 1987
55. Wolkind S: Fostering the disturbed child. J Child Psychol Psychiatry 19:393–397, 1978

The Henry J. Kaiser Family Foundation
525 Middlefield Road—Suite 200
Menlo Park, California 94025

0031-3955/88 $0.00 + .20

School Absence—A Health Perspective

Lorraine V. Klerman, DrPH*

For most families, school absence is a trivial problem. The student misses a few days at infrequent intervals and there are only minor inconveniences—a note must be sent to the school and the academic work must be made up. For a few students, however, absence is a major problem. Their absences are frequent and prolonged; as a consequence, these students find it difficult if not impossible to complete their academic work. They may perform poorly in class, be retained in grade, or even drop out, behaviors that have important consequences for adult life. Excessive school absenteeism should be of interest to physicians not only because of its impact on school and adult performance, but also because much absence is either caused by a physical or psychological health problem or is associated with other risk-taking behaviors that may have a direct effect on health.

This article will review recent studies of the causes of school absence and of programs that are attempting to ameliorate this problem. The emphasis will be on health-related causes and medically based programs, although other factors and programs will be discussed when they are particularly relevant. The review will focus on studies published since 1980, although a few earlier, landmark investigations will be noted. Also, American studies will be highlighted, with a few references to British ones. (For reviews of previous studies see references.[44, 22])

EPIDEMIOLOGY OF SCHOOL ABSENCE

Relatively few analyses have been conducted of the characteristics of children who are absent from school, and even fewer of children whose absences are frequent or prolonged.

Definitions

The first issue in an epidemiological analysis is definition. Among the parameters that should be considered are the causes of the absence, particularly whether or not they are health-related, and the duration and frequency of the absences.

Health-related causes include not only physical illnesses and injuries, but also psychological problems, of which refusal to attend school and school phobia are probably the best known. Truancy often is cited as a cause of absence, particularly

---

*Professor, Public Health, Department of Epidemiology and Public Health, Yale School of Medicine, New Haven, Connecticut

Table 1. *School-Loss Days per Person (1980–1986)**

	ACUTE AND CHRONIC CONDITIONS	ACUTE CONDITIONS ONLY
1986	5.0	4.2
1985	4.8	3.9
1984	5.1	4.1
1983	5.0	4.2
1982	4.7	3.7
1981	4.9	4.4
1980	5.3	4.9

*From National Health Interview Survey. In 1980 and 1981, the National Center for Health Statistics calculated these data for children and youth ages 6–16. From 1982 through 1986, they were calculated for 5–17 year olds.

excessive absence. Truancy usually is defined as absence without an acceptable or justifiable reason and, some investigators add, without parental knowledge or approval.

These types of causes overlap significantly. Emotional factors may contribute to absences that are basically attributable to physical health reasons. Students may develop psychological problems as a result of an illness or injury and thus increase the duration of the absence. Truancy, usually considered a form of social deviance, may have its origins in an underlying physical problem, making it difficult for the student to achieve in school. Hearing loss and dyslexia are examples of conditions that might lead to inability to keep up with one's peers and cause antisocial reactions. Some investigators have found truancy associated with neurotic symptoms.[15]

Parents' physical or emotional problems may contribute to absence. They may react inappropriately to a condition, encouraging a student to stay home when a condition, such as dysmenorrhea, does not warrant it; or extending an absence unnecessarily, as for an asthmatic attack. A parent's reaction to a young child's reluctance to attend school may make the condition more serious. In addition, a student may be required to stay home because the physical or emotional illness of a parent, a sibling, or another relative requires a caretaker.

The duration and frequency of the absence also need to be considered. Absences that are infrequent or of short duration probably have little consequence unless they follow a significant pattern. For example, a sequence of Monday absences in a junior or senior high school student might suggest an alcohol or drug problem, and two or three consecutive days absence in each month in a teenage girl might indicate menstrual difficulties. Educators believe that students who miss more than 10 days in a 90-day semester (11 per cent of school days) have difficulty in staying at grade level.

National Health Interview Survey

The major source of data on the extent of school absence is the National Health Interview Survey (NHIS), which counts as a school-loss day only those caused by an acute or chronic health condition in children 5 to 17 years of age. The NHIS does not note the number of absences or length of absence for the individual respondent.

The NHIS estimated that in 1986 health conditions caused 226.4 million days of school to be lost, or 5.0 days per child 5 to 17 years of age. This rate has remained relatively constant over the past 7 years[26–29] (Table 1). The rate for females is slightly higher than for males, the white rate is somewhat higher than the black, and the rate is highest for those with the least income (Table 2).

Table 2. *School-Loss Days Per Person by Sex, Race, and Income (1986)*

	ACUTE AND CHRONIC CONDITIONS	ACUTE CONDITIONS ONLY
Sex		
Male	4.3	3.7
Female	5.8	4.8
Race		
White	5.3	4.5
Black	4.0	2.9
Income		
Less than $10,000	5.8	3.8
$10,000–$19,999	4.5	3.8
$20,000–$34,999	5.1	4.5
$35,000–or more	5.2	4.5
All	5.0	4.2

From National Health Interview Survey.

Most of the school-loss days are due to acute conditions, defined as "a type of illness or injury that ordinarily lasts less than 3 months, was first noticed less than 3 months before the reference date of the interview, and was serious enough to have had an impact on behavior." The illness or injury is considered to have had an impact if the person reduced the things usually done for at least a half day or if a physician was contacted. School-loss days associated with acute conditions for children 5 to 17 years old were estimated to average 4.2 in 1986. There has been a slight decline in this rate since 1980 (see Table 1).

The demographic characteristics of those with school-loss days associated with acute conditions are similar to those with school-loss days due to acute and chronic conditions (see Table 2). The most frequent cause of school-loss days due to acute conditions is respiratory conditions, particularly influenza. This is followed by infective and parasitic diseases, including the common childhood diseases. Injuries are the third most common cause, followed by digestive system conditions and ear infections. Female rates are higher than those among males for most major categories except injuries; and white rates are higher than those among blacks for most major categories except injuries and digestive system conditions.

Adolescent School Health Program (Boston)

As part of the Adolescent School Health Program, a Boston-based demonstration project, absence in six inner-city middle schools was studied in 1983.[41] All students enrolled in those schools were categorized as problem absent students (PASs) if they had been absent in the study quarter or any of the three preceding ones: (1) six or more consecutive days (a quarter or more of an academic quarter), (2) 10 or more nonconsecutive days, or (3) half or more of any particular weekday (a patterned absence). Just over a third (33.4 per cent) of the 3246 students in the study met one or more of these criteria. The PASs were compared with the non-PASs on the variables available on the standard school record (sex, race, age, bused or not, and special education and bilingual status). In addition, appropriate grade for age was derived from the data using the Bureau of the Census criteria.

All the study variables except sex were found to be highly associated with absence. White students were more likely to be PASs than black or Hispanic ones and older students were more likely than younger ones. Being behind in grade, in a special education class, or bused were positively associated with being a PAS, but being in a bilingual class was negatively associated. Rates of PAS were significantly higher in some schools than in others. A multiple logistic regression revealed that increasing age, being behind in grade, being white, or attending certain schools were significantly associated with PAS status. Special education status was marginally significant.

The six middle schools study described above was not limited to health-related causes of absence. In a study undertaken in the 1982 to 1983 and 1983 to 1984 academic years,[42] PASs were matched with regular attenders in another Boston inner-city middle school to determine the contribution of health-related factors to excessive absence. No differences were found in self-reported health status, chronic health conditions, recent injuries, menstrual history, or average number of medical conditions in the household. The two groups were similar in health habits (smoking or alcohol and illegal drug use) and utilization of physicians, emergency departments, and hospitalization. The two studies suggest that educational and demographic factors have a greater impact on excess absence than does health.

RISK FACTORS

Certain factors place students at higher than average risk of being absent from school. These include physical or psychological problems in the student, physical or psychological problems in other family members, socioeconomic conditions, and the characteristics of the schools attended. Several recent studies have analyzed the effect of chronic illnesses, especially asthma, on school attendance. Among the psychological problems, school phobia often has been studied but will not be reviewed here. The impact of family health or socioeconomic conditions on school absence is still little understood, although clearly they have an important influence. Finally, while it is obvious that the atmosphere of the school itself may cause students to decide to attend or stay away, little has been done to isolate and measure this variable.

Student Physical Health

Most studies focus on the impact of specific health problems on absence or its inverse, attendance. A few, however, examine such problems generically. As part of the Adolescent School Health Program, the reasons Boston inner-city middle school students and their parents/guardians gave for non-attendance were examined in 1980 to 1983.[21] The study was limited to students classified as *problem absent students*. In response to an open-ended question, almost half of the PASs gave health-related reasons for absence, primarily their own physical health rather than their emotional health or a physical or emotional health problem of a family member. The physical health reasons given most often were colds, menstrual pain, and accidents. When the students were given a list of 15 reasons that might have contributed to their absence, 69 per cent checked a common, acute physical illness, such as a cold or diarrhea, 49 per cent mentioned headaches or stomach aches, 45 per cent cited an ache or pain, such as earache, toothache, or menstrual cramps, and 17 per cent listed injuries. (Multiple answers were permitted.)

The parents gave similar responses to the open-ended question. Over half believed that a health problem, almost always the student's physical health problem, caused the absence. In contrast, when parents were shown the list, they were more likely to select emotional health reasons, such as nervousness or sadness, than were students and less likely to mention illnesses, various types of aches, or injuries.

Some studies group chronic illnesses and look at their effect on absence. For example, Wolfe,[43] in a 1970s study of chronically ill children in Rochester, New York, reported that the largest negative effect on attendance was caused by health problems that made strenuous physical activities difficult to perform. These problems increased days missed by 150 per cent. Health problems that interfered with classroom communications and group physical activities increased days missed by 70 per cent. Unexpectedly, children who suffered from moderate to severe psychological discomfort missed fewer days.

Another study of chronic illness was conducted by Weitzman et al.[40] in Berkshire County, Massachusetts, during the 1979 to 1980 school year. They found that among children 6 to 17 years of age, those with chronic conditions missed significantly more days of school than those without (8.7 versus 5.8). Conditions leading to 12 or more mean days absent were mental retardation, cerebral palsy, asthma, arthritis, seizures, and permanent stiffness, although the number of children in some of these categories was very small. In addition, among children with chronic conditions, functional impairment increased absence: those with no functional impairment lost an average of 8.1 days and those with none, 11.0. The presence of psychosocial problems also increased the number of days absent among children with chronic conditions. This was true for all types of problems studied (e.g., school, learning, social, behavioral, and family), but the difference reached significance only for the school and learning problems.

Stein and Jessop[36] also examined the effect of psychological adjustment on school absence among children 5 to 10 years of age with chronic physical conditions treated at a university-affiliated municipal hospital in New York. Psychological adjustment was measured using the Personality Adjustment and Role Skills Scale. Although there was no relationship between psychological adjustment and days in bed or hospitalized, a significant relationship was found between psychological adjustment and both number of days absent from school and functional status.

In 1983 to 1984, Cook et al.[5] studied over 300 chronically ill children under 17 years of age who were receiving care from Florida's Children's Medical Services and were Medicaid eligible. The mean number of days absent in the previous year was 16.9 and the mean percentage of days absent was 9.4. Among children with specific diagnoses, the relatively few children receiving care for injuries and poisonings had the highest mean days absent (23.9) followed by those with congenital anomalies (20.1), those with diseases of the circulatory system (17.8), those with diseases of the respiratory tract (17.4), neoplasms (16.9), and diseases of the nervous system and sense organs (16.7). A stepwise linear regression found education of the parents and participation in physical activities to be predictive of number of days absent. Diagnosis was not a significant predictor.

Several studies have examined the effect of allergies, especially asthma, on school attendance. Freudenberg et al.[9] studied 200 low-income families in New York with asthmatic children 4 to 16 years of age. The parents reported that their children missed an average of 3 school days a month and 20 per cent were absent 6 or more days per month. A comparison of the school records of 50 of these children with the average for the district revealed a 24 per cent higher rate among the asthmatic children (26 days versus 21 days per year). Seventeen per cent of the children had to repeat the school year.

Mak et al.[21] surveyed almost 3000 first and sixth grade students in the Baltimore public schools in the 1978 to 1979 school year. Over 10 per cent of the parents reported that their children had asthma, described as a condition that causes difficulty breathing, with wheezing noises in the chest. Among those who reported wheezing in the previous 12 months, 52 per cent of the first and 41 per cent of the sixth graders missed 6 days or more of school (3.3 per cent of the total school year) and 15 per cent of the first and 6 per cent of the sixth graders missed 20 days or more. Unfortunately, the days missed by nonwheezers is not provided. Asthmatic children using the emergency department as a primary source of care were absent more frequently than those who used a private physician or a pediatric clinic (14 per cent of the former and 4 per cent of the latter were absent 20 days or more).

McLoughlin et al.[22] surveyed parents of nursery through 12th grade students who visited allergists in the Louisville, Kentucky, area in 1982, using as controls parents of nonallergic children visiting pediatricians or clinics in the same neighborhoods. They reported that allergic children had significantly more absences than did nonallergic children (between 1 and 3 days monthly). Absence also was related significantly to the use of bronchodilators.

Anderson et al.,[1] in a study of 9-year-old school children in London with asthma or wheezing illnesses, found that 12 per cent had been absent more than 30 days, 19 per cent had experienced 5 or more periods of absence, and 7 per cent had experienced a period of over 10 days absence in the past year. Compared with controls, children with wheezing illness were more likely to have experienced eczema, allergic nose problems, frequent headaches, and frequent episodes of abdominal pain. All of these, except eczema, significantly increased the amount of absence.

Klein and Litt[18] analyzed the data collected in 1966 to 1970 by Cycle III of the National Health Examination Survey. Of the 2699 menarcheal girls, 60 per cent reported discomfort or pain in connection with their menstrual period. Overall, 14 per cent of the sample frequently missed school because of cramps: 17 per cent of those with mild and 50 per cent of those with severe symptoms. Black adolescents did not suffer from dysmenorrhea more than whites, but they were almost twice as likely to be absent from school because of their symptoms, even when socioeconomic status was held constant.

Student Psychological Health

Several of the studies already reviewed examined the impact of psychological problems on children with chronic conditions. Weitzman et al.[42] and Stein and Jessop,[36] found that these problems increased absence; Wolfe did not. Relatively few studies, however, have examined the effect of psychological variables on absence in physically healthy children.

Swearingen and Cohen[37] analyzed the relationship between adolescents' life events as measured by the Junior High Life Experiences Survey and absence in a sample of over 200 seventh and eighth grade students in 1981. They found that the number of negative uncontrollable events was significantly correlated with number of days absent.

Eagleston et al.[6] studied the relationship between the type A behavior pattern (competitiveness, time urgency, and hostility) and school absence, as well as personal and family health among almost 200 fifth, seventh, and ninth grade students. Although those with high type A behavior scores reported more physical symptoms, they did not miss more school because of illness than those with low scores; nor did they use medical services more often. Among students with low type A behavior scores, however, physical symptoms and absence were related. The authors believe that these findings suggest that children with high type A scores may deny the severity or meaning of their symptoms.

Galloway[10] studied students 5 to 15 years of age in inner-city districts of Sheffield, New Zealand, who had "illegally" missed at least half of the previous autumn term or had been referred to a psychological service over a 2-year period for advice about poor school attendance. He divided them into *truants*, whose parents claimed to seldom or only occasionally know where they were during school absences, and *other absentees*, whose parents claimed generally to know where their absent children were, which usually meant at home. No significant differences were found in the the medical histories of the two types of students or their siblings. Over the subsequent five terms, the mean attendance of the truants ranged between 44 and 50 per cent and of the other absentees between 43 and 49 per cent. The parents of other absentees were significantly more likely to report behavior associated with anxiety and reluctance to leave home, suggesting that some of the other absentees were suffering from school phobia.

The Adolescent School Health Program study of reasons for absence[21] found that students or parents rarely mentioned an emotional problem of the students in response to an open-ended question. When given a list of 15 possible reasons for absence, however, 9 per cent of the students agreed that nervousness had contributed to their absence and 10 per cent that sadness had. Parents were more likely to check these items: 19 per cent for nervousness and 20 per cent for sadness. Agreement between students and their parents on these items was close to chance.

Family Health

The influence of the physical and emotional health of other family members on absence is seldom explored, although students and teachers report that children are sometimes expected to stay home to care for an ill sibling or even an incapacitated adult. This possibility was explored in the Adolescent School Health Program study of reasons for absence.[21] These reasons were mentioned infrequently in response to the open-ended question. In response to the list of possible reasons for absence, however, 25 per cent of the students and 7 per cent of the parents cited "need to care for younger member of the household" and 24 per cent of the students and 9 per cent of the parents cited "need to care for adult in household." Agreement between students and parents on these items was very low, suggesting that the parents were denying a cause of absence they believed was unacceptable or that the students were distorting the truth.

Galloway's study[10] found that 64 per cent of the other absentees' mothers were suffering from a chronic illness in comparison to 33 per cent of the truants' mothers. In addition, many parents in both the truant and the other absentees group were in poor psychiatric health.

Anderson et al.[1] found a maternal history of treatment for nerves or depression associated with higher rates of absence among his 9-year-old British students with asthma and wheezing conditions.

Socioeconomic Conditions

None of the studies reviewed focused exclusively on socioeconomic conditions, although many included it as a possible mediating factor. Cook et al.[5] found parental education related to school absence in their sample of chronically ill children. Anderson et al.[1] noted that households missing one or both parents or with more than three children, rental housing, lack of access to a car, and a maternal nonmanual occupation were related to absence among children with asthma and wheezing illnesses. Stein and Jessop[36] reported that psychological adjustment in children with chronic physical conditions was less likely to affect absence if both parents were present and more likely if the mother was living with an adult other than the child's father, usually a grandmother or other female relative.

Institutional Characteristics

Perhaps the strongest case for the influence on absence of the school as a social institution was made by Rutter et al.[33] Considerable variation in rates of absence was found in the 12 secondary schools studied in an inner London borough in the mid-1970s. Pupils of below average intellectual ability or from families of low occupational status were the most likely to have poor attendance records. When these variables were controlled, however, large and statistically significant differences in attendance by school persisted. These differences were not related to the physical plant, that is, the size or age of the school, space available, or administrative status or organization. They were systematically related to the schools' characteristics as social institutions. The investigators report that secondary schools do have an important influence on their students' behavior and attainments. Specifically, "factors as varied as the degree of academic emphasis, teacher actions in lessons, the availability of incentives and rewards, good conditions for pupils, and the extent to which children were able to take responsibility were all significantly associated with outcome differences among schools."

Two components of the Adolescent School Health Program showed school influences. In the six-school study[41] comparing problem absent and non–problem absent students, the school attended affected absence even when demographic and educational characteristics were controlled through multiple logistic regression. In the reasons for absence study,[21] 39 per cent of the students' and 36 per cent of the parents' responses to the open-ended question were school related, including attitudes toward education (dislike of school, poor relationship with teachers, etc), laziness, missing the bus, waking up late, and educational problems (suspensions, failures, inappropriate age for grade, etc). Similar items in the list also elicited positive responses: missed bus frequently (students 43 per cent; parents 38 per cent), dislike school (students 40 per cent; parents 41 per cent), no one woke me up (students 39 per cent; parents 17 per cent), violence in school (students 23 per cent; parents 32 per cent), and racial problems (students 9 per cent; parents 16 per cent).

In the fall of 1987 *The New York Times*[29] reported that only half of the approximately 6000 school-aged homeless children living in hotels in New York City were known to be attending schools. An executive assistant to the School Chancellor stated that she had received attendance reports for about 3300 children, indicating that they were attending school, though not always regularly. She had not received attendance records from local schools for 2000 other children whom she suspected were having "severe attendance problems." Seven hundred additional children had "fallen through the cracks." She attributed the problem to the Board of Education's reliance on the hotel management, rather than the records of the city's Human Resources Administration, to tell Board workers when families with school-aged children moved in and out of hotels. A second problem cited was the failure of the Board to develop a plan under which its family workers and attendance teachers would follow up homeless children.

ASSOCIATION BETWEEN EXCESSIVE ABSENCE AND OTHER RISK-TAKING BEHAVIORS

Research findings are making it increasingly clear that children, especially adolescents, are unlikely to adopt only one behavior that puts their health in jeopardy or is socially deviant. The first such activity may be relatively innocuous, such as smoking a cigarette or drinking a beer. If such activities are rewarded by peers and not strongly censured by parents, teachers, or other adults, however, they may be repeated and other potentially harmful behaviors adopted. These findings have major implications for program planning. They suggest that smoking, alcohol and drug abuse, premature or unprotected sexual activity, delinquency, and similar problem behaviors should not be targeted independently for preventive services, since they appear to be imbedded in a constellation of behaviors that are well protected through the selection of peers who approve of them and who engage in similar ones. Rather, programs need to focus on the early signs of risk-taking behavior to find the underlying causes of the behaviors, prevent the formation of peer groups that share the behaviors, and provide models for more constructive activity.

Excessive school absence, without an underlying physical health problem, is one of the behaviors now included in the group of risk-taking or deviant behaviors that often result in health and social problems during adolescent or in adult years. Thus, excessive school absence without a clear physical cause is a symptom that should be explored by physicians. The child manifesting this behavior also may be involved in early sexual activity, smoke, or use alcohol or drugs, or may be associating with peers who do. Early intervention by physicians, parents, and school officials may prevent the sequelae of these behaviors.

Some of the earliest work in this area was conducted by Jessor and Jessor[15] in the late 1960s and early 1970s, using a Boulder, Colorado, sample. These investigators were able to show associations between problem drinking, illicit drug use, delinquent-type behavior, and precocious sexual intercourse, but they did not consider absenteeism.

Similarly, Robins and Ratcliff[31] have reported the results of a study of black school boys born between 1930 and 1934 who attended St. Louis, Missouri, schools for at least 6 years and had IQs of 85 or higher. They found that truancy (absences of more than 20 per cent of the school days in a quarter) often began in the first or second grade and that elementary school truancy strongly predicted high school truancy. Moreover, 35 per cent of those often truant in elementary school had four or more of 11 juvenile deviant behaviors as compared to 14 per cent of those not truant or mildly truant. The average number of such behaviors for the sample was 2.3. The investigators also reported that truancy was associated with dropping out of school, low earnings as an adult, and a variety of adult deviant behaviors.

In the period from 1980 to 1981, Kandel, Raveis, and Kandel[16] interviewed a group of young adults who had been studied 9 years earlier as 10th and 11th grade students in New York public high schools. They compared "absentees," or students who had been absent on both original survey days and who averaged 19.5 days absent in the 1970–1971 school year, to "regular" students, who averaged 12 days absent during the same period. Unfortunately, this study did not provide data on other problem behaviors during the school years; but, like the Robins and Ratcliffe study,[31] it found excess absence to be associated with such behaviors in early adulthood. The absentees were more likely to have dropped out of school, to have experienced a divorce or separation, or to have had at least one abortion. They were also more likely, especially if women, to have spent more post–high-school time "loafing," that is, not working, not looking for a job, not going to school, or not being a housewife. Absentees reported poorer subjective health status and, among women, a higher rate of medical hospitalization, even after pregnancies were excluded. Male absentees were more likely to have been arrested and less likely to register to vote. There were few differences in lifetime experience with the legal or illegal drugs studied. Daily cigarette smoking was much higher, however, among male absentees than regular students.

Young and Rogers[44] found a relationship between absence and subsequent smoking behavior. Almost a quarter (23.5 per cent) of the over 1400 ninth through twelfth grade students studied were smokers. The difference in mean days absent between eventual smokers and eventual nonsmokers was significant in second, third, and fifth grades and in high school. Also, heavy smokers were absent more than light ones and early-onset smokers more than late onset, but these differences were not statistically significant.

Other investigators have found relationships among problem behaviors but unfortunately have not included school absence among their variables. For example, Barnes and Welte[2] found heavy drinking in seventh through twelfth grade students associated with frequent school misconduct and poor grades. In a sample of inner-city junior and senior high school students, Zabin et al.[45] reported that sexually active teenagers rated higher on an index of substance abuse than did virgins. Those high on this index were also more likely to be behind in grade. Robinson et al.[32] found the level of substance abuse among tenth grade students was associated with school performance, perceived safety of cigarette smoking, and use of diet pills, laxatives, or diuretics for weight control.

PROGRAMS FOR REDUCING SCHOOL ABSENCE

Programs that attempt to reduce excessive school absence, or programs directed at other problems that use absence as an outcome measure, are of several types. Perhaps best known are those whose objective is to reduce rates of school dropout. These programs, frequently involve counseling, work-study activities, remedial courses, and alternative schools. They focus on intermediate and high school students who are believed to be at high risk of leaving school before high school graduation.

Another smaller group of programs is concerned with socioeconomically deprived families who appear not to be functioning in ways that would maximize child development or are at risk of inadequate functioning. These programs offer a variety of support services to families. A reduction in rates of absence among children in these families or a lower rate than in comparison families is used as one of many criteria of success.

Another group of programs targets the schools and how their activities affect not only students' academic performance, but also their attendance and behavior. These programs usually focus on teaching school administrators, teachers, and support staff how to improve their interactions with students and their families.

Finally, there are programs that focus on the health-related conditions of students and their families. These programs are of two major types: (1) those that provide primary medical care directly or that refer students to it and provide support services to ensure that the care is used appropriately; and (2) those that target specific health conditions and teach students and parents how to manage them and assist school staff to understand and cope with them.

This section will be devoted primarily to programs that focus on health problems. A school improvement program and a family development program will be briefly described to provide a perspective on the impact of broader based efforts.

Health-Related Programs: Primary Care

The Adolescent School Health Program[41] was an experimental study that examined the effect of an intervention with problem absence students in two inner-city, Boston intermediate schools. The intervention involved placing a nurse in each experimental school, creating school-based teams that included the nurse, a full-time outreach worker, a part-time pediatrician, and mental health workers. Medical care was not provided at the school; rather the team assisted the family in selecting a primary care provider (office- or clinic-based physician), helped the provider design an intervention plan to meet the student's or family's health care needs, and assisted the student or family in implementing the plan. Interventions included primary care provider and medical subspecialty activities, mental health and social services, and school-based services such as classroom or school changes, tutoring, in-school counseling, and behavior modification. The intervention was limited to those students (1) whose reason for excessive absence was a health problem, their own or a member of their families; (2) who agreed to participate; and (3) whose parents or guardians also consented.

It had been hypothesized that overall attendance in the two experimental schools would improve because the presence of the school-based teams would affect all students including those who were not excessively absent. A statistically significant increase in attendance was found in both experimental schools, but was also found in the matched control schools. Although the changes were greatest in the experimental schools, the differences between the experimental and the control schools were not statistically significant.

Similarly, the problem absent students who were enrolled in the intervention program, and for whom student and parent interviews were available, showed a slight decrease in the average percentage absence while the students meeting the same absence criteria in the control schools showed a slight increase, but these differences were not statistically significant. The authors conclude, on the basis of this study as well as the others described earlier in the article,[39, 40] that (1) student- or family-based health problems or unmet needs are not major contributors to excessive absence among inner-city, middle school students; and (2) a health-oriented approach is not effective in reducing absence even among those students who give a health problem as a major or contributing cause for their absences.

The Adolescent School Health Program differed appreciably from the school-based clinics currently generating considerable controversy because of their linkage to school-age sexuality and pregnancy. Unlike the Adolescent School Health Program, school-based clinics provide medical care in the schools. Although the model for school-based clinics, the St. Paul–Minneapolis program[8] was originally developed with the intention of reducing the birth rate among female students and improving the outcomes of school girl pregnancies; the objectives of these clinics have broadened to improving the overall health status of students, particularly those in medically underserved areas.[19]

Unfortunately, despite several attempts to document the impact of school-based clinics on attendance, there is no firm evidence that their presence reduces rates of absence overall or among clinic users. The school-based clinic experience may parallel the early findings of studies of new primary care facilities where, shortly after the facilities open, previously unknown health problems are detected and rates of utilization increase. Rates later decline as preventive measures begin to have an effect. Similarly, it may require a longer period of operation before school-based clinics begin to influence absence. Evaluation will be difficult, however, since students usually spend only 3 years in high school. During this period, conditions will need to be detected and treated and health habits changed. It may not be possible to accomplish this in 2 years so that an effect can be shown in the third.

Health-Related Programs: Targeted at Specific Conditions

Because asthma is a common chronic condition among children, it is not surprising that many school-based programs have been developed to help control its symptoms and that absence is often used as a measure of success. Colver[4a] described a childhood asthma campaign that operated through existing health services in an inner city area of Newcastle on Tyne. The program attempted to identify children with asthma in the nursery and primary schools, initiate or improve management, and increase awareness and knowledge of asthma among parents, teachers, and the primary health care team. Among those families who thought their child's asthma had improved as a result of the program (77 per cent), there was a reduction in days absent due to wheezing. This was not true in the unimproved group, many of whom had not visited their family physician, or, if they had, had not received new medication. The design and analysis of this study make its results questionable. But the observations about the reluctance of family physicians to use asthma medications and the lack of information about the relationship between asthma and wheezy bronchitis among parents, teachers, and physicians suggest that a community-based program can have a positive impact.

Another British study by Speight et al.[35] found that childhood asthma was underdiagnosed and undertreated. They reported a tenfold drop in school absenteeism among children placed on continuous prophylactic treatment. In this and the Colver study, physicians expressed fear that a diagnosis of asthma would cause anxiety among parents and therefore were reluctant to make such diagnoses. Underdiagnosis was associated with a failure to prescribe appropriate medication. Results in both studies indicate that most parents were relieved to have the cause of their children's wheezes finally determined and to receive medication for it.

Although these British programs stress the identification of unknown, untreated, or undertreated cases and placement on adequate treatment regimens, the American literature devotes more attention to self-care and teacher education. In 1981 a conference was held to discuss the findings of 11 studies of the self-management of childhood asthma. These studies have been summarized by Bruhn.[4] Five include attendance or absence as a variable. In 1983 the National Institute of Allergy and Infectious Diseases and the National Heart, Lung, and Blood Institute sponsored another conference on the subject, stressing the theoretic issues as well as implementation and evaluation.[13]

In addition, several programs have reported the results of self-management programs on school attendance. In a Pittsburgh program, Fireman et al.[8] found that children and their families who were assigned to a nurse-educator for individual instruction, group sessions, and telephone monitoring experienced significantly fewer days of absence than did a control group. Lungs Unlimited was a self-management program developed by the American Lung Association of Northwestern Ohio[32] to teach asthmatic children and their families breathing and relaxation techniques. Parents reported a reduction in asthma-related school absences, hospitalization, and visits to physicians and emergency departments, as well as decreased fear of asthma and increased self confidence in managing the disease. Parents of Asthmatic Kids (PAK)[9] is another program, often sponsored by state lung associations or universities, that helps parents to learn more about the disease through interactions with each other and from guest speakers. Teachers also may be involved since parents express concern that teachers are unaware of what might trigger an attack, the signs and symptoms of asthma, how to control attacks, or the possible side effects of medication.

Juvenile diabetes, another potential source of absence, has also been targeted by several programs. The Minnesota Diabetes in Youth Program[25] has attempted to improve the functioning of diabetic children by providing clinical services and working with the children, their families, and community organizations. Parents in a community served by this program reported that their children missed less school than parents in a control community. The sample size, however, was small and demographic and other characteristics were not controlled. Orr et al.[28] also reported a reduction in absence among adolescents whose diabetes had been poorly controlled following referral to a tertiary treatment center. Treatment included not only insulin readjustment but also individual and group counseling for the adolescents and their families and an educational and peer support group for the adolescents. Again, the sample size was very small.

School Improvement Programs

The School Development Program[14] is an example of a program that attempted to improve the climate of the schools and that used attendance among its indicators of success. The Program created a governance and management group in each school composed of the school principal, teachers, parents, and a member of the school mental health team. In addition, a parent participation program and curriculum and staff development were established to create "a positive, supportive and caring environment." In a study of this program over 300 third through fifth grade students were randomly selected from seven experimental, four control, and three special schools in low socioeconomic areas. Also studied were the almost 100 teachers of these children and over 200 of their parents. After 1 full year of the program, the percentage of days absent among children in the experimental schools had dropped significantly. The experimental children and their parents' assessment of their classrooms' climate improved, but the teachers' did not. Reading scores also improved. These changes were not generally found in the control or special schools.

(The oft-cited report on the effects of a preschool program, Changed Lives,[3] notes that those who attended the program had fewer absences per year in elementary school than the control group [12 versus 16 days].)

Family Development Programs

In the late 1960s, Provence and fellow workers at Yale's Child Study Center[34] developed a family support program for a group of 17 new families in a depressed inner city area. The program included social work, pediatric care, day care, and psychological services tailored to family need. The team, which provided care beginning during pregnancy and continuing until 30 months' postpartum, consisted of home visitors, pediatricians, primary day care workers, and developmental examiners. A control sample of children was drawn later from among women who would have met the original selection criteria. Followup evaluations were conducted at 5 and 10 years after the evaluation ended. At 10 years, 15 pairs of children were available for study. Experimental children were significantly less likely to be truant (i.e., missing 20 or more days of school without a valid excuse). The experimental boys were rated less negatively by their teachers and received fewer remedial or supportive school services than did the control boys.

THE IMPACT OF SCHOOL ABSENCE ON THE MEDICAL CARE SYSTEM

For many reasons, school absence deserves more attention from medical care professionals than it currently receives. A frequent or prolonged school absence may be an indicator of a physical or emotional health problem in the student or his or her family. Truancy may be an indicator of present or future problem behaviors. Therefore, pediatricians and other health professionals who examine children should routinely ask the students and parents about school performance. This should include not only how well the students are doing academically but also whether they attend school regularly. Reports of prolonged or frequent absences should be explored as indicators of possible health problems in the student or her/his family that may be amenable to change.

One example of such a problem is dysmenorrhea. Many young women regularly miss one or two days a month because of "painful periods." They and their mothers apparently believe that this problem cannot be prevented and consequently the student is allowed to miss school. However, this condition usually can be corrected by medication and absence can be prevented.

Frequent or prolonged absence also can alert the schools to a possible health problem that may require referral to a physician. Unfortunately, many schools view school attendance as an administrative matter and assign clerical staff to the task of checking on absent students. Those responsible for school health care should urge that attendance monitoring and remediation be conducted by health personnel who are trained to probe for underlying health-related factors and know how to initiate the assistance-seeking process.

Another reason for professional health attention to the problem of school absence is the potential availability within the schools of assistance with health problems. Almost all schools have some form of health service. In small schools, a school nurse may be present for limited periods; in larger ones, she may be in the school building whenever school is in session; and, in a few but growing number of schools, a school-based clinic may operate on a part- or full-time basis. Clearly, the number of staff and the availability of time will affect how much attention can be paid to the health problems of particular students. Nevertheless, particularly in the era of P. L. 94–142, the school should be viewed as an ally in the treatment of children's health problems.[16]

Finally, the sensitivity of excessive, unexplained school absence among elementary school children as an indicator of later problems, as well as the association of truancy with other problem behaviors in all grades, makes it imperative that physicians and other health personnel investigate this phenomenon whenever it is presented. Early and concentrated attention to the problem may prevent later health and social problems of considerable magnitude.

CONCLUSION

Most excessive school absence, particularly in the intermediate and high schools, is probably the result of factors outside the health care sphere. Chaotic family environments, lack of achievement motivation, understaffed and uninviting schools, and other societal problems are undoubtedly the major reasons for absenteeism and early school leaving in those grades. In addition, these factors contribute to excessive absence and underachievement in the lower grades. Nevertheless, there is a role for the health care system both in detecting and treating absence problems that are health related and in assisting those programs that attempt to solve the larger problems.

The societal problems are not hopeless, as several of the studies reviewed make clear. Nor does the absence of a clear health problem preclude the involvement of health personnel in their solutions. Families can be helped to provide physically and emotionally healthy environments for growing children by using support staffs that include health personnel. Schools can be made more challenging and appealing, again with well-designed programs that include health personnel. It is noteworthy that three programs described earlier, the School Development Program,[14] the family support program,[34] and the Adolescent School Health Program,[43] were all developed by physicians (pediatricians and child psychiatrists). This shows the need for the skills of health specialists, as well as those of educators and community development and welfare specialists, to bring about the changes essential for healthy child development.

In addition, health professionals should be aware of the educational implications of the treatment of children with special health care needs. P. L. 94–142 requires that all children, regardless of health condition, receive a free and appropriate education and in the least restrictive environment. Physicians and other health professionals must consider the effects of their therapy on the school day. Teachers and other school personnel, as well as parents, should be alerted to potential problems and taught how to manage them. Health care professionals should be full partners in programs that teach self-management or that educate school staff. They should not restrict their activities to offices and clinics, but should view the family household and the school as sites for the care of their student patients.

Many students who formerly could not or were not allowed to attend school are now participating in educational activities, but unfortunately many students who could benefit from education are leaving school prior to graduation. For both groups, excessive absence may be an indicator of their need for assistance. Health care professionals can play an important role in improving the life prospects of both these groups of children.

The support of the Robert Wood Johnson Foundation for the initial studies in this area is gratefully acknowledged, as is the expert assistance of Linda White in the preparation of this review.

REFERENCES

1. Anderson R, Bailey PA, Cooper JS et al: Morbidity and school absence caused by asthma and wheezing illness. Arch Dis Child 58:777, 1983
2. Barnes GM, Welte JW: Patterns and predictors of alcohol use among 7–12th grade students in New York state. J Stud Alcohol 47:53, 1986
3. Berrueta-Clement JR, Schweinhart LJ, Barnett WS et al: Changed Lives: The Effects of the Perry Preschool Program on Youths Through Age 19. Ypsilanti, Michigan, High/Scope Press, 1984, p 25
4. Bruhn JG: The application of theory of childhood asthma self-help programs, Part 2. J Allergy Clin Immunol 72:561, 1983
4a. Colver AF: Community campaign against asthma. Arch Dis Child 59:449, 1984
5. Cook BA, Schaller K, Krischer JP: School absence among children with chronic illness. J School Health 55:265, 1985
6. Eagleston JR, Kirmil-Gray K, Thoresen CE: Physical health correlates of type A behavior in children and adolescents. J Behav Med 9:341, 1986
6a. Edwards LE, Steinman ME, Harkanson EY: An experimental comprehensive high school clinic. Am J Public Health 87:765, 1977
7. Esquibel KP, Foster CR, Garnier VJ et al: A program to help asthmatic students reach their potential. Public Health Rep 99:606, 1984
8. Fireman P, Friday GA, Gira C et al: Teaching self-management skills to asthmatic children and their parents in an ambulatory care setting. Pediatrics 68:341, 1981
9. Freudenberg N, Feldman CH, Clark NM et al: The impact of bronchial asthma on school attendance and performance. J School Health 50:522, 1980
10. Galloway D: Research note: Truants and other absentees. J Child Psych Psychiatr 24:607, 1983
11. Green LW, Goldstein RA, Parker SR eds: Workshop proceedings on self-management of childhood asthma. J Allergy Clin Immunol 72: 1983
12. Haynes NM, Comer JP, Hamilton-Lee M et al: School development effects on perceived climate, achievement and attendance. Yale University Child Study Center, 1987. Paper presented at the annual meeting of the American Educational Research Association, Washington, D.C., April 1987
13. Hersov L, Berg I (eds): Out of School: Modern Perspectives in Truancy and School Refusal. New York, John Wiley & Sons, 1980, pp 1–6
14. Jacobs FH, Walker DK: Pediatricians and the Education for All Handicapped Children Act of 1975. Pediatrics 61:135, 1978
15. Jessor R, Jessor SL: Problem Behavior and Psychosocial Development: A Longitudinal Study of Youth. New York, Academic Press, 1977, p 19
16. Kandel DB, Ravies VH, Kandel PI: Continuity in discontinuities: adjustment in young adulthood of former school absentees. Youth and Society 15:325, 1984
17. Kirby D, Lovick S, Levin-Epstein J et al: School-Based Health Clinics: An Emerging Approach to Improving Adolescent Health and Addressing Teen-age Pregnancy. Washington, D.C., Center for Population Options, 1985
18. Klein JR, Litt IF: Epidemiology of adolescent dysmenorrhea. Pediatrics 68:661, 1981

19. Klerman LV, Weitzman M, Alpert JJ et al: Why adolescents do not attend school: The views of students and parents. J Adolesc Health Care 8:425, 1987
20. Klerman LV, Weitzman M, Alpert JJ et al: School absence: Can it be used to monitor child health? In Walker DK, Richmond JB (eds): Monitoring Child Health in the United States: Selected Issues and Policies. Cambridge, Massachusetts, Harvard University Press, 1984, pp 143–152
21. Mak H, Johnston P, Abbey H et al: Prevalence of asthma and health service utilization of asthmatic children in an inner city. J Allergy Clin Immunol 70:367, 1982
22. McLoughlin J, Nall M, Isaacs B et al: The relationship of allergies and allergy treatment to school performance and student behavior. Ann Allergy 51:506, 1983
23. Minnesota Diabetes in Youth Program: Evaluation Report, 1984–1985
24. National Center for Health Statistics, Bloom B: Current Estimates from the National Health Interview Survey, United States, 1981. Vital and Health Statistics. Series 10, No. 141. DHHS Pub. No. (PHS) 83–1569. Public Health Service. Washington, D.C., U.S. Government Printing Office, October, 1982
25. National Center for Health Statistics: Current Estimates from the National Interview Survey, United States, 1982. Vital and Health Statistics. Series 10, No. 150. DHHS Pub No. (PHS) 85–1578. Public Health Service. Washington, D.C., U.S. Government Printing Office, September, 1985
26. National Center for Health Statistics, Moss AJ, Parsons VL: Current Estimates from the National Interview Survey, United States, 1985. Vital and Health Statistics. Series 10, No. 160. DHHS Pub No. (PHS) 86–1588. Public Health Service. Washington, D.C., U.S. Government Printing Office, September, 1986
27. National Center for Health Statistics: Dawson DA, Adams PF: Current Estimates from the National Health Interview Survey, United States, 1986. Vital and Health Statistics. Series 10, No. 164. DHHS Pub. No. (PHS) 87–1592. Public Health Service, Washington, D.C., U.S. Government Printing Office, October, 1987
28. Orr DP, Golden MP, Myers G et al: Characteristics of adolescents with poorly controlled diabetes referred to a tertiary care center. Diabetes Care 6:170, 1983
29. Perlez J: Thousands of pupils living in hotels skip school in New York. The New York Times, November 12, 1987
30. Pituch M, Bruggeman J: Lungs Unlimited: A self-care program for asthmatic children and their families. Children Today 11:6, 1982
31. Robins LN, Ratcliff KS: The long-term outcome of truancy. In Hersov L, Berg I (eds): Out Of School: A Modern Perspectives in Truancy and School Refusal. New York, John Wiley & Sons, 1980, pp 65–83
32. Robinson TN, Killen JD, Taylor B, et al: Perspectives on adolescent substance use: A defined population study. JAMA 258:2078, 1987
33. Rutter M, Maughan B, Mortimore P et al: Fifteen Thousand Hours: Secondary Schools and Their Effects on Children. Cambridge, Massachusetts, Harvard University Press, 1979
34. Seitz V, Rosenbaum LK, Apfel NH: Effects of family support intervention: A ten-year follow-up. Child Dev 56:376, 1985
35. Speight ANP, Lee DA, Hey EN: Underdiagnosis and undertreatment of asthma in childhood. Br Med J 286:1253, 1983
36. Stein REK, Jessop DJ: Relationship between health status and psychological adjustment among children with chronic conditions. Pediatrics 73:169, 1984
37. Swearingen EM, Cohen LH: Measurements of adolescents' life events: the junior high life experience survey. Am J Commun Psychol 13:69, 1985
38. Weitzman M, Walker DK, Gortmaker S: Chronic illness, psychosocial problems and school absences: Results of a survey of one county. Clin Pediatr 25:137, 1986
39. Weitzman M, Klerman LV, Lamb GA et al: Demographic and educational characteristics of inner city middle school problem absence students. Am J Orthopsychiatry 55:378, 1985
40. Weitzman M, Klerman LV, Albert JJ et al: Factors associated with excessive school absence. Pediatrician 13:74, 1986
41. Weitzman M, Alpert JJ, Klerman LV et al: High-risk youth and health: The case of excessive school absence. Pediatrics 78:313, 1986
42. Weitzman M, Klerman LV, Lamb G et al: School absence: A problem for the pediatrician. Pediatrics 69:739, 1982

43. Wolfe BL: The influence of health on school outcomes: A multivariate approach. Medical Care 23:1127, 1985
44. Young TL, Rogers KD: School performance and characteristics preceding onset of smoking in high school students. Am J Dis Child 140:257, 1986
45. Zabin LS, Hardy JB, Smith EA et al: Substance use and its relation to sexual activity among inner city adolescents. J Adolesc Health Care 7:326, 1986

Department of Epidemiology and Public Health
60 College Street
P.O. Box 3333
New Haven, Connecticut 06510

0031–3955/88 $0.00 + .20

Adolescent Sexuality

Linda M. Grant, MD, MPH,* and Efstratios Demetriou, MD†

Adolescent sexuality has received increasing public attention over the past 25 years. Sexuality is not unique to the adolescent period, but is a phenomenon that spans the entire life cycle. What is remarkable about adolescence are the complex physical, cognitive, and psychosocial changes that affect how sexuality is expressed. Physical maturity and the ability to engage in sexual activity does not necessarily imply sufficient cognitive maturity to understand and anticipate undesirable consequences such as pregnancy and sexually transmitted disease. Health providers who care for this age group must understand adolescents' evolving sexuality and be prepared to help them make responsible decisions. This article reviews the epidemiology of adolescent sexual behavior, the risk factors related to adverse outcomes of adolescent sexual behavior, and potential interventions that pediatric practitioners working with their adolescent patients, parents, and the community may undertake to foster the healthy sexual development of young people.

EPIDEMIOLOGY OF ADOLESCENT SEXUAL BEHAVIOR

Sexual Activity

Several contemporary surveys have provided a glimpse of adolescent sexual behavior in the United States. In 1973, Sorensen studied a national sample of 411 teenagers from urban, suburban, and rural areas regarding their sexual attitudes and behaviors.[66] The National Survey of Young Women, conducted by Kantner and Zelnik, studied a national sample of metropolitan area young women in 1971, 1976, and 1979.[88] In 1979, these investigators also conducted the National Survey of Young Men. Haas, in 1979, interviewed 625 15- to 18-year-old adolescents, mostly from southern California.[29] The 1982 National Survey of Family Growth, Cycle III contains reports of sexual and contraceptive behavior among young women.[30] In 1985, Coles and Stokes published the results of their survey of over 1000 randomly

*Assistant Professor of Pediatrics, Boston University School of Medicine, Boston, Massachusetts
†Clinical Assistant Professor of Pediatrics, Boston University School of Medicine, Boston, Massachusetts

From the Adolescent Center, Boston City Hospital, and the Department of Pediatrics, Boston University School of Medicine, Boston, Massachusetts.

selected adolescents from urban, suburban, and rural areas regarding their sexual knowledge, attitudes, and behaviors.[12] The data that will be presented highlight significant sexual behaviors and major trends in these behaviors, based on those studies.

Sorensen reported that 58 per cent of all boys and 39 per cent of all girls surveyed had masturbated at least once.[66] Coles and Stokes found that 46 per cent of all teenage boys and 24 per cent of all teenage girls reported engaging in this behavior.[12] Masturbation often begins prior to adolescence[12, 66]; 72 per cent of females and 75 per cent of males who had masturbated had first done so by age 13.[66]

Kissing and petting are the traditional first steps in the sequence of heterosexual activity for most adolescents. Kissing is common prior to early adolescence, and girls begin at an earlier age than boys.[12] Coles and Stokes reported that 73 per cent of 13-year-old girls and 60 per cent of 13-year-old boys had kissed at least once.[12] The pattern for breast touching is similar. Because young adolescent girls date older boys, a higher percentage engage in this activity at an earlier age. Twenty per cent of 13-year-old boys reported touching a girl's breast, whereas 25 per cent of 13-year-old girls had had their breasts touched.[12] As boys begin to date more, the pattern changes: 54 per cent of 14-year-old boys, but only 31 per cent of the girls had engaged in breast touching.[12]

Younger teenage boys are more likely to engage in vaginal touching than comparably aged girls; 50 per cent of 14-year-old boys but only 21 per cent of 14-year-old girls reported this behavior. As teenagers become older and involved in more serious relationships, both sexes are equally active; by 18 years, 61 per cent of the boys and 60 per cent of the girls reported vaginal touching.[12] Similarly, of all 17- to 18-year-old boys, 77 per cent reported having their penis touched by a girl; 78 per cent of all comparably aged girls had engaged in this behavior.[29]

Haas reported that among 17 to 18 year olds, 59 per cent of girls and 56 per cent of boys had engaged in oral sex.[29] Oral sex for many teenagers precedes intercourse: 16 per cent who had engaged in oral sex had never had intercourse.[12]

Several studies have examined the epidemiology of adolescent heterosexual intercourse. The National Survey of Young Women is the best known,[88] although its findings are limited because only adolescents living in large metropolitan areas were surveyed. This study indicated that less than half of all never-married 15- to 19-year-old adolescent girls had experienced sexual intercourse. It also documented the remarkable increase in sexual activity among this group during the 1970s, from 28 per cent in 1971, to 39 per cent in 1976, and 46 per cent in 1979.[88] Data from the National Survey of Family Growth in 1982 indicated a slight decline, to 42 per cent.[30] Zelnik and Kantner's 1979 survey for the first time examined sexual activity among male subjects aged 17 to 21 years; 69 per cent of never-married males reported premarital sexual activity, including 78 per cent of never-married 19 year olds.[88]

Black females have higher levels of sexual experience than do white females. The disparity was greatest in 1971, when 23 per cent of never-married 15- to 19-year-old whites and 52 per cent of blacks were sexually experienced. The proportion of sexually experienced white females increased dramatically, to 34 per cent in 1976, and 42 per cent in 1979, before falling slightly to 40 per cent in 1982. Sexual experience among black adolescent females peaked at 64 per cent in 1976, remained at 64 per cent in 1979, and fell to 53 per cent in 1982.[30, 88] The 13 per cent difference between whites and blacks in 1982 was the lowest over this 11-year period. The 1979 survey found that black girls initiate intercourse about 1 year earlier (15.5 years) than do white girls (16.4 years).[88]

As expected, a greater proportion of adolescents are sexually experienced with each successive year of age. The 1983 National Longitudinal Survey of Youth reported that 17 per cent of boys and 5 per cent of girls had had intercourse by 15 years of age; 48 per cent of the boys and 27 per cent of the girls had done so by their 17th birthday, and 83 per cent of the boys and 74 per cent of the girls by 20 years of age.[30] Boys initiate sexual activity earlier than girls, but by late adolescence, the proportion of girls who are sexually experienced approaches that of boys.[12, 30]

Despite the high proportion of teenagers who are sexually experienced, many have intercourse infrequently. Data from Kantner and Zelnik's 1979 study found that 12 per cent of sexually experienced 15- to 19-year-old young women had had intercourse only once. Only 42 per cent reported intercourse in the preceding four weeks.[87] Adolescent girls had a limited number of premarital sex partners: 49 per cent reported one lifetime partner; only 16 per cent reported four or more partners.[87]

Kantner and Zelnik's 1979 survey examined the relationship a young woman had with her first sexual partner.[91] About 80 per cent reported they were going steady with or dating their initial partner. Only 9 per cent reported they were engaged to be married to their first partner. Even among those who reported first intercourse at age 15 or less, 73 per cent reported they were dating or going steady with their first partner. At least one consequence of early dating may be the early initiation of sexual activity.[91] Black adolescents are more likely to have sex for the first time with someone they are dating or friends with, whereas whites are more likely to report they are going steady with their first partner.[91] Another study supports the notion that white adolescents are more likely than are blacks to engage in a series of noncoital behaviors for a period prior to their first sexual experience.[64] These precipitous sexual behaviors among black adolescents may place them at greater risk for unplanned pregnancy.[64]

Homosexual behavior is common during adolescence, particularly early adolescence.[26, 54] A large number of teenagers will have a homosexual experience as part of their normal sexual development. Those young people who will adopt a homosexual lifestyle as adults often have their first sexual contact during adolescence. Kinsey, 35 years ago, reported that 33 per cent of girls and 60 per cent of boys had a homosexual experience by the age of 15 years.[38, 39] Sorensen, in his survey conducted some 20 years later, found that among 16 to 19 year olds, only 17 per cent of the boys and 6 per cent of the girls reported one or more such experiences.[66]

Contraceptive Use

The use of contraceptives by adolescents in the United States is relatively low and inconsistent. According to the Alan Guttmacher Institute, more consistent use of family planning methods could prevent an additional 313,000 pregnancies among teenagers each year.[75] The National Survey of Young Women and the National Survey of Family Growth demonstrated increased contraceptive use during the 1970s and early 1980s. In 1982, 85 per cent of sexually active girls reported they had used a contraceptive at some time in their lives, compared to 73 per cent in 1979 and 66 per cent in 1976.[30] Unfortunately, contraceptive use by adolescent girls is inconsistent; in 1979, 34 per cent reported they always used contraception, 39 per cent sometimes used contraception, and 27 per cent never used any form of birth control.[88] Blacks are less likely than whites to ever have used contraceptives[30]; they are also less likely to have used contraceptives at first intercourse.[30] Blacks, when they do use contraception, more frequently use a prescription method as their first method of birth control (41 per cent vs 17 per cent in 1979), and their most recent contraceptive method (56 per cent vs 44 per cent in 1979).[88]

Data indicate that age is a strong determinant of contraceptive use.[30, 91] Kantner and Zelnik's 1979 survey found that only 31 per cent of girls under 15 used a contraceptive at first intercourse, compared to 52 per cent of the 15 to 17 year olds, and 62 per cent of the 18 to 19 year olds. Younger teenagers were also more likely to use nonprescription methods.[91] Similar patterns were found for men, with 59 per cent of those over the age of 18 years when they initiated sexual activity reporting the use of some contraceptive method, compared with 49 per cent of 15 to 17 year olds, and 34 per cent of those under 15 years of age.[91]

In 1979, 51 per cent of all never-married 15- to 19-year-old women reported use of contraception at first intercourse. Among contraceptive users, condoms were most often chosen (38 per cent), followed by withdrawal (36 per cent), and oral contraceptives (18 per cent). Whereas many teenage girls who use contraception at first intercourse rely on male methods, they later switch to more effective prescription methods. Data from the 1982 National Survey of Family Growth indicated that 68 per cent of all never-married sexually active 15- to 19-year-old women were using some method of contraception; of the contraceptive users, 62 per cent were using oral contraceptives, 1 per cent intrauterine devices (IUDs), 6 per cent diaphragms, and 22 per cent condoms. Vaginal spermicides, douching, rhythm, and withdrawal accounted for 8 per cent of all other methods used.[3]

Adolescents' use of effective contraceptive methods has increased since the early 1970s. Oral contraceptive use increased from 1971 to 1976, fell in 1979 because of concern regarding medical risks associated with their use, but increased substantially by 1982. IUD use increased in the early 1970s but has declined since 1976 because of medical risks. The popularity of the diaphragm has increased since the mid-1970s. Condom use decreased between 1971 and 1976, increased in 1979, but leveled between 1979 and 1982. The use of least effective methods increased substantially between 1976 and 1979, and then fell between 1979 and 1982.[3, 30]

Teenage girls delay seeking contraceptive services an average of 16.6 months from first intercourse. Younger teenage girls wait the longest before making their initial visit.[84] Unfortunately, half of all first premarital pregnancies occur during the first 6 months of sexual activity, more than 20 per cent in the first month alone.[86]

Pregnancy and Abortion

The adverse outcomes of adolescent sexual behavior, particularly pregnancy, are of considerable consequence to society. Disrupted educations, reduced employment opportunities, low incomes, unstable marriages, health and developmental risks to the children of adolescent mothers, as well as the substantial public costs are among the most obvious concerns.[30]

In 1984, there were just over 1 million pregnancies to women less than 20 years of age in the United States; nearly 470,000 gave birth, and just over 400,000 obtained abortions.[30] Almost 40 per cent of these births were to girls less than 18 years of age.[30] Over 80 per cent of nonmarital pregnancies were unintended.[88] Almost 1 in 12 adolescents become pregnant each year; about 43 per cent of all adolescent girls (40 per cent of white teenagers and 63 per cent of black teenagers) will become pregnant at least once before their 20th birthday.[30]

The number of adolescent pregnancies increased during the 1970s, from 950,000 in 1972 to 1,142,000 in 1978, and subsequently declined to 1,005,000 in 1984.[30] This decline was in part due to a decrease in the adolescent population. The adolescent pregnancy rate, which stood at 94 per 1000 women 15 to 19 years old in 1972, increased until 1980, and subsequently has leveled off; it was 109 per 1000 women in 1984. When adjusted for sexual activity, the pregnancy rate actually has declined from 272 per 1000 women 15 to 19 years of age in 1972, to 233 per 1000 women in 1984. This decline is attributable to the improved use of contraceptives by adolescent girls.[30]

In spite of the increased number of adolescent pregnancies, the number of births to teenagers declined, from 628,000 in 1972 to 470,000 in 1984.[30] The declining adolescent population again contributed to this decrease, but increased use of abortion was also a factor. Birth rates for black 15 to 19 year old women are more than double those of comparably aged whites.[30, 48] Adolescent birth rates remain considerably higher in the United States than in most other developed countries.[75]

In 1971, women 15 to 19 years of age obtained over 150,000 abortions; in 1973, when abortion was legalized, this number increased to 280,000. In 1984, just over 400,000 abortions were performed.[30] About 30 per cent of all abortions performed in the United States each year are for women less than 20 years of age.[30]

The proportion of out of wedlock births to teenage girls has increased steadily since 1970. In that year, 30 per cent of live births to teenagers occurred outside of marriage; by 1984, this proportion had increased to 56 per cent.[30] Although the birth rate for unmarried teenagers was four times higher among nonwhites as compared to whites in 1983, this difference had decreased significantly since 1955 when it was nearly 13 times higher among nonwhites.[48]

Outcomes for Adolescent Parents and Their Children

Adolescent childbearing poses significant medical and social risks for both the adolescent mother and her child. Early studies reported increased obstetric risks for adolescent mothers, such as toxemia, anemia, cephalopelvic disproportion, and abrupt or prolonged labor.[30, 44, 48] Recent research indicates that many of these medical risks may be due to socioeconomic factors that were not adequately controlled for.[30, 44, 48] Other characteristics of adolescent mothers, including low socioeconomic status,[30, 48, 93] poor nutritional status,[30, 48, 93] late onset of prenatal care,[30, 48, 75, 93] and use of cigarettes, alcohol, or illicit drugs[48, 93] may account for their increased risk. Despite the fact that many problems associated with adolescent pregnancy and childbearing can be significantly reduced with early, appropriate prenatal care,[30] adolescent mothers less than 15 years of age do appear to have a higher rate of obstetric complications[30, 48] and are more likely to have low birth weight infants.[30, 42, 48] Children of adolescent parents have higher infant mortality rates, are at higher risk of dying from SIDS, have impaired socioemotional development, and appear more likely to suffer deficits in cognitive function during their school years.[48]

The social and economic consequences of teenage pregnancy and childbearing are considerable. Adolescents who give birth prior to completing high school are less likely to earn a high school diploma and complete college than women who delay childbearing into their twenties.[68, 75] Women who first give birth as teenagers are more likely to have a greater number of children, more closely spaced births, and a higher proportion of unintended births.[30, 68, 75] Adolescent mothers who do marry have higher rates of separation and divorce.[30, 48, 68, 75] As a result, adolescent mothers often are confronted by economic hardship. As young adults, they are more likely to be unemployed or when they are employed, receive lower hourly wages and have low status positions.[30, 68] Families headed by young mothers are seven times more likely to be living below the poverty level.[48, 68] Many are dependent on public assistance for financial support.[6, 68] In 1985, Aid to Families with Dependent Children (AFDC), food stamps, and Medicaid for women who first gave birth as teenagers cost taxpayers $16.65 billion.[6]

Sexually Transmitted Diseases

Many teenagers contract sexually transmitted diseases (STDs). The highest incidence of reportable STDs occurs in those 20 to 24 years of age, but is closely followed by the 15- to 19-year-old age group.[51] This is largely due to biologic and behavioral factors characteristic of adolescence.[36] Teenagers also less frequently use barrier contraceptives, which prevent transmission of many STDs, and prefer the use of oral contraceptives, which appear to render women more susceptible to chlamydial infection.[23, 28, 60]

The consequences of STDs are particularly significant since adolescents are just entering their reproductive years. These consequences include pelvic inflammatory disease, infertility, ectopic pregnancy, cervical intraepithelial neoplasia, spontaneous abortion, and neonatal morbidity.[36, 50]

Genital infections caused by *Chlamydia trachomatis* are now recognized as the most prevalent and potentially damaging of all STDs in the United States today,[10] and affect 3 to 4 million individuals each year.[10] This organism is a common cause of endocervicitis, endometritis, and pelvic inflammatory disease in women, and urethritis and epididymitis in men.[77] Sexually active women less than 20 years of age have chlamydial infection rates two to three times higher than women 20 years of age or older.[10, 28] Similarly, rates of urethral infection with chlamydia among teenage males are higher than those 20 years of age or older.[69] Studies have found the prevalence of chlamydial infections in nonpregnant adolescent women to range between 8 per cent and 23 per cent.[8, 23, 25, 56, 60] Most show chlamydial infection to be more prevalent than gonorrhea.[8, 25, 56, 60]

Gonorrhea is the most common reportable STD. It is a major cause of urethritis in men and cervicitis and pelvic inflammatory disease in women. In 1985, 911,419 cases were reported to the Centers for Disease Control; 218,821 cases, 24 per cent of the total, occurred in adolescents 15 to 19 years of age.[73] Age-specific incidence of gonorrhea in sexually experienced 15- to 19-year-old females was estimated to be twice that for 20- to 24-year-old women.[4]

Pelvic inflammatory disease (PID) is the most prevalent and serious complication of sexually acquired infection. Following infection, a young woman is at increased risk for recurrent PID, ectopic pregnancy, infertility, and chronic pelvic pain.[79] One million American women experience an episode of PID each year; 16 to 20 per cent of these cases occur in teenagers.[79] Rates for hospitalized PID in the United States for 15-year-old girls, adjusted for sexual activity, were twice those for 25-year-old women in one study.[81] Westrom estimated the incidence of PID in 15-year-old Swedish girls to be one in eight annually, ten times the annual incidence for 24-year-old women.[81]

Cervical intraepithelial neoplasia (CIN) among adolescent women, once regarded as a gynecologic curiosity, is a significant problem today.[55] CIN includes a continuum of neoplastic alterations, from mild dysplasia to carcinoma in situ. One large study found the prevalence of dysplasia and carcinoma in situ in 15- to 19-year-old women to be almost 2 per cent.[55] Risk factors for the development of CIN include early age at first coitus, multiple sex partners, male partners who have had multiple sex partners, and viral sexually transmitted agents, particularly herpes and human papillomavirus.[47] Human papillomavirus infections are among the most common STDs[36]; most of those infected are between 14 and 24 years of age.[57]

DETERMINANTS OF SEXUAL RISK-TAKING BEHAVIOR

Adolescence is a period of high-risk health behavior.[34] Drug use, violence, accidents, pregnancy, and STDs potentially can compromise an adolescent's ability to lead a full, productive, and healthy life. The risks are immediate or deferred, behaviorally or environmentally mediated, and often interrelated.[34] To understand and deal with the risks posed by adolescent sexual behavior, one needs to appreciate (1) the complexity of adolescence as a stage where behaviors are emerging in response to developmental needs, (2) the biologic and physiologic uniqueness of adolescence, (3) the personal attributes of the individual, and (4) the influence of the environment.

Developmental Characteristics

Adolescence begins with the first physical changes of puberty; the endpoint is less clearly defined. A series of developmental tasks must be accomplished during adolescence to enter adulthood successfully.[21] Tasks that relate to sexual development are (1) achieving comfort with one's body, (2) developing an identity separate from the family, (3) realizing the capacity to develop intimate, meaningful relationships, and (4) developing an ability to think abstractly and in futuristic terms. The ease with which an adolescent negotiates these tasks determines the degree of sexual risk taking behavior.

Puberty. To achieve comfort with their bodies, adolescents must come to terms with a changing body image, hormonal influences, disproportionate development, and new physiologic manifestations such as menstruation and ejaculation. Puberty begins between years 10 and 11 for most girls and about a year and a half later for boys. These changes span 2 to 4 years, and are measured by the Tanner staging system, a method of developmentally grading pubic hair growth and breast or genital development.[74]

Evidence suggests that early pubertal development is associated with early initiation of sexual activity.[80, 89] Reasons for this are unclear. Hormonal influences may be responsible for early sexual motivation and behavior, particularly in boys.[30] Early pubertal development in girls is associated with greater heterosexual interests and behavior, more concern with personal physical appearance, and lower self-esteem.[62] Consequently, the early maturing female adolescent may be more susceptible to peer pressure to begin sexual activity. In male adolescents, early maturation may be associated with high self-esteem.[16] Clearly, not all early maturers are sexually active, while some prepubertal boys are sexually experienced.[11] A clearer understanding of the interrelationships of physical changes, sexual activity, and social influences is needed to further assess the sexual risk posed by pubertal changes.

Even when physical development occurs at an average pace and onset, the degree to which adolescents feel comfortable with their bodies may affect fertility-related behaviors. A sexually active 13 year old who is unable to use tampons or look at her genitalia in a mirror during a pelvic examination is unlikely to use a diaphragm successfully. Use of oral contraceptives or condoms is more appropriate for her at this point in her development, with the diaphragm becoming an option as she moves into later adolescence and becomes more comfortable with her body.

Identity. As adolescents develop a new physical identity, they must also develop a new emotional, spiritual, and social identity, separate from that of their family or caretakers. One of the first steps in achieving this new identity is resolution of conflict and confusion about sexual orientation. The earliest sexual experiences of many teenagers are same-sex experiences.[26, 54] As proposed by Glasser,[24] the young adolescent is looking for friends who mirror his or her own narcissistic characteristics. Relationships at this stage may involve physical intimacy as a means of comparison and reassurance. This is normal behavior and poses no risks, unless the youth has no outlet to discuss these behaviors or overcompensates with heterosexual activity.

The movement toward independence and identity development involves the separation from family, yet it is the family that has provided the adolescent with a moral and ethical foundation on which to build his or her own ethical code. It is unclear whether the separation process is related to coital behavior and whether decreasing family closeness precedes or follows coital initiation.[31]

There are multiple, at times conflicting, studies that examine the relationship between the family and adolescent sexual behavior. In general, families in which there is mutual closeness, consistency of values between parent and child, and an intact family structure are more likely to have adolescents who delay sexual activity.[32, 35] There is also conflicting evidence as to whether parental communication on sexual issues actually delays sexual activity.[31, 32, 35] The relationship of family communication to sexual behavior seems to vary with the sex of parent and child.

In counseling their sons, mothers appear to be effective in delaying sexual activity while fathers appear to promote it.[31] Sexual discussions with daughters by either parent do not seem to delay sexual activity.[31]

The nature and quality of communication are also important. Adolescents want more than prescriptions and admonitions for sexual behavior from their parents. In Sorensen's study, 50 per cent of males and 63 per cent of females wanted to discuss sex with their parents.[66] Parents, however, have a number of barriers to overcome in providing sexual information. In one study, only 45 per cent of mothers correctly knew the time of the month that pregnancy is most likely to occur.[75] Parents may also be uncomfortable with their own sexuality. As the prime socializers of their children, parents teach them how to share, how to cooperate with others, and how to respond politely to adults but are generally uncomfortable in teaching a child how to be sexual. Indeed, most of a parent's direction in this matter involves teaching children *not* to be sexual. Masturbation, a normal behavior which starts in infancy, provides a child with enjoyment of his or her body, yet parents rarely feel comfortable observing this behavior. Even the youngest child may sense a parent's discomfort about sexual issues and learns not to ask questions. Therefore, sexual behavior in children develops with much less parental input than other behaviors.

As children move away from their family, they normally move toward developing replacement relationships with their peers. A strong association with a peer group is part of the process of achieving a new identity separate from the family. Some studies find a positive correlation between having sexually permissive friends and being sexually active.[9] Peer influence varies with gender, race, and age, however. Whites tend to be more influenced by peers than blacks, females more than males, and young adolescents more than older ones.[30] Male and female adolescents use their peer groups differently. Boys seek peer support for decisions; females may be influenced by what they perceive as their female peers' sexual activity, but it is their male partner that they rely on for sexual decisions.[17] Other studies suggest that young sexually active girls are more likely to engage in sexual behavior to please their boyfriends, without actual enjoyment of sex.[9] For both sexes, peers are a major source of sex information.[26, 78] In early adolescence, parental influences are strongest, whereas in later adolescence peers' influences are most prevalent.[30] The extent to which adolescents can balance these two influences contributes to their sexual risk-taking behavior.

Intimacy. Another task is the development of a shared intimacy outside of the family. This capacity develops in middle to late adolescence and involves more than physical intimacy. Sexual intimacy includes a blending of eroticism, emotional closeness, mutual caring, vulnerability, and trust.[58] This is usually spoken of as "commitment." The level of commitment may be important in determining coital initiation, STD protection, and contraceptive practices. However, there is no good method of measuring commitment.[45] Teens who engage in sexual activity before they reach this developmental level are at high risk for the undesirable consequences of sexual activity.

Whether adolescent or adult, a couple brings to a relationship two individual levels of development and two different moral and ideologic frameworks that need to be merged. Individual decision making becomes less important than couple decision making.[45] This suggests that the strength of a "couple-identity" may be a more powerful antecedent to outcomes such as pregnancy than peer or family influences.

The interpersonal decision-making process of the couple is of particular importance to adolescents, whose decision-making skills are often poorly developed. In addition, individual decisions regarding sexual behavior often are overcome by couple dynamics. For example, a female may understand the need for and prefer her partner to use a condom, but if he refuses, her intent is nullified. Further study of couple dynamics is needed to develop effective intervention strategies.

Cognitive Development. While the physical and emotional changes of adolescence are occurring, cognitive development is beginning to move from concrete operational thinking to formal operational thinking, as described by Piaget.[52] Formal operational thinking in sexual matters allows the adolescent to convert erotic thoughts into symbolic abstractions, which helps to resolve potential guilt conflicts.[41] Fantasies are recognized as such and no action is taken on them. Without formal operational thinking, the adolescent is unable to develop a decision-making tree; there is no understanding of potential consequences as a result of certain behaviors. Unfortunately, there is evidence that about a third of the adult population never fully achieves formal operational thinking.[52]

Concrete operational thinking or incomplete development of formal operations results in adolescents believing they are omnipotent and infallible. Misfortunes happen to someone else. There is a sense that they alone are immune from mishaps.[20] This thinking results in excessive risk taking that, when coupled with sexual behavior, results in unwanted pregnancies and STDs.

Biologic Determinants

Biologic characteristics make sexually active teenagers more vulnerable to pregnancy and STDs than sexually active adults. The age of menarche in the United States has decreased over time, extending the period of sexual maturity to a portion of the life cycle when cognitive and decision-making skills are less mature.[83] Teenage girls less than 15 years old and their offspring are at increased perinatal risk.[30, 42, 48] Changes in the epithelium of the uterine cervix during adolescence also increase the risk for developing STDs. In early adolescence, the columnar epithelium extends from the endocervical canal onto the exocervix, where it is not protected by cervical mucus from potential pathogens introduced during sexual intercourse.[7, 36] Exposure of columnar epithelial cells to the vaginal environment may increase susceptibility to *Neisseria gonorrhoeae* and *Chlamydia trachomatis*, which selectively infect these cells.[36] Moreover, exposure of cells undergoing squamous metaplasia at the squamocolumnar junction at an early age to potential infectious carcinogens such as herpes and human papillomavirus may produce cervical cytologic changes earlier in adulthood.[82] One study found that women who developed human papillomavirus infection before the age of 25 years were almost 40 times more likely to develop cervical carcinoma in situ compared to the general population of women less than 25 years old.[46] Adolescents also have a relatively unchallenged immune system because they have had little prior exposure to most sexually transmissible agents. With age and sexual experience, their local and systemic immune systems mature and may provide some degree of protection from these agents.[79]

Individual Characteristics

In general, the future- and achievement-oriented adolescent is more likely to delay intercourse and use contraception once sexual activity begins.[9] High self-esteem, a sense of directedness, and goal orientation are all associated with delayed sexual activity and effective contraceptive use.[32] McAnarney[45] suggests further research is needed to determine if there are social antecedents that determine the nature of adolescent's self-esteem and locus of control, and the impact that these characteristics have on sexual behavior.

Religiosity. Religion appears to be an important factor that distinguishes early from later initiators of sexual activity.[30] Those who view religion as important to them and who attend services regularly appear to be more likely to abstain from sexual activity.[33, 35, 89] Individual denominations do not seem to be as powerful as the perceived importance of religion.[30]

The Environment

Race and Socioeconomic Status. Statistics indicate that blacks are more likely to engage in intercourse earlier and in larger numbers than whites.[49, 88] Studies attempting to explain these racial differences are confounded by variables linking socioeconomic status with race. More blacks than whites are of a lower socioeconomic status, making it difficult to separate out what may be inherent cultural differences. Hofferth suggests that it may be more appropriate to think in terms of community norms of sexuality when planning intervention strategies.[30]

Media and Society. Compared with other countries, the United States gives its young people many more mixed messages about sexuality.[37] Although sexual images are pervasive in our society, Americans fantasize about sex rather than handling it realistically and responsibly. Popular magazines prominently depict a social connection between sex and drugs. Liquor and cigarette advertisements invariably display men and women in romantic settings. Movie portrayal of sexual relations have moved from innuendos to explicit demonstrations. In the face of all this sexual exposure, our society expects adolescents to practice chastity. In recent years, television has begun to assume responsibility for its sexual messages. Couples are mentioning "safe sex," and adolescents are discussing their options and choosing abstinence or contraceptive use. However, there remains a large amount of sexual material on television for which there is no forum for discussion. Cable TV is a particular concern. On some music stations drug use and sexual encounters mingle with overtones of violence. Many cable systems have "blue stations," on which explicit sexual depictions not subject to censorship can be viewed. The advent of VCRs also has allowed pornographic movies to move from theatres into the living room.

THE ROLE OF THE PEDIATRIC PRACTITIONER

It is not an easy task for the pediatric practitioner simultaneously to protect adolescents from the negative consequences of their sexuality and promote healthy sexual development. Sex education is effective in imparting knowledge, yet knowledge alone does not change attitudes and behaviors. Potential interventions include counseling both adolescents and their parents, as well as promoting responsible changes on a community and national level.

Counseling Adolescents and Parents

The practitioner who cares for children is in a unique position to not only provide sexual information directly to adolescents but also to support parents as the major sexual socializers of their children. The guidelines that follow represent concrete ways in which the pediatric practitioner can intervene to prevent adolescent pregnancy and sexually transmitted disease.

1. *The practitioner needs to be comfortable with his or her own sexuality.* The practitioner needs to be aware of his or her own attitudes and values. What these values are is less important than how they are managed by the practitioner in the counseling situation. The adolescent needs information and guidance, not moralistic admonitions and directives. However, objectivity should not outweigh the need to provide age-appropriate guidance. Adolescents need to hear that (1) sex should never be forced on anyone; (2) it is better to delay childbearing beyond adolescence; and (3) it is acceptable to abstain from sexual activity. Practitioners have an obligation to address their adolescent patients' needs either directly or through an appropriate referral.

2. *The practitioner must be adequately trained in the fundamentals of*

adolescent health care. Although over 15 years ago the American Academy of Pediatrics expanded the scope of pediatrics to include young people up to 21 years,[2] pediatricians care for only 25 per cent of all adolescents.[76] In 1978, 66 per cent of responding pediatricians felt their training in adolescent medicine to be insufficient.[76] A recent survey found that 26 per cent felt they lacked adequate knowledge in adolescent medicine.[13] Several methods for gaining proficiency and comfort in adolescent health are available to the practitioner through continuing medical education. Practitioners need training in the following areas related to adolescence: physical growth and development, cognitive development, common medical problems, including sexually transmitted diseases, adolescent gynecology, and common behavioral and psychological problems.[1]

3. *Sexuality issues should be included in anticipatory guidance beginning at the first pediatric visit.* Throughout childhood, each well-child visit should include discussions of sexuality related issues appropriate to the child's level of development (Table 1). Expectations for male–female behavior are present even before birth. Awareness of this allows for later dialogue on expression of individuality. Likewise, using appropriate names (e.g., penis, clitoris, vagina) during the well-child visit makes it easier to facilitate discussions as the child grows older. When discussions regarding sexuality are initiated early, parents and children are more comfortable talking about sexually related issues.

4. *The practitioner should know the community norms and expectations.* Sexual activity and practices vary with different cultures. Urban adolescents exposed to socioeconomic disadvantage may present with different patterns of behavior and sexual attitudes than suburban adolescents. The sexual issues that both groups are handling are the same; it is their response to them that varies.

Parental expectations may also differ. It is important for the pediatric practitioner to have a sense of the community's values on adolescent sexual issues to maximize effectiveness of interventions. A conservative community with strong religious beliefs may require a different approach than a more liberal community. A practitioner who anticipates and responds to parental concerns is assured that there will be a minimum of resistance to sexual counseling.

5. *Prior to puberty, the practitioner–patient–parent relationship needs to be redefined.* Through the child's infancy and latency, the pediatric practitioner has obtained information primarily from the parent. As the child enters adolescence, he or she becomes the principal historian and helps to establish the agenda during the visit. The issue of confidentiality is paramount to teenagers and often difficult to negotiate with parents. The practitioner can help the parent accept the adolescent's need for privacy while encouraging the adolescent to speak with his or her parents. If the rules of communication are clearly established, there should be no misunderstanding when contraception is discussed.

Many practitioners see the teenager and parent together at the beginning of the visit. The practitioner can obtain information at this time about specific parental concerns and subjects the parent will know more about, such as medical history, immunizations, and family medical history. Both the parent and the teenager are told that anything the teenager subsequently tells the practitioner will remain confidential. After the parent has left the room, the patient is told he or she will be asked a series of questions, some of which are of a personal nature, and that all responses will remain confidential.

6. *The practitioner must establish him- or herself as "askable."* Initiation of sexual discussions, presence of sex education materials in the waiting room, and separate teen office hours indicate the practitioner recognizes that adolescents have their special needs and concerns.

7. *The provider should ask the appropriate questions if the patient has not initiated any sexual questions.* All adolescents need to have a sexual history taken

Table 1. *Sexuality and Routine Health Care Maintenance*

AGE	SEXUAL AREAS OF CONCERN	RISK FACTORS	ANTICIPATORY GUIDANCE
Prepubertal 6–10 years	Out of home influences on sexuality	Irresponsible media depiction of sexuality	Isolated censorship generally does not work. Open discussion of sexual scenarios in movies, magazines, and songs can help parents open conversations about attitudes they are uncomfortable with.
	Homosexual encounters	Heterosexual overcompensation	Same sex crushes are a normal part of development for both males and females and help consolidate and reaffirm his/her gender identity. Discussion of this helps both child and parent appreciate normal development.
Early Adolescence Early Puberty 10–12 years	Pubertal changes	Self-image	Gynecomastia is normal in adolescent males as is breast asynchrony in females. Such body disproportions distort adolescents' image of themselves. Early maturers, particularly females, need special guidance to avoid low self-esteem and premature sexual advances.
		Hormonal influences	Masturbation is a normal behavior which relieves sexual tension. Fantasies are normal while masturbating. Masturbation is a choice—teens can choose to do it or not.
Late Puberty 12–14 years	Initiation of sexual activity without intimacy	Concrete thought Cannot perceive long-range implications of current actions	Discussions of sexual choices should emphasize that it is alright to say "no"; discussions regarding contraceptive use need to emphasize more immediate as well long-term benefits—i.e., in addition to pregnancy prevention, oral contraceptives may relieve dysmenorrhea.
Midadolescence 14–17 years	Intimacy related to sexual romanticism rather than genuine commitment	Looks to peer group for support as he/she separates from family	Parents should be encouraged to continue sexual dialogue begun in latency. They should know their own values (what is sex for; who is it for; what makes it enjoyable; what makes it exploitive?). Parental values should be shared with opinions, rather than judgments. Parents should respect teens' decisions.
	Sporadic or absent use of birth control; sexual experimentation	Formal operational thinking, variably applied	Teens begin to understand future implications of current actions; they know that use of birth control will protect from unwanted pregnancy, condoms will protect from STDs.
		Risk taking and sense of omnipotence	Risk taking should be discussed. Once a young woman risks unprotected intercourse without becoming pregnant, she is liable to risk it again. Other risk behaviors such as drunk driving and drug use may have a negative interactive effect on sexual decision making.
Late Adolescence 17–21 years	Intimacy involves commitment	Family conflicts resolving as independence established	Teen begins to plan for future, including marriage and family.
		Comfort with bodies and gender identity	Relationships involve a mutual reciprocity. Counseling involves understanding of female sexual response, couple discussions of feelings.

Table 2. *The Sexual History*

1. Have you ever had romantic feelings toward someone of the opposite sex? The same sex?
2. Have you ever dated?
3. Have you ever had sexual intercourse with someone of the opposite sex? The same sex?
4. Have you ever had a sexual relationship with someone where it was forced upon you?
5. Do you enjoy sex?
6. If you have not had sex, what are your feelings about it?
7. Are you using birth control? How do you feel about it? How does your boy(girl)friend feel about it?
8. What methods of birth control do you know about?
9. Do you know where to get condoms? Do you know how to use them?
10. Have you ever been pregnant? Have you ever fathered a baby? What happened to the pregnancy? How did you feel about it?
11. Have you ever masturbated? How did you feel about it?
12. Can you talk to your parents about sex? Have you?
13. Have you ever had a sexually transmitted disease? Have you asked your partner if he(she) has ever had a sexually transmitted disease?
14. How many different people have you had sex with?
15. Have you ever had oral sex?
16. Have you ever had anal sex?
17. Do you have any questions or concerns about sex that you would like to discuss?

when they are seen for routine health care and for certain emergent problems. A list of questions that are helpful in obtaining the sexual history, based on our and other's experience, is presented in Table 2.[5, 63, 70] The practitioner plays an essential role in addressing fears and myths, interpreting sexual encounters, and providing accurate information on sexual feelings, family planning, sexually transmitted diseases, masturbation, homosexuality, relationships, and normal physiology. In addition to providing individual counseling, some physicians or their office nurses provide sex education for adolescents in small group sessions.[61]

For those adolescents who wish to postpone intercourse, it is helpful for the practitioner to support their decision and to emphasize it is their choice when to have intercourse.[63] It is important to realize that not all adolescents are sexually active. Many teens feel stigmatized by their virginal status because of the perceptions that "everyone is doing it."

Younger teens should be asked about incest. Teens who reply affirmatively should be referred to an appropriate mental health professional for treatment.

Homosexual experiences are common during adolescence, and many teenagers wonder if they are homosexual. Because of the negative response to homosexuality by society in general,[70] and family and peers in particular,[53] it is important to discuss these feelings and experiences with the adolescent in a supportive and nonjudgmental manner.

8. The sexual history needs to be much more detailed than it has traditionally been in the past. With the rising incidence of AIDS, sexual history taking must be more explicit to assess a sexually active adolescent's risk for acquiring AIDS and other STDs. Asking "Are you sexually active?" is no longer sufficient. Information regarding the number of sexual partners, age of first intercourse, and practice of oral or anal sex is necessary to care for the sexually active teenager adequately.

9. The provider should encourage the parent to discuss sexual issues. Practitioners can help educate parents about sexuality, clarify values, and help them to guide their children's decision making. Parents can be reassured they need not be sex experts to discuss sexuality with their children.

The American Academy of Pediatrics recently published a bibliography of educational materials on sex education[59] from which the practitioner can select

Table 3. *Recommended Books for Parents and Patients*

For Parents
1. Marilyn Ratnor and Susan Chamlin: *Straight Talk–Sexuality Education for Parents and Kids 4–7.* New York, Penguin Books, 1985.
2. Mary Calderone and James Ramey: *Talking with Your Child About Sex.* New York, Pocket Books, 1979.
3. Mary Calderone and Eric W. Johnson: *The Family Book About Sexuality.* New York, Harper and Row, 1981.
4. Sol Gordon and Judith Gordon: *Raising a Child Conservatively in a Sexually Permissive World.* New York, Simon and Schuster, 1985.
5. Ruth Bell and Leni Zeiger Wildflower: *Talking with Your Teenager.* New York, Random House, 1984.

For Preadolescents
1. Sam Gitchel and Lorri Foster: *Let's Talk About. . . . S-E-X. A Read and Discuss Guide for People 9–12 and Their Parents.* Fresno, CA, Planned Parenthood of Fresno, 1982.
2. Peter Mayle: *What's Happening to Me?* Secaucus, NJ, Lyle Stuart, Inc., 1975.
3. Margaret Sheffield: *Where Do Babies Come From?* New York, Alfred A. Knopf, 1973.
4. Kathy McCoy and Charles Wibbelsman: *Growing and Changing, A Handbook for Preteens.* New York, Pedigree Books, 1986.

For Adolescents
1. Ruth Bell: *Changing Bodies, Changing Lives.* New York, Random House, 1980.
2. Kathy McCoy and Charles Wibbleman: *The Teenage Body Book.* New York, Pocket Books, 1979.
3. Sol Gordon: *Facts About Sex for Today's Youth.* Fayetteville, NC, Ed-U Press, 1987.
4. Alex Comfort and Jane Comfort: *The Facts of Love, Living, Loving and Growing Up.* New York, Crown Publishers, Inc., 1979.
5. Eleanor Hamilton: *Sex with Love: A Guide for Young People.* Boston, Beacon Press, 1978.

pamphlets that are suitable to his specific practice setting and community. A list of suggested readings for use by parents and patients can be prepared and sample materials made available for review in the office. A list of suggested books is presented in Table 3.

Practitioners can also conduct group sessions for parents to teach the knowledge and skills that parents need to become competent sex educators of their children. The preadolescent and early adolescent can also be involved in these sessions, which can focus on imparting knowledge, developing decision-making skills, and improving communication with parents. Several studies suggest that improved communication may enhance contraceptive use by adolescent girls.[22, 67] Large group practices and health maintenance organizations often have health promotion departments that can organize and run such programs with the support of an interested practitioner.

10. *The developmental stage of the adolescent should be acknowledged at all times.* A teen who has not reached formal operational thinking is not going to understand the cause and effect of sexual behavior in the same way that an adult does. This does not mean that she cannot use contraception or practice abstinence, but rather that the guidance provided needs to be concrete and geared to the present rather than to the future.

Practitioner–patient interactions also vary with age and gender. The young adolescent male, for example, may have more difficulty accepting a genital examination by a female practitioner than the older adolescent male. This is related to his developmental stage and comfort with his body.

11. *Sexuality involves more than just intercourse.* Sexuality involves feelings and relationships. Teens need an opportunity to discuss their feelings as part of a partnership. It is very helpful to see sexually active couples together and facilitate their joint sexual decision making.

12. *Sexuality is only one aspect of an adolescent's life.* To focus exclusively on sexual issues is as shortsighted as not addressing them at all. The acronym HEADS (*H* for home, *E* for education, *A* for activities, *D* for drugs, and *S* for sexuality) is helpful in remembering the information that is needed to evaluate how effectively an adolescent is dealing with the developmental tasks of adolescence.[5] This series of questions demonstrates to the adolescent patient that the practitioner is interested in all aspects of his or her life, and not just sexuality.[63]

The Community

Pediatric practitioners are in an ideal position to work with their local school system and parent–teacher groups to ensure that adequate and effective sex education programs are available in the public schools.[19, 61, 71] Unfortunately, though three quarters of all junior and senior high schools offer sex education, most programs are very brief, usually 10 hours or less; fewer than 10 per cent cover the full spectrum of sexuality-related issues.[27, 30] Pediatric practitioners can clear up misconceptions that may be responsible for parents' and school administrators' hesitation about sex education. Sex education programs increase knowledge, change attitudes, and may increase contraceptive use.[18, 40, 43, 90] They have not been shown to promote earlier or more frequent sexual activity or increase the risk of pregnancy.[18, 40, 43, 90] Practitioners should be aware of these findings and be able to communicate this information effectively. Practitioners also may serve as a resource for sex education teachers by being knowledgeable of recent advances, helping update education materials, and participating in selected classroom sessions.[19] Where availability of health services for adolescents is limited, school-based health clinics have increased access to care, and also may improve contraceptive use and decrease pregnancy rates.[30, 85] Those practitioners located near such areas are in an excellent position to advocate for these clinics with local school boards.

National Advocacy

Physicians, through their local, regional, and national professional organizations, make ideal political advocates for adolescents' health care needs. The American Academy of Pediatrics' Committee on Youth and the Society for Adolescent Medicine in 1973 drafted a model act providing for consent of minors for health services.[15, 65] Interested physicians played an important role in several states in having features from these model bills enacted into law.[72] The Department of Health and Human Services' parental notification rule was withdrawn in 1983 in part because of organized opposition from health professionals.[71] Pediatricians, through their individual and collective lobbying efforts through the American Academy of Pediatrics, were instrumental several years ago in rescinding budgetary cuts proposed by the Reagan administration and later expanding Medicaid and the Maternal and Child Health block grants, which included funds for maternal and child health services and adolescent pregnancy. The American Academy of Pediatrics' Committee on Adolescence recently published a policy statement supporting the advertisement of nonprescription contraceptives on radio and television, decreased use of suggestive sexual messages in product advertising, and portrayal of sexuality in a manner that will promote responsible sexual behavior.[14]

SUMMARY

The consequences of adolescent sexual behavior are an enormous burden both for the adolescent and society. The problem is not that teens are sexually active but rather that they have little preparation and guidance in developing responsible sexual behavior. Developmentally, adolescents reach physical maturity before they are cognitively able to appreciate the consequences of their behavior. A teenager's primary source of information regarding sexuality is his or her peer group, all of whom are experiencing and reinforcing the same behaviors. The family, the major socializer of other behaviors, is not as powerful a force in shaping responsible sexual behavior because of parental discomfort with sex education and sexual discussions. This is the result of a social milieu in which sex is frequently portrayed but rarely linked with responsible behavior or accurate, nonjudgmental information.

The pediatric practitioner is in an ideal position to intervene in these dynamics. In the office, the practitioner can provide accurate sexual information to both parents and adolescents, support parental–child communication on sexual issues, and provide appropriate services or referral. In the community, the practitioner can advocate for school-based sex education as well as act as an information resource. Finally, the practitioner can advocate for the health care needs for adolescents on a national level, supporting legislation that provides adolescents with information and access to services necessary to make responsible sexual decisions.

REFERENCES

1. American Academy of Pediatrics: Policy statement: Preparing for adolescent medicine. AAP News: May, 1985, p 11
2. American Academy of Pediatrics: Policy statement. Pediatrics 49:463, 1972
3. Bachrach CA, Mosher WD: Use of contraception in the United States, 1982. Advance Data from Vital and Health Statistics, No. 102. DHHS Publication No. (PHS) 85–1250. Public Health Service, Hyattsville, Maryland, Dec. 4, 1984
4. Bell TA, Holmes KK: Age-specific risks of syphilis, gonorrhea and hospitalized pelvic inflammatory disease in sexually experienced U.S. women. Sex Transm Dis 11:291, 1984
5. Berman HS: Talking HEADS: Interviewing adolescents. HMO Pract 1:3, 1987
6. Burt MR: Estimating the public costs of teenage childbearing. Fam Plann Perspect 18:221, 1986
7. Cates W, Rauh JL: Adolescents and sexually transmitted diseases: An expanding problem. J Adol Health Care 6:257, 1985
8. Chacko MR, Lovchik JC: *Chlamydia trachomatis* infection in sexually active adolescents: Prevalence and risk factors. Pediatrics 73:836, 1984
9. Chilman CS: Adolescent Sexuality in a Changing American Society: Social and Psychological Perspectives. U.S. Dept. of Health, Education and Welfare publication No. (NIH) 79–1426. Washington, D.C., U.S. Government Printing Office, 1978
10. *Chlamydia trachomatis* infections: Policy guidelines for prevention and control. MMWR 34 (Suppl 3):53S, 1985
11. Clark SD, Zabin LS, Hardy JB: Sex, contraception, and parenthood: Experience and attitudes among urban black young men. Fam Plann Perspect 16:77, 1984
12. Coles R, Stokes G: Sex and the American Teenager. New York, Harper & Row, 1985
13. Comerci G: Adolescent Medicine and the Pediatrician: Changes and Controversies. Presented at the American Academy of Pediatrics, San Francisco, October 24, 1983
14. Committee on Adolescence: Sexuality, contraception, and the media. Pediatrics 78:535, 1986
15. Committee on Youth: A model act providing for consent of minors for health services. Pediatrics 51:293, 1973
16. Gross RT, Duke PM: The effect of early versus late physical maturation on adolescent behavior. Pediatr Clin North Am 27:71, 1980
17. Cvetkovich G, Grote B: Psychosocial development and the social problems of teenage illegitimacy. In Chilman CS (ed): Adolescent Pregnancy and Childbearing: Findings from Research. U.S. Dept. of Health and Human Services publication No. (NIH) 81–2077. Washington, D.C., U.S. Government Printing Office, 1980, pp 15–41
18. Dawson DA: The effects of sex education on adolescent behavior. Fam Plann Perspect 18:162, 1986

19. Duke PM: Adolescent sexuality. Pediatr Rev 4:44, 1982
20. Elkind D, Weiner I: Development of the Child. New York, John Wiley & Sons, 1975
21. Felice ME, Friedman SB: Behavioral considerations in the health care of adolescents. Pediatr Clin North Am 29:399, 1982
22. Fox GL: The family's role in adolescent sexual behavior. In Ooms T (ed): Teenage Pregnancy in a Family Context. Philadelphia, Temple University Press, 1981, pp 73–130
23. Fraser JJ, Rettig PJ, Kaplan DW: Prevalence of cervical *Chlamydia trachomatis* and *Neisseria gonorrhoeae* in female adolescents. Pediatrics 71:333, 1983
24. Glasser M: Homosexuality in adolescence. Br J Med Psychlol 50:217, 1977
25. Golden N, Hammerschlag M, Neuhoff S, Gleyzer A: Prevalence of *Chlamydia trachomatis* cervical infection in female adolescents. Am J Dis Child 138:562, 1984
26. Greydanus DE: Adolescent sexuality: An overview and perspective for the 1980s. Pediatr Ann 11:714, 1982
27. Haffner D, Casey S: Approaches to adolescent pregnancy prevention. Semin Adol Med 2:259, 1986
28. Handsfield HH, Jasman LL, Roberts PL et al: Criteria for selective screening for *Chlamydia trachomatis* infection in women attending family planning clinics. JAMA 255:1730, 1986
29. Haas A: Teenage Sexuality–A Survey of Teenage Sexual Behavior. New York, Macmillan, 1979
30. Hayes CD (ed): Risking the Future: Adolescent Sexuality, Pregnancy, and Childbearing, Vol 1. Washington, D.C., National Academy Press, 1987
31. Hayes CD (ed): Risking the Future: Adolescent Sexuality, Pregnancy, and Childbearing, Vol 2. Washington, DC, National Academy Press, 1987
32. Herold E, Goodwin MS, Lero AS: Self-esteem, locus of control and adolescent contraception. J Psychol 101:83, 1979
33. Inazu JK, Fox GL: Maternal influence on the sexual behavior of teenage daughters. J Fam Issues 1:81, 1980
34. Jessor R: Adolescent development and behavioral health. In Matarazzo JK (ed): Behavioral Health: A Handbook of Health Enhancement and Disease Prevention. New York, John Wiley & Sons, 1984, pp 69–90
35. Jessor SL, Jessor R: Transition from virginity to nonvirginity among youth: A social-psychological study over time. Dev Psychol 11:473, 1975
36. Johnson J: Sexually transmitted diseases in adolescents. Primary Care 14:101, 1987
37. Jones EF, Forrest JD, Goldman N et al: Teenage pregnancy in developed countries: Determinants and policy implications. Fam Plann Perspect 17:53, 1985
38. Kinsey AC, Pomeroy WB, Martin CE: Sexual Behavior in the Human Male. Philadelphia, WB Saunders, 1948
39. Kinsey AC, Pomeroy WB, Martin CE: Sexual Behavior in the Human Female. Philadelphia, WB Saunders Co, 1953
40. Kirby D: Sexuality Education: An Evaluation of Programs and Their Effects. Santa Cruz, California, Network Publications, 1984
41. Kohlberg L, Gilligan C: The adolescent as philosopher: The discovery of the self in a post conventional world. In Kagan J, Colers R (eds): 12 to 16: Early Adolescence. New York, W.W. Norton & Co, 1972, pp 144–179
42. Makinson C: The health consequences of teenage fertility. Fam Plann Perspect 17:132, 1985
43. Marsiglio W, Mott FL: The impact of sex education on sexual activity, contraceptive use and premarital pregnancy among American teenagers. Fam Plann Perspect 18:151, 1986
44. McAnarney ER, Roghmann KJ, Adams BN et al: Obstetric, neonatal, and psychosocial outcome of pregnant adolescents. Pediatrics 61:199, 1978
45. McAnarney ER, Schreider C: Identifying Social and Psychological Antecedents of Adolescent Pregnancy. New York, William T. Grant Foundation, 1984
46. Mitchell H, Drake M, Medley G: Prospective evaluation of risk of cervical cancer after cytological evidence of human papillomavirus infection. Lancet 1:573, 1986
47. Nelson JH, Averette HE, Richart RM: Dysplasia, carcinoma in situ, and early invasive cervical carcinoma. CA 34:306, 1984

48. Newberger CM, Melnicoe LH, Newberger EH: The American family in crisis: Implications for children. Curr Probl Pediatr 16:674, 1986
49. Newcomer SF, Udry JR: Adolescent sexual behavior and popularity. Adolescence 18:515, 1983
50. O'Reilly KR, Aral SO: Adolescence and sexual behavior: Trends and implications for STD. J Adolesc Health Care 6:262, 1985
51. Perrine PL: Epidemiology of the sexually transmitted diseases. Ann Rev Public Health 6:85, 1985
52. Piaget J: Intellectual evolution from adolescence to adulthood. Human Dev 15:1, 1972
53. Remafedi G: Male homosexuality: The adolescent's perspective. Pediatrics 79:326, 1987
54. Rigg CA: Homosexuality in adolescence. Pediatr Ann 11:826, 1982
55. Sadeghi SB, Hsieh EW, Gunn SW: Prevalence of cervical intraepithelial neoplasia in sexually active teenagers and young adults: Results of data analysis of mass Papanicolaou screening of 796,337 women in the United States in 1981. Am J Obstet Gynecol 148:726, 1984
56. Saltz GR, Linnemann CC, Brookman RR et al: *Chlamydia trachomatis* cervical infections in female adolescents. J Pediatr 98:981, 1981
57. Sanz LE, Gurdian J: Human papillomavirus and cervical intraepithelial neoplasia as sexually transmitted diseases. Semin Adolesc Med 2:121, 1986
58. Sarrel LJ, Sarrel PM: Sexual unfolding. J Adolesc Health Care 2:93, 1981
59. Sex Education: A Bibliography of Educational Materials for Children, Adolescents, and Their Families. Elk Grove Village, Illinois, American Academy of Pediatrics, 1986
60. Shafer M-A, Beck A, Blain B et al: *Chlamydia trachomatis:* Important relationships to race, contraception, lower genital tract infection, and Papanicolaou smear. J Pediatr 104:141, 1984
61. Shenker IR, Nussbaum M, Kaplan E: Sex and the pediatrician, letter. Pediatrics 61:160, 1978
62. Simmons RG, Blyth D, VanCleave EG et al: Entry into early adolescence: the impact of school structure, puberty, and early dating on self-esteem. Am Sociol Rev 44:948, 1979
63. Sladkin KR: Counseling adolescents about sexuality. Semin Adolesc Med 1:223, 1985
64. Smith EA, Udry JR: Coital and non-coital sexual behaviors of white and black adolescents. Am J Public Health 75:1200, 1985
65. Society for Adolescent Medicine: A model bill for minors' consent to health services. Pediatrics 52:750, 1975
66. Sorensen RC: Adolescent Sexuality in Contemporary America. New York, World Publishing Co, 1972
67. Spanier QB: Sources of sex information and parental sexual behavior. J Sex Res 13:73, 1977
68. Spivak H, Weitzman M: Social barriers faced by adolescent parents and their children. JAMA 258:1500, 1987
69. Stamm WE, Koutsky LA, Benedetti JK et al: *Chlamydia trachomatis* urethral infections in men: Prevalence, risk factors, and clinical manifestations. Ann Intern Med 100:47, 1984
70. Stewart DC: Sexuality and the adolescent: Issues for the clinician. Primary Care 14:83, 1987
71. Strasburger VC: Normal adolescent sexuality: A physician's perspective. Semin Adolesc Med 1:101, 1985
72. Strasburger VC, Eisner JM, Tilson JQ et al: Teenagers, physicians, and the law in New England. J Adolesc Health Care 6:377, 1985
73. Summary of notifiable diseases, United States, 1985. MMWR 34(54):10, 1987
74. Tanner JM: Growth at Adolescence, ed 2. Oxford, Blackwell Scientific Publications, 1962
75. Teenage Pregnancy: The Problem That Hasn't Gone Away. New York, Alan Guttmacher Institute, 1981
76. The Task Force on Pediatric Education: The Future of Pediatric Education. Evanston, Illinois, American Academy of Pediatrics, 1978
77. Thompson SE, Washington AE: Epidemiology of sexually transmitted *Chlamydia trachomatis* infections. Epidemiol Rev 5:96, 1983
78. Thornberg HD: Adolescent sources of initial sex information. Psychiatr Ann 8:419, 1978
79. Washington AE, Sweet RL, Shafer M-A: Pelvic inflammatory disease and its sequelae in adolescents. J Adol Health Care 6:298, 1985

80. Westney OE, Jenkins RR, Benjamin CM: Sociosexual development of preadolescents. In Brooks-Gunn J, Peterson J (eds): Girls at Puberty. New York, Plenum Press, 1983

81. Westrom L: Incidence, prevalence, and trends of acute pelvic inflammatory disease and its consequences in industrialized countries. Am J Obstet Gynecol 138:880, 1980

82. Wright VC, Riopelle MA: Age at beginning of coitus versus chronologic age as a basis for Papanicolaou smear screening: An analysis of 747 cases of preinvasive disease. Am J Obstet Gynecol 149:824, 1984

83. Wyshak G, Frisch RE: Evidence for a secular trend in age of menarche. N Engl J Med 306:1033, 1982

84. Zabin LS, Clark SD: Why they delay: A study of teenage family planning clinic patients. Fam Plann Perspect 13:205, 1981

85. Zabin LS, Hirsch MB, Smith EA et al: Evaluation of a pregnancy prevention program for urban teenagers. Fam Plann Perspect 18:119, 1986

86. Zabin LS, Kantner JF, Zelnik M: The risk of adolescent pregnancy in the first months of intercourse. Fam Plann Perspect 11:215, 1979

87. Zelnik M: Sexual activity among adolescents: Perspective of a decade. In McAnarney ER (ed): Premature Adolescent Pregnancy and Parenthood. New York, Grune & Stratton, 1983, pp 21–33

88. Zelnik M, Kantner JF: Sexual activity, contraceptive use and pregnancy among metropolitan-area teenagers: 1971–1979. Fam Plann Perspect 12:230, 1980

89. Zelnik M, Kantner JF, Ford K: Sex and Pregnancy in Adolescence. Beverly Hills, California, Sage Publications, 1981

90. Zelnik M, Kim YJ: Sex education and its association with teenage sexual activity, pregnancy, and contraceptive use. Fam Plann Perspect 14:117, 1982

91. Zelnik M, Shah FK: First intercourse among young Americans. Fam Plann Perspect 15:64, 1983

92. Zuckerman BS, Walker DK, Frank DA et al: Adolescent pregnancy: Biobehavioral determinants of outcome. J Pediatr 105:857, 1984

Adolescent Center
Boston City Hospital
818 Harrison Avenue, ACC 5
Boston, Massachusetts 02118

The Changing American Family

Howard Dubowitz, MD,* Carolyn Moore Newberger, EdD,†
Lora H. Melnicoe, MD,‡ and Eli H. Newberger, MD§

What is a "typical" American family? The description in our first grade primers of father at work and mother at home caring for their children applied to only 22 per cent of American families in 1981.[49] A spiraling divorce rate, increasing poverty, pregnancies to unmarried teenagers, and changing work patterns are among the factors that contribute to a dramatically different portrait of the American family today.

At the same time, developments such as readily available birth control that enable the planning of families, an increased awareness of the needs and rights of children, and the institution of "family-sensitive" public policies may enhance the quality of family life. As some old problems are being resolved, new ones emerge, however.

The life of a family is complex and vulnerable to forces within and outside the family. This complexity can only be captured imperfectly by summary statistics of social and demographic trends, and our knowledge of the impact of these trends on family life is limited. We know that enormous heterogeneity exists among American families. Nonetheless, recent changes in the profile of American families have profound implications not only for society, but also for individual families.

This article examines several of the major developments in American families in recent decades, with particular attention to their effects on children and the roles of the pediatrician. Four of these developments, involving divorce, poverty, teen pregnancy, and homelessness, are addressed in separate articles in this volume and will be covered here only briefly to illustrate how they fit into a pattern of increasing poverty for women and children.

*Assistant Professor of Pediatrics, University of Maryland Medical School; Co-Director, Child Protection Team, University Hospital, Division of Pediatric Medicine, Baltimore, Maryland

†Instructor in Psychology, Department of Psychiatry, Harvard Medical School; Director, Victim Recovery Study and Associate in Medicine and Psychiatry, The Children's Hospital, Boston, Massachusetts

‡Medical Director, Las Animas-Huerfano Counties District Health Department, Trinidad, Colorado

§Assistant Professor of Pediatrics, Harvard Medical School; Director, Family Development Study; Senior Associate in Medicine, The Children's Hospital, Boston, Massachusetts

DIVORCE

Between 1955 and 1980, the incidence of divorce rose from about 400,000 to nearly 1,200,000 a year.[75] Since 1980, the rate of divorce has stabilized at approximately one divorce for every two marriages.[75] Rates for children involved in divorce have similarly skyrocketed. Between 1960 and 1984, the number of children involved in divorce each year increased from 460,000 to 1,100,000.[79]

Although divorce may resolve some conflicts, it invariably is associated with considerable stress for the children. The year following divorce is typically marked by chaos in the home, and parents may exhibit compromised coping and parenting skills.[61] Custodial mothers tend to become increasingly restrictive, while noncustodial fathers become more permissive with their children. This can be confusing to children and exacerbate tensions between the parents.

Preschoolers appear to be most vulnerable, particularly in the first year after divorce. Feelings of guilt, abandonment, and grief may manifest in regressive behaviors, depressed play patterns, nightmares, sleep and eating problems, and difficulties with toilet training.[109] Young school-aged children may display "pervasive sadness," with a decline in school performance,[58] whereas older children may feel shame and anger and may develop somatic symptoms.[110] Adolescents experience considerable pain and anger in the immediate postdivorce period but make a relatively rapid recovery.

Children are helped in the postdivorce period if they can maintain a good relationship with both parents.[60] The maintenance of an enduring tie between a boy and his father is especially crucial but is all too infrequent. The pediatrician can play a valuable role by helping the parents deal with their divorce in ways that minimize the traumatic effects on their children. For example, parents must be urged to keep children out of their spousal conflict, and to minimize parental conflict whenever possible. A stable routine of activities in the household also has been associated with improved psychological outcomes.[43]

ADOLESCENT PARENTHOOD

Contrary to public perceptions, there has been a slight decline in the birth rate among adolescents since 1970, although the rate of approximately one half million births per year has been stable over the last decade.[20] In 1983, nearly 14 per cent of all births in the United States were to adolescents.[70] Among adolescents, white girls between the ages of 10 and 14 are the only group that has had an increased birth rate in recent years: a rate of 0.6 births per 1000 girls in 1983 compared to half that number in 1955.[78] The overall rate of childbearing among older teenagers who are *unmarried* also has increased, from 15.1 births per 1000 unmarried 15 to 19 year olds in 1955 to 29.7 in 1983.[78] A gradual decrease in the adolescent birthrate is associated with increasing rates of abortion. Were it not for the availability of abortion, adolescent birthrates would have increased over the past 15 years.

Spivak and Weitzman recently reviewed the deleterious outcomes associated with adolescent pregnancies and conclude that many of the findings are confounded by low social class, making it difficult to separate the effects associated with poverty from those due to the pregnancy per se.[101] The incidence of low birth weight babies is highest among mothers under 15 years,[77] and the infant mortality rate is highest for the offspring of adolescent mothers.[104] This is largely a result of the social and behavioral factors associated with poverty.[67]

Infants of adolescent mothers are at increased risk for sudden infant death syndrome,[5] hospitalization for gastroenteritis, noninflicted injuries, and cognitive deficits.[92, 102] It is uncertain whether they have a higher likelihood of physical abuse.[1] Greater family instability due to the higher rates of marital separation, divorce, and remarriage of adolescent mothers may also contribute to poor outcomes.[104]

The high abortion rates suggest that many of these teenage pregnancies are unintended and unwanted. The pediatrician should inquire about sexual activity and counsel the adolescent about contraception. More attention needs to be paid to adolescent males concerning their contraceptive responsibilities. Pediatricians can also play a valuable role by advocating appropriate sex education for teenagers and facilitating their access to family planning services. In addition, pediatricians need to recognize potential risks to adolescent mothers and their offspring and should provide anticipatory counseling and referrals to diminish those risks.

THE SINGLE PARENT FAMILY

Demographic Trends

Over the last three decades there has been a marked increase in the number of single-parent families, accompanied by a decline since 1970 in the number of families headed by two parents.[39] In 1984, nearly 26 per cent of children were living in single-parent homes, compared with 13 per cent in 1970.[106] Most (89 per cent) of the 6.7 million children in single-parent homes in 1984 were living with their mothers. If current patterns continue, nearly 60 per cent of children born in 1982 will spend at least 1 year living in a single-parent home before they reach 18 years of age,[81] and children who spend their entire childhood in two-parent families will be the minority.[38]

"Single parents" represent a variety of marital patterns. Among female headed households in 1984, 42 per cent of mothers were divorced, 23 per cent were separated, and 7 per cent were widows.[106] However, the segment that has shown the most rapid increase among single-parent households is the "never married," who accounted for 28 per cent of mother-headed families in 1984. It is apparent that the dramatic increase in female-headed households has resulted from increases both in the proportion of never-married mothers (1 per cent of all families in 1970 to 7 per cent in 1984) and from increases in divorced and separated women (8 per cent of all families in 1970 to 21 per cent in 1984).[81]

Another changing pattern in single parent families is a decline in maternal age, from a median of 37.2 years in 1970, to 34.6 years in 1984.[81] This decline in age is due to the increase in younger, never-married mothers as well as to the higher divorce rate among women who marry at very young ages. Fathers who head households tend to be approximately 5 years older than single women heads of households.

Racial differences can also be seen in the distribution of single parent families. In 1984, over one half of black children (59 per cent) lived with a single parent, compared to 20 per cent of white children.[106]

Single Parenthood and Poverty

Single-parent households, and particularly female-headed households, are at a considerable economic disadvantage in comparison with two-parent households. In 1983, the median income for two-parent families was $27,286, for father-headed families $21,845, and for mother-headed families $11,789.[105] Although only a small minority (9 per cent) of two-parent families fall into the lowest income category of under $10,000 a year, most (55 per cent) mother-headed families fall into this income category.[81] Fewer than 20 per cent of mother-headed families have yearly incomes above $20,000.

The implication of these statistics is that *families headed by a woman are likely to be poor,* and, because most children in single-parent families live with their mothers, they too, are poor. In 1983, 22 per cent of all children under 18 years were classified as living below the poverty level. In single-parent families, however, 60 per cent of children in mother-headed households were classified as poor, compared to 26 per cent of children in father-headed households. The increasing prevalence of mother-headed families among those below the poverty level has been referred to as the "feminization of poverty."

The higher income for male subjects reflects both their greater participation in the work force and their higher earning potential, partly as a consequence of differences in educational levels of single mothers and fathers. In 1984, 88 per cent of single fathers, compared to 69 per cent of single mothers, were employed.[81] For women, employment rates are higher for mothers with older children and for divorced women (80 per cent employed) compared to women who have never married (51 per cent employed).

Single-Parent Families and Children's Health

Little is known about the child health consequences of living in a single-parent family. A survey of growth in primary school children in Great Britain reveals shorter stature in children from single-parent families, although this finding diminishes after adjustments are made for parental height and for the children's lower birth weights.[36] A tendency toward obesity in children from single parent families was also detected. However, a recent review of the literature on this topic in the United States and Great Britain concludes that there are *no* demonstrable differences in health status between children in single-parent and two-parent families after other socioeconomic factors are controlled.[53]

In 1984, 37 per cent of families reported for child maltreatment were headed by a single mother, whereas single women headed only 23 per cent of all U.S. families with children under age 18 years.[4] A retrospective study of a random sample of adults found that those raised in single-parent families reported twice the frequency of physical punishment when they were children compared to those from two parent families.[95] While other research has yielded conflicting findings,[13, 25] most of the evidence suggests that single parenthood is a risk factor for child maltreatment. This is not surprising, since childrearing can be extremely stressful without another adult to share the many responsibilities.

Do single parents model different health habits or health-seeking behaviors to their children? A recent survey of middle class families found no significant differences in sleep, exercise, dental hygiene, smoking, alcohol consumption, or dietary habits between single and two-parent families.[62] However, there is a need for preventive education for single parents, as with all parents, and opinion surveys have indicated that single parents desire additional information to help them keep their children safe and healthy.[85]

Functional Consequences for Children in Single-Parent Families

Single-parent families vary greatly, as do other families. Family life varies in relation to the parent's sex, the ages, sexes, and characteristics of the children, and the educational and employment status of the parent. The circumstances that preceded single-parent status are also important; single parenthood following a conflictual divorce and a decline in family income may be quite different for an educated woman in her thirties than single parenthood for a young, unskilled, never-married woman. It is clear that *economic hardship* is a unifying feature for most single-parent families, and many of the consequences for children appear to be linked to this reality. In the past, both clinicians and researchers have viewed single parenthood as deviant, even pathologic, with a focus on negative child outcomes associated with the absence of a father. More recently, attempts have been made to understand the many kinds of single-parent families, to identify strengths as well as weaknesses, and to evaluate the social supports that bolster the family structure.

Surveys of single-parent families have compared daily activities in single and two-parent homes. Although members of households headed by single, employed parents are reported to spend less time on household tasks and personal care, the amount of time spent in parent–child interaction is not significantly different from two-parent families.[96] When socioeconomic status is taken into account, there is no evidence of adverse psychological outcomes in children from single parent homes.[11, 100]

There appears to be a relationship between growing up in a single-parent family and deleterious economic and educational outcomes. In a recent survey of 1448 young adults, individuals raised in single parent homes are found to have *lower educational, occupational, and economic* attainment when compared to young adults raised in two-parent homes, even after controlling for the economic disadvantages associated with single parent families.[70] Similarly, a second study comparing young adult men from single and two-parent homes suggested that coming from single parent homes may be associated with *lower levels of education and income*.[59] This pattern appeared to be most pronounced for the men who lived in single-parent homes during their preschool years. At higher income levels, the difference in educational attainment between the two groups was reduced.

The evidence to date therefore suggests that single-family status, especially when the family is poor, may be stressful for children and may often be associated with lower educational and economic status later in life. Children from single-parent homes, however, are not doomed to lives of failure. There are many mediating factors that can ameliorate these outcomes. One task of future research is to identify factors associated with positive outcomes, in order to develop services more effectively for families headed by single parents. The importance of adequate income is clear, as is the significance of social support to the well-being of single-parent families. Pediatricians and others can function as sources of support; they can also enhance parents' opportunities and abilities to form supportive social networks of their own. Effective means of obtaining child support payments from absent fathers are needed to reduce the number of children living with their mothers in poverty.

STEPFAMILIES

A stepfamily is a family in which at least one adult is a step-parent. Although families with stepfathers are the most common form, there is considerable heterogeneity. There may be stepsiblings from previous marriages, continued involvement of a biologic parent, and varying custody and visiting arrangements. Earlier in this century, stepfamilies were most frequently formed after the death of a parent; currently, most stepfamilies result from remarriage following divorce. Rather than being substitutes, step-parents today are more likely to be added parents.

Each year approximately half a million adults become step-parents, and one out of six American children is a stepchild.[89] This is not surprising given that almost half of marriages since 1980 are ending in divorce[75]; approximately 80 per cent of those who divorce will remarry, and half of those who remarry will marry previously divorced persons. Many of these divorced persons bring children into their remarriages.[89]

What are the effects on children of living in stepfamilies? In the past, a popular assumption has been that living with a step-parent had negative consequences for the child. This has perhaps been fueled by fairy tales portraying wicked stepmothers behaving cruelly toward their stepchildren.[35] This view is reflected in the popular use of the term "stepchild" as a metaphor for unwanted or of low status.

Ganong and Coleman have reviewed the available data on the effects of remarriage on children.[35] Most studies found no differences between stepchildren and children in nuclear or in single-parent families. It is interesting that this was particularly so in the more recent studies, suggesting that the stigma attached to stepfamilies may be diminishing.

Studies of the mental health of stepchildren demonstrate conflicting results. For example, two studies failed to show that stepfathers' presence helped ameliorate negative effects of father absence.[21, 57] In another study, however, the negative effects of father absence were reduced when the stepsons lived for long periods with their stepfathers.[84]

Stepchildren do not appear to differ from other children in their personality characteristics, or in their cognitive and intellectual achievements.[35] Similarly, family relationships among individual members in stepfamilies differed little from other families in perceptions of parental happiness and family conflict,[90] reciprocal confiding, supportiveness, and trust between mothers and daughters,[32] and observed step-parent–child and parent–child interactions.[97] Most stepchildren reported liking their step-parents and getting along well with them.[22] Although a few studies found stepchildren to have problems in their social behavior, these studies were conducted early in the development of these children's new stepfamilies.[21, 57] Most of the data suggest no differences compared to children in other families.

Lutz interviewed 103 students between the ages of 12 and 18 years in an attempt to identify potential stresses associated with living in stepfamilies.[63] The adolescents reported relatively low levels of stress; in 9 out of 11 potentially stressful areas they more frequently marked "nonstressful" than "stressful." The areas causing the most difficulty were those of divided loyalty and discipline.

Divided loyalty refers to conflicted or negative feelings because of conflict or guilt about their positive feelings for another person.[91] "Experiencing one natural parent talking negatively about the other natural parent" and "feeling caught in the middle between two parents" were especially painful for the adolescents. Discipline referred to the establishment and enforcement of family rules. "Adjusting to living with a new set of rules from your step-parent" and "accepting discipline from a step-parent" were reported as being particularly stressful. Lutz suggests that it might be difficult for adolescents to accept rules from an "outsider," but adds that discipline is often a problem during adolescence and is hardly unique to stepfamilies. Most importantly, living in stepfamilies was not felt to be particularly stressful as reflected by the overall scores.

Several studies demonstrate that children living with stepfathers are more likely to be maltreated by them.[65, 111] However, this body of research was conducted only on *reported* cases of child maltreatment, with the potential problem of biased diagnoses and reporting by professionals maintaining negative stereotypes of step-fathers. The National Incidence Study (1981) offers more useful findings because it is based on both reported cases of child maltreatment and cases that were known to professionals and agencies but had not necessarily been reported to child protection services.[76] In this study, stepfathers were the perpetrators in 30 per cent of cases involving sexual abuse and in 18 per cent of cases of maltreatment. Glick has estimated that in 1978, the year in which data for the Incidence Study were collected, 1 in 10 children lived with a step-parent, usually a stepfather.[38] This indicates that stepfathers *are* significantly over-represented as perpertrators of maltreatment, particularly of sexual abuse. However, Giles-Sims and Finkelhor have pointed out that Glick did not include step-parents not living with their children in his estimate, and did not control for the increased likelihood that poor children have for living in a stepfamily. They conclude that "adequate testing of whether children are at an unusually high risk of abuse from stepparents requires data on rates of abuse in different family structures controlling for many socio-demographic characteristics."[37]

What are the factors that appear to influence how children adjust to stepfamily life? The age of the child is understandably important, and preadolescent, school-aged children have been found to be especially vulnerable to the stresses associated with remarriage of the resident parent.[108] The step-parent–stepchild relationship is crucial and has been found to be a better predictor of the child's adjustment than the quality of the relationship with the nonresident natural parent.[33] Still, most studies suggest that regular contact with the nonresident father helps post-divorce adjustment,[48] although it is unclear whether this continues after the resident parent remarries.

Girls have been found to have more difficult relationships with stepfathers than do boys.[17] It is important to recognize that these relationships are dynamic processes and are likely to change over time; short-term adjustment problems may be resolved as an equilibrium of family roles and relationships is established.[18] Timing is an important factor; if the remarriage occurs abruptly or before the child is ready to accept a new parent, this can be stressful; if, on the other hand, a substantial period has elapsed with the child living with a single parent, a close bond might have formed, making it difficult for the child to share the natural resident parent.

Ganong and Coleman are careful to point out the methodologic shortcomings in much of the research on stepfamilies, and the significant limitations in our knowledge.[35] It is striking that while research on nonclinical populations presents a rather favorable picture of stepfamilies, this is not the case in the clinical studies. Since clinical research is conducted on people who are sufficiently distressed to seek or be referred for professional help, it is to be expected that significantly more problems would be encountered.

It is important that pediatricians abandon stereotypes of stepfamilies. Stepfamilies vary greatly and the effects on children, particularly in the long term, are not necessarily negative. Indeed there can be substantial benefits if an absent parent is replaced, the natural parent gains the love and support of a new spouse, and the economic difficulties of single-parent families are alleviated.

There are a number of ways that pediatricians can facilitate adjustment in stepfamilies. Many children might still be unaware that many of their friends also live in stepfamilies. Discussing this with them can be comforting, and children should be encouraged to express their feelings and thoughts about their stepfamilies, especially regarding divided loyalties and discipline. The pediatrician is then able to assess whether any problems can be addressed adequately by counseling in the office or whether a referral is needed.

Parents need to appreciate that it is very important that their children be excluded from spousal conflict, and that the more effective their communication with each other, the better for their children. Pediatricians can help families to clearly define the caregiving roles of different family members. Young children in particular require a clear understanding of family roles. Step-parents are often uncertain of their roles and may feel awkward, for example, concerning such issues as discipline. It seems advisable that they conform to the approaches used by the parent with custody, especially in the early phase of the new family. There are a variety of written materials for helping both adults and children in stepfamilies[89]; the pediatrician ought to be familiar with some of these to make appropiate recommendations. As always, pediatricians need to recognize situations that are beyond his or her abilities to manage, and to make suitable referrals.

MATERNAL EMPLOYMENT

In preindustrial U.S. society, it was common for women to work. With industrialization, work and home were separated, and men had jobs outside the home while a woman's place was "in the home." This was the situation during the Victorian period; few women were employed in the first part of this century. The number of employed women increased during World War II, with governmental support and encouragement, and by 1947, 19 per cent of women with children under age 18 were in the labor force.[54, 81] By 1984, this figure had more than tripled, with 61 per cent of women with children under age 18 years employed outside the home.* Nearly 50 per cent of women with children under 3 years and almost 60 per cent with children under 6 were working in 1984; women with young children are the fastest growing segment of the female work force. More women who are separated or divorced are likely to work than are those who are currently married.[66] It is, however, among married women with children that the increase has been most marked; from 1960 to 1985 the number of married women with children under 6 years who were employed full-time rose from 19 to 53 per cent.[103]

There are a number of reasons why more women are working today. Marital instability and the high divorce rate have led to many single-parent families, where the mothers' earnings are often the sole source of family income. In married families, mothers working full-time contributed 40 per cent of the family income, and the median family income in 1983 was $32,110 if both parents worked, compared to $21,890 if the mother did not work.[105] In short, many women work because of financial necessity.

It is also evident that many women work because of career aspirations and the satisfaction and sense of achievement that they derive through work. In 1976, 76 per cent of a national sample of working women said that they would continue working even if they did not have to.[23] Hoffman has suggested that a decrease in the amount of time required for homemaking and in the number of children per family, have made employment more psychologically important for the mother.[50] Even when work is not that satisfying, the personal interactions can be a valuable relief from the social isolation and loneliness that many homemakers experience. It is in this context that the views expressed by the women's movement have influenced women to aspire to the range of opportunities that men have long enjoyed. One result of the increased proportion of working women has been a sense of inadequacy felt by mothers who remain at home with their children, feeling that they "should" go out to work.[12]

Women's participation in the labor force has generated concern about possible ill effects on children. Prior to 1960, many assumed that maternal employment resulted in negative outcomes and research in the field attempted to prove or disprove this hypothesis. More recently, researchers have begun to consider potential benefits for children whose mothers work.

Several extensive reviews of the literature on the effects of maternal employment on children have led to a consensus that there is not a direct causal effect between a mother working and a particular child outcome.[46, 113] Quality of substitute care and maternal role satisfaction,[52] family stability and paternal attitude toward maternal employment,[86] and quality of time spent with children[28] appear to be more important factors than maternal employment per se in determining child outcomes. A panel supported by the National Institute of Education concluded that maternal employment cannot be viewed as a single, uniform phenomenon. Many intervening

---

*The authors readily acknowledge that housework and child care are certainly types of work. To conform with popular usage, employment and work refer to out-of-home-work in this article.

factors such as the type of work, the woman's reason for working, maternal and paternal attitudes towards a mother's work, and the family's adaptation to the work all affect children's adaptation, development, and behavior.[9, 54]

At this time, no clear conclusions can be drawn about the effects of maternal employment on children. The child's age and developmental level are important factors. We will briefly review what is known about the effects of maternal employment at different stages.

Prenatal Period

Zuckerman et al. examined the impact of pregnant women's work outside the home on neonatal outcome.[115] Of 1507 low income women, 55 per cent did not work outside the home or attend school, 7 per cent worked into the third trimester in a standing position, and 38 per cent had other work histories or attended school. Possible confounding factors such as the mothers' health habits were controlled. No adverse effects of any type of work were found on the length of gestation or on the newborn's weight and head circumference.

According to Zuckerman and his colleagues, these findings are consistent with research findings from Europe, although two earlier American studies showed lower birth weights resulting from maternal employment: a 150- to 400-gm decrease in the first study[71] and 31- to 61-gm in the second.[64] These discrepancies may be due to changes in the work force, working conditions, obstetrical care, and womens' health, and methodologic differences. They conclude that low income women who are healthy, have apparently low-risk pregnancies, and feel well enough to work may do so into the third trimester without jeopardizing the health of their infants.

There has been little research examining the impact of specific types of work on pregnancy outcome. Obviously, particular occupations present certain hazards or toxic exposures that can endanger the fetus. One study found a significantly increased rate of fetal deaths associated with work in textile mills and in printing and publishing industries.[99] Presumably, these increased risks pertain to specific jobs within these industries where women are exposed to certain toxins. Results of one study suggest an increased risk of spontaneous abortion may be associated with working more than 20 hours per week in front of video display terminals.[15] More information is needed to identify the pregnancy risks of specific types of work.

Early Childhood

There has been relatively little research on the effects of maternal employment on infants and children. Controversy has surrounded the issue of attachment between mother and child, which is thought to be an important developmental precursor of trust, a sense of security, and later abilities to relate well interpersonally. This question will be addressed in the section on substitute care. The quality and consistency of child care during early childhood may be a greater predictor of a child's development than whether or not the mother is working.

It is important that the mother's work not be so stressful or exhausting that it compromises her ability to nurture her infant.[12] There is research evidence that the quality of time spent together with the child may be more important than the amount of time. For example, a study of middle-class preschoolers found that they had similar amounts of one-to-one contact with their working or nonworking mothers,[114] and it appears that many working mothers make extra efforts to set aside time for their children, rather than pursuing other individual interests. Working mothers may be more likely to overindulge and underdiscipline their children, however.[50]

Zimmerman and Bernstein followed a group of 200 white, middle-class mothers and infants to examine the impact of different maternal work patterns on the development of the children.[114] The mothers were either working part time or full time, or not employed, and the childrens' social, emotional, and cognitive development were assessed at 1, 3, and 6 years of age. There was no evidence of negative effects associated with maternal employment. Other research has indicated that the social adjustment and competence of preschoolers may be enhanced by having working mothers.[40]

School-aged Children

During this period, the father becomes increasingly important in the socialization of the child. Research demonstrates that husbands of employed women help more with house work and child care, although the women continue to carry the bulk of these responsibilities.[46] Consequently, the children of employed mothers have less rigid, traditional stereotypes of sex roles, particularly if the mother performs work that is not traditionally associated with females.

Daughters of employed women are more likely to admire their mothers and to hold the female role in high esteem compared to girls whose mothers are not employed.[51] In her review of the literature, Hoffman concluded that there is a fairly consistent picture that daughters of employed mothers are higher achievers than daughters of nonworking mothers.[50] Other researchers have found that children whose mothers do not work outside the home tend to be more adult oriented and to conform to adult standards, compared to children of working mothers, who appear to be more peer oriented and nonconformist.[30] This is particularly so for boys.

Sons of employed mothers have been found to see women as more competent and men as warmer than sons of mothers who remain at home.[51] Hoffman and others have found that in low-income families, maternal employment has been associated with a strain in the father–son relationship, perhaps reflecting the sons' perceptions that the inadequacy of their fathers' earnings requires their mothers to work.[50] No impact has been found regarding the boys' cognitive abilities, and both sons and daughters of employed, lower class mothers do better in school. The relationship between full-time mothering and the sons' academic achievements *in middle-class families* is not clear. Although most studies show no effect of maternal employment, lower IQs and academic scores have been reported.[50]

Adolescence

Maternal employment has been shown to be beneficial for both adolescent sons and daughters. For example, the adolescents in one study were found to show better social adjustment, a greater sense of personal worth, more feeling of belonging, and better relationships with family members and peers at school.[41] While the focus thus far has been on the effects of maternal employment on children, it is apparent that maternal employment is an important influence on the parents and the family system.

Hoffman points out that many of the needs of adolescents mesh well with their mother's need to work. The adolescent is becoming increasingly independent and spending a decreasing amount of time at home; parents are often undergoing their own developmental crises, with concerns about aging, anticipation of the empty nest, and possible marital difficulties. In a study comparing educated full-time mothers to professionally employed mothers, the former were found to have lower self-esteem, perceived themselves as less attractive and more lonely, felt less competent, and expressed more concern over identity issues.[10] Being a full-time mother with an adolescent child(ren) can be very stressful, and employment might offer a satisfying solution. The mother's satisfaction with her role appears to increase her effectiveness as a parent.

At the family level, the socioeconomic status of the family is a significant contributor to children's overall well-being.[50] Although higher income does not guarantee a better developmental outcome, poverty is often associated with adverse effects on children and families. The mother's earnings may be particularly important to poorer families,[30] enabling them to rise above the poverty level, and to two-parent families, in which the additional income alleviates financial worries and offers the children greater opportunities.

In summary, maternal employment alone does not appear to exert significant negative effects on children, and adolescents appear to benefit substantially from having their mothers employed. No clear harm has been found in the infancy period, although concerns related to substitute care are unresolved. There are multiple and interacting factors influencing the development of children, and maternal employment is but one of them.

What is an appropriate role for a pediatrician in advising a mother regarding the impact on her children of working outside her home? It is critical to recognize that maternal employment has become increasingly common and to appreciate the reasons for this, and the pediatrician needs to convey accurate information on the effects of work on the family. In addition, it is necessary to cast aside personal bias and to assist the mother in making the decision that is right for her and her family. A national survey of 5758 pediatricians found that there were generally positive attitudes toward maternal employment, and that they were supportive of women working outside the home.[47] However, older pediatricians, men, and those with unemployed spouses had less favorable attitudes.

The American Academy of Pediatrics has issued guidelines for pediatricians advising mothers about employment.[3] These include (1) evaluating the availability of quality substitute care for the child, the mother's satisfaction with her work, support of her family, and her residual vitality to nurture her child; (2) assessing the adequacy of the substitute care; (3) alerting the mother to possible ill effects on the child; (4) counseling the mother with regard to the timing of a return to work following the birth of her baby; and (5) anticipatory guidance of feelings and reactions that may arise in her or her family due to her working. In addition, the Academy suggests that pediatricians can make a valuable contribution by supporting subsidized parental leave after the birth of a newborn baby and by encouraging the involvement of fathers in child care and household work.

CHILD CARE

As maternal participation in the work force has increased, so has the demand for substitute child care. In the past, women relied primarily on members of their extended families to provide this service, but the increasing mobility of American families has led to the decreasing availability of such help. In 1985, 45 per cent of children under 3 in substitute care were cared for by a relative (27 per cent in their own home, 18 per cent in a relative's) and 24 per cent were cared for in family day care.[55] A minority of children attended day care centers.

A major difficulty confronting many families is the shortage of quality and affordable child care.[56] According to Census Bureau statistics, 45 per cent of single mothers not in the work force reported that they would work if affordable child care were available.[16] In single-parent families, maternal employment is more likely if child care by extended family members is an option.

An important question related to maternal employment concerns the possible effects on children who spend a substantial amount of time in substitute care. Whereas there have been good experience and research data regarding substitute care for children over 3 years of age in out of home settings, less information is available concerning infants and toddlers. There are nurseries that accept infants as young as 3 weeks of age, and increasingly mothers are returning to work within 2 or 3 months after delivering. An increasing number of American infants and toddlers are being raised jointly in their natural families and by substitute caregivers.

As in the case of maternal employment, it has been difficult to discern specific effects of child care on children. Firstly, there exists enormous heterogeneity both within and among different types of child care; the nurturant qualities of the caregivers, the ratio of infants to caregivers, and the quality and safety of the facility are some of the factors likely to be influential. There is obviously a difference if the child is cared for by one sitter in the family home compared to attending a center with multiple caregivers and a significant turnover of staff (as is frequently the case).

Secondly, the type of child care is only one of many factors that influences the child's development. Accordingly, one view holds that any single factor, such as type of care, is unlikely to have a great influence.[6] In contrast, Belsky, perhaps differing more in perspective than in basic ideas, sees early child care as a major influence during an important period in the young child's life, with significant short-term and long-term ramifications.[8] More empiric research is needed to assess these hypotheses.

In addition to the methodologic shortcomings of many studies of the impact of infant care, most of the research has been conducted on stable, middle-class families using high-quality centers. There is limited generalizability of these findings to the wide range of poor to excellent day care centers. Relatively little is known about the effects of family day care and sitter arrangements, which is where most infants are in care, and these should be compared to infants not in substitute care.

There have been several reviews of studies on the effects of infant day care, but there is no consensus whether infants who experience regular nonparental care have negative psychological outcomes.[34, 94] Research has focused on the attachment relationship between mothers and their infants, which is thought to reflect a sense of emotional security and to be important for developing trust and interpersonal relationships. A number of studies have not found any impact of infant day care on this relationship. Still, failure to demonstrate ill effects is not proof that none exist. Reviewers such as Rutter have been cautious to conclude "although day-care for very young children is not likely to result in serious emotional disturbances, it would be misleading to conclude that it is without risks or effect. Much depends on the quality of the day-care, and on the age, characteristics, and family circumstances of the child."[94]

Most recently, Gamble and Zigler reviewed studies in which deleterious effects have been found.[34] One study reported that infants of mothers employed full time were more likely to avoid their mothers compared to those who were home reared, and infants of mothers working part time had an intermediate response.[98] In another study, infants were examined at 12 and 18 months of age, and a disproportionate number of infants whose mothers had returned to work before their first birthdays were found to be anxious and avoidant with their mothers.[107]

Another area that has been examined concerns children's social interactions with peers and adults. Again, a number of studies have not found any differences between infants who attended day care and those who were home reared,[93] whereas others have shown effects.[29] An example of the latter is a study that found lower social class males in group care were less enthusiastic, less compliant, and had a more negative affect than peers who remained at home or who started care after 18 months.[29] Another study of over 400 low-income children in family, group, and home care found that the group care children fared as well or better than those reared at home, but children in family day care were more competent linguistically, emotionally, and in social interactions with adults than were children in group care.[42] Gamble and Zigler conclude that children who have experienced early group care tend toward assertiveness, aggression, and peer orientation rather than adult orientation. A number of studies have demonstrated these characteristics to be more common for boys.[34]

Infants in group care have been found to have an increased incidence of intestinal infections, influenza, and colds.[45] Careful hygiene and handwashing are key to reducing these risks. There have been a fair number of widely publicized instances of sexual abuse of children in day care settings. At times, this has involved reputable centers and instances in which the abuse was occurring over years, apparently unsuspected by any parents. It seems likely that this is a problem in a very small minority of facilities.

At this time, the effects of infant day care are not conclusive and several studies yield contradictory findings that are difficult to reconcile. Nevertheless, there is some indication that group care is not optimal for infants and that it might place some infants at risk for problems in their socioemotional development. This does not mean that there will necessarily be negative outcomes; rather, it suggests that certain infants in vulnerable circumstances are more likely to have particular difficulties in group care.

The uncertain effects of infant day care make it difficult for pediatricians to advise families. Ultimately, each situation needs to be weighed individually. It appears that there might be some risk associated with group care for infants, but this is just one factor, albeit an important one, in considering a family's situation. There might be other over-riding considerations requiring the infant to be in care. Perhaps the optimal alternative to parental care is having a nurturing person care for just one or two infants. However, the costs for this care may make such care a luxury beyond the means of most families.

There are helpful guidelines on substitute care, such as those issued by the American Academy of Pediatrics.[2] A spirit of sharing in the care of an infant between the substitute provider(s) and the parents, the ability of parents to drop in at any time, an appropriate ratio of staff to children, a pleasant and safe facility, and the nurturant qualities of the provider(s) are all important aspects of day care. In addition, consideration of the parents' needs and feelings is critical in helping a family make the decision that is best for them.

Substitute care is also an issue for many school-aged children. It is estimated that between 2 and 5 million children 6 to 13 years of age regularly return home from school to an empty home; these are called "latch-key" children.[31] Some communities have attempted to address the problem with after-school programs, but these are not adequate to meet current needs. One strategy has been telephone hotlines that allow children in self-care to call an adult if they are bored, lonely, afraid, or injured. The quality of these services varies substantially. The long-term psychological effects of self-care are unknown and given the possible risks, research in this area is needed.

POVERTY

During the 1960s, the rate of children living in poverty decreased from 25 to approximately 15 per cent.[20] It began to rise in the late 1970s, and approximately one in four U.S. children is now living in poverty.[16] Children living in households headed by single women, while constituting 20 per cent of the nation's children, included nearly half (49 per cent) of all poor children in 1983.[82] Similarly, minority children comprise one quarter of U.S. children, but account for nearly one half of poor children.[20] In 1983, 70 per cent of children living in households headed by minority, single females were poor.

Low birth weight and an increased infant mortality rate are significantly correlated with poverty,[112] as is childhood mortality.[80] One study showed that children in families on welfare had a risk of death three times greater than those not on welfare.[80] There is also a significant morbidity associated with poverty, reflected in the risks for lead poisoning,[68] iron deficiency anemia,[24] growth deficits,[68] and psychosocial and psychosomatic illnesses.[68] Immunization rates are significantly lower in impoverished areas; in 1982, 66 per cent of black preschoolers were not properly immunized.[68]

Poverty also exerts tremendous influences on the mental health and development of children. One major study found that poverty more than any other single factor was associated with psychological problems and with a variety of learning difficulties.[74] A longitudinal study of physically abused children showed that their poor outcomes were similar to the comparison group.[27] Both groups of children were poor, and the conclusion of the study was that the abuse did not appear to add further harm beyond the damaging impact of poverty.

Helping families grappling with poverty presents a difficult challenge to pediatricians. Pediatricians hold positions of influence in society, and they can become effective advocates for social and health policies and programs that will enhance the health of children. An example is the area of health insurance; in 1982, 16 per cent of children had no coverage.[73] In addition, pediatricians should be aware of and refer families to available resources such as the Women, Infants and Children (WIC) Nutrition Program; voluntary social support services; and the Headstart Program because these help prevent some of the poor outcomes associated with poverty.

HOMELESS FAMILIES

Although precise numbers of homeless families have been difficult to estimate, a 1986 hearing in the U.S. House of Representatives drew attention to striking increases in this population.[19] Approximately 25 per cent of the homeless population consists of families, typically single mothers with two or three, usually preschool, children.[7] Mowbray has delineated several of the realities concerning the homeless: most homeless people are desperately looking for a place to live, the contribution by deinstitutionalization of the mentally ill is not clear, the extent of the problem is a new development, although the underpinning poverty is obviously not, and long term solutions are needed, not more shelter beds.[69]

Bassuk and Rubin have reported a study on 82 homeless Massachusetts families and their 156 children.[7] Results of the Denver Developmental Screening Test indicated that 47 per cent of the 81 preschoolers had at least one developmental delay, 33 per cent had two or more, and 14 per cent had four. The children manifested increased sleep problems, shyness, withdrawal, and aggression. Over half of the 42 school-aged children were sufficiently depressed to warrant a psychiatric evaluation, and a majority had thought about suicide. At school, 43 per cent were reported as failing or below average, 25 per cent were in special classes, and 43 per cent had repeated a grade.

The enormous stress confronting these children and their families is not difficult to imagine. Pediatricians must attend to the special health and psychological vulnerabilities of these children, referring to mental health professionals when necessary, and assisting the family in securing access to resources in the community. It is apparent that homelessness is a complex and devastating problem. Pediatricians can be advocates for efforts to find decent, long-term solutions.

ADDITIONAL CHANGES IN THE AMERICAN FAMILY

There are several additional changes in the American family that warrant mention, although little is known of their effects on children.

The ready availability of birth control and family planning clinics, and the legalization of abortion, should result in most babies being planned and wanted. However, these options are not always used. Of all births to *married* women in 1982, 10 per cent were "unwanted" around the time of conception, compared to 14 per cent in 1973.[88] Twenty-five per cent of births to *never married* women were "unwanted," and only 21 per cent were deliberately conceived by stopping or not using contraceptives.

There has been an increasing acceptance of the needs and rights of children in American society. This has been part of the Civil Rights movement, which began in the 1950s and gained momentum in the ensuing decades. This movement drew public attention to the predicament of the disempowered and dispossessed: the poor, minorities, and children. Public awareness was increased and consciousness raised, and consequently a new appreciation of children's rights evolved. An example of the application of this are the federal and state laws to protect children from maltreatment. Children now have the right to be protected from maltreatment, and each state is mandated to intervene on their behalf. Still, it is clear to child advocates that much work remains. It can be argued that despite rhetoric to the contrary, the limited resources allocated to children and families reflects the low priority of children in this society.

A related issue is the growth in knowledge regarding the influence of physical and environmental factors on the health and development of children. This new information has been very accessible through coverage by the popular media, and entire sections in book stores also are devoted to topics on childhood and parenting. It might be expected that parents today are more knowledgeable and competent in their parenting as a result of this information. However, knowledge is only one facet of parenting, and changes in parenting across generations are difficult to measure.

In his book, "The Hurried Child," David Elkind has described the high expectations that parents may impose on children to acquire a variety of skills at early ages.[26] This may result in substantial stress and pressure, with deleterious psychological outcomes for the children who are unable to meet these demands. Examples include endeavors that provide exercise classes for toddlers, aggressively encourage academic achievement in preschoolers, and the immense pressures on school athletes. Although some children might benefit from this stimulation, others may not. The nature of childhood, Elkind argues, is sometimes drastically altered, with much of the fun being replaced by the aggressive pursuit of academic and athletic achievements.

From 1957 to 1976, the average number of births per woman decreased from 3.7 to 1.8, and family size decreased.[87] This could lead to a greater investment in these children, but the many possible reasons for smaller families make it unclear whether this is so. In addition, smaller families mean fewer siblings and smaller extended families. This may contribute to the loss of important support.

In addition, there has been a trend toward marriage at a later age for women and men, and correspondingly, childbearing has been deferred. This is illustrated by examining birth rates according to maternal age from 1955 to 1983.[73] Birth rates for women of all ages have decreased, except for increases for women in their thirties, and particularly for those 30 to 34 years of age. There has also been a decline in first birth rates for women in their twenties.

Marriage at an older age has been associated with a decreased likelihood of divorce. In addition, parents who are older may be better established in their work and more secure financially, and thus may diminish the risk of poverty for their offspring. The statistics on divorce and on poverty cited earlier, however, indicate that the positive impact of marriage at an older age has not been sufficient to counter other influences leading to the increasing number of divorced couples and impoverished children.

The mobility of Americans is a striking feature of this society. Between 1980 and 1985, 40 per cent of the population moved, including 50 per cent of 5 to 9 year olds.[14] This diminishes the ability of extended family to sustain contact and provide support. In addition, frequent moves may make it difficult to develop deep and enduring friendships, which require time and shared experiences. Although it is often noted how children appear to adapt more easily than adults, it is not known how family mobility affects them.

CONCLUSION

It is evident that there have been dramatic changes in the American family in recent decades. Some of these, such as poverty, divorce, single-parent families, and adolescent pregnancies, clearly exert negative impacts on the lives of many families and their children. Other trends, toward smaller family size, the increased awareness of the rights of children, and our greater understanding of their needs, offer hope for a positive outlook for children. However, all changes demand major adjustments and present our society with formidable challenges to find strategies that facilitate the healthy growth and development of children and families.

Families are our most basic and precious social unit, and there has been an increasing appreciation of the relationship between families and institutions, including government.[83] Ooms argues that the myth of family self-sufficiency has been dispelled, and that most critical family functions are now shared on a day-to-day basis with a variety of public and private institutions.[83] Rather than labeling families as functional (healthy) or dysfunctional (problematic), she sees a continuum of need for connection and support. The question then is how can our society, through its institutions (primarily local, state, and federal governments), appropriately support families?

In the public sector, there is a need for a family-oriented approach in the development and implementation of policies and programs that impact, directly and indirectly, upon families. The partial elimination of the marriage penalty in the income tax code, the strengthening of the dependent care tax credit, and a current bill in Congress for parental leave after the birth or adoption of a baby are some examples of policies helpful to families. In contrast, inadequate federal support by the present administration for programs that administer Food Stamps, Medicaid, Aid for Families with Dependent Children (AFDC), school lunch, and day care has seriously hurt many families.[16]

The principle that needs to be established as a priority is the importance of families and children, and the constructive role that institutions should play in supporting them. Some issues such as divorce are not amenable to governmental remedy. Others, including homelessness, poverty, and the shortage of substitute child care, require a substantial commitment by local, state, and federal governments. In addition, the private sector should contribute; employment practices that include comprehensive health benefits for the family, reasonable parental leave policies, and the provision of day care facilities are a few examples.

How can the pediatrician help to strengthen the changing American family? Much of what has been described in this article pertains to "the new morbidity," the psychosocial problems confronting many families that are an increasing concern for pediatricians.[44] The Task Force on Pediatric Education confirmed that pediatricians frequently are confronted with these problems in clinical practice and are interested in learning more about them. There is a definite need at both the residency and postresidency levels for training that will enhance the competency of pediatricians in the psychosocial domain.

Pediatricians need to be sensitive to signs and symptoms that children might manifest in connection with issues such as divorce, father absence, and homelessness. Often the pediatrician can make a useful contribution by counseling families on how to deal with these problems. In addition, it is necessary to be familiar with other resources in the community and to facilitate referrals when appropriate. Finally, pediatricians can be effective advocates for children. Whether at the family, community, state, or federal level, we can work for practices, policies, and programs that will enhance the lives of children.

ACKNOWLEDGMENTS

The authors would like to thank the editors and Diana Zuckerman for their helpful comments, and Lynn Menefee, Ann Lazur, and Jan Roberts for their assistance in preparing the manuscript for the article.

REFERENCES

1. Altemeier WA, O'Connor S, Vietze PM et al: Antecedents of child abuse. J Pediatr 100:823, 1982
2. American Academy of Pediatrics: Tips on selecting the "right" day care facility. Elk Grove Village, Illinois, American Academy of Pediatrics, 1985
3. American Academy of Pediatrics: The mother working outside the home. Pediatrics 73:874–875, 1984
4. American Association for Protecting Children: Highlights of Official Child Neglect and Abuse Reporting 1984. Denver, The American Humane Association, 1986
5. Babson SG, Clarke NG: Relationship between infant death and maternal age. J Pediatr 103:391, 1983
6. Barglow P: Some further comments about infant day-care research. Zero to Three 7:26–28, 1987
7. Bassuk E, Rubin L: Homeless children: A neglected population. Am J Orthopsychiatry 57:279–286, 1987
8. Belsky J: Infant day-care: A cause for concern? Zero to Three 7:1–7, 1986
9. Benedek RS, Benedek EP: Children of divorce: Can we meet their needs? J Soc Issues 35:155, 1979
10. Birnbaum JA: Life patterns and self-esteem in gifted family oriented and career committed women. In Mednick MS, Tangri SS, Hoffman LW (eds): Women and Achievement. Washington, D.C., Hemisphere, 1975
11. Blechman EA: Are children with one parent at psychological risk? A methodological review. J Marriage Fam 44:179, 1982
12. Brazelton TB: Issues for working parents. Am J Orthopsychiatry 56:14–25, 1986
13. Brunnquell D, et al.: Maternal personality and attitude in disturbances of child rearing. Am J Orthopsychiatry 51:680, 1981
14. Bureau of Census: U.S.A. Statistics in Brief. Washington, D.C., U.S. Department of Commerce, 1987
15. Butler WJ, Brix KA: Video display terminal work and pregnancy outcome in Michigan clerical workers. Unpublished data
16. Children's Defense Fund: A Children's Defense Budget: An Analysis of the President's FY 1986 Budget and Children. Washington, D.C., Children's Defense Fund, 1985
17. Clingempeel WG, Segal S: Stepparent-stepchild relationships and the psychological adjustment of children in stepmother and stepfather families. Child Dev 57:474–484, 1986
18. Clingempeel WG, Brand E, Ievoli R: Stepparent-stepchild relationships in stepmother and stepfather families: A multi-method study. Fam Relat 33:465–473, 1984

19. Committee on Government Operations. U.S. House of Representatives: Homeless Families: A Neglected Crisis. Washington, D.C., Government Printing Office, 1986
20. Congress of the United States Congressional Budget Office: Reducing Poverty Among Children. Washington, D.C., Congressional Budget Office, 1985
21. Dahl BB, McCubbin HL, Lester GR: War-induced father absence: Comparing the adjustment of children in reunited, non-reunited, and reconstituted families. Int J Soc Fam 6:99–108, 1976
22. Duberman L: Step-kin relationships. J Marriage Fam 35:283–292, 1973
23. Dubnoff SJ, Veroff J, Kulka RA: Adjustment to work: 1957–1976. Paper presented at the meeting of the American Psychological Association, Toronto, August, 1978
24. Egbuone L, Starfield B: Child health and social status. Pediatrics 69:550, 1982
25. Egeland B et al: A prospective study of the antecedents of child abuse. Minneapolis, University of Minnesota, 1979
26. Elkind D: The Hurried Child: Growing Up Too Fast Too Soon. Reading, Mass, Addison-Wesley, 1981
27. Elmer E: Follow-up study of traumatized children. Pediatrics 59:273, 1977
28. Etaugh C: Effects of maternal employment on children: Review of recent research. Merrill Palmer Q 20:71, 1974
29. Farber E, Egeland B: Developmental consequences of out-of-home care for infants in a low income population. In Zigler E, Gorden E (eds): Day Care: Scientific and Social Policy Issues. Boston, Auburn House, 1982
30. Ferber MA, Birnbaum B: The impact of mothers' work on the family as an economic system. In Kamerman SB, Hayes CD (eds): Families That Work: Children in a Changing World. Washington, D.C., National Academy Press, 1983
31. Fosarelli P: Children in self-care: A new priority for pediatricians. Pediatrics 77:548, 1986
32. Fox GL, Inazu JK: The influence of mothers' marital history on the mother-daughter relationship in black and white households. J Marriage Fam 44:143–153, 1982
33. Furstenberg FF, Seltzer JA: Divorce and child development. Paper presented at the meeting of the Orthopsychiatric Association, Boston, 1983
34. Gamble TJ, Zigler E: Effects of infant day care: Another look at the evidence. Am J Orthopsychiatry 56:26–42, 1986
35. Ganong LH, Coleman M: The effects of remarriage on children: A review of the empirical literature. Fam Relat 33:389–406, 1984
36. Garman AR, Chinn S, Rona RJ: Comparative growth of private school children from one and two-parent families. Arch Dis Child 57:453, 1982
37. Giles-Sims J, Finkelhor D: Child abuse in step-families. Fam Relat 33:407–413, 1984
38. Glick PC: Marriage, divorce, and living arrangements. J Fam Issues 5:7, 1984
39. Glick PC: The American household structure in transition. Fam Plann Perspect 16:205, 1984
40. Gold D, Andres D: Relations between maternal employment and development of nursery school children. Can J Behav Sc 10:116–129, 1978
41. Gold D, Andres D: Developmental comparisons between adolescent children with employed and non-employed mothers. Merrill-Palmer Q 24:243, 1978
42. Golden M, et al: The New York Infant Day Care Study. New York, Medical and Health Research Association of New York, 1978
43. Guidubaldi J, Cleminshaw H: Divorce, family health, and child adjustment. Fam Relat 34:35, 1985
44. Haggerty RJ: The changing role of the physician in child health care. Am J Dis Child 127:545–549, 1974
45. Haskins R, Kotch J: Day-care and illness: Evidence, costs, and public policy. Pediatrics 77(Suppl):951–982, 1986
46. Hayes CD, Kamerman SD (eds): Children of Working Parents: Experiences and Outcomes. Washington, D.C., National Academy Press, 1983
47. Heins M, Stillman P, Sabers D et al: Attitudes of pediatricians toward maternal employment. Pediatrics 72:283–290, 1983
48. Hess RD, Camara KA: Post-divorce relationships as mediating factors in the consequences of divorce for children. J Soc Issues 35:79–96, 1979
49. Hill MS: Trends in the economic situation of U.S. families and children: 1970–1981. In

Nelson RR, Skidmore F (eds): American Families and the Economy: The High Cost of Living. Washington, D.C., National Academy Press, 1983

50. Hoffman LW: Effects of maternal employment on the child: A review of the research. Dev Psych 10:204–228, 1974

51. Hoffman LW: Maternal employment: 1979. Am Psych 34:859–865, 1979

52. Howell M: Effects of maternal employment on the child: II. Pediatrics 52:327, 1973

53. Jennings AJ, Sheldon MG: Review of the health of children in one-parent families. JR Coll Gen Pract 35:478, 1985

54. Kamerman SB, Hayes CD (eds): Families That Work: Children in a Changing World. Washington, D.C., National Academy Press, 1982

55. Kamerman SB: Child-care services: The national picture. Mon Labor Rev 106:35, 1983

56. Kamerman S: Infant care usage in the United States. Report presented to the National Academy of Sciences Ad hoc Committee on Policy Issues in Child Care for Infants and Toddlers. Washington, D.C., 1986

57. Kellam SG, Ensminger ME, Turner J: Family structure and the mental health of children: Concurrent and longitudinal community-wide studies. Arch Gen Psych 34:1012–1022, 1977

58. Kelly JB, Wallerstein JS: The effects of parental divorce: Experiences of the child in early latency. Am J Orthopsychiatry 46:20, 1976

59. Krein SF: Growing up in a single-parent family: The effect on education and earnings of young men. Fam Relat 35:161, 1986

60. Kurdek LA, Berg B: Correlates of children's adjustment to their parents' divorces. In Kurdek LA (ed): Children and Divorce. San Francisco, Jossey-Bass, 1983

61. Levitin TE: Children of divorce: An introduction. J Soc Issues 35:1, 1979

62. Loveland-Cherry CJ: Personal health practices in single-parent and two-parent families. Fam Relat 35:133, 1986

63. Lutz P: The step-family: An adolescent perspective. Fam Relat 32:367–375, 1983

64. Marbury MC, Linn S, Monson RR et al: Work and pregnancy. J Occup Med 26:415–421, 1984

65. Martin MJ, Walters J: Familial correlates of selected types of child abuse and neglect. J Marriage Fam 44:267–276, 1982

66. Masnick G, Bayne MJ: The Nation's Families: 1960–1990. Boston, Auburn House Publishing Company, 1980

67. McAnarney ER, Roghmann KJ, Adams BN et al: Obstetric, neonatal and psychosocial outcome of pregnant adolescents. Pediatrics 61:199, 1978

68. Miller CA, Fine A, Adama-Taylor S, et al: Monitoring children's health: Key indicators. Washington, DC, American Public Health Association, 1986

69. Mowbray CT: Homelessness in America: Myths and realities. Am J Orthopsychiatry 55:4–8, 1985

70. Mueller DP, Cooper PW: Children of single parent families: How they fare as young adults. Fam Relat 35:169, 1986

71. Naeye RL, Peters EC: What you do in pregnancy: Effects on the fetus. Pediatrics 69:724–727, 1982

72. National Center for Health Statistics: Advanced Report of Final Natality Statistics, 1983. Hyattsville, Maryland, Monthly Vital Statistics Report, Vol 34, No 6(Suppl), 1985

73. National Center for Health Statistics: Health, United States, 1985. Public Health Services. Washington, D.C., U.S. Government Printing Office, 1985

74. National Academy of Sciences: Toward a National Policy for Children and Families. Washington, D.C., U.S. Government Printing Office, 1976

75. National Center for Health Statistics: Annual Summary of Births, Marriages, Divorces and Deaths, 1984. Hyattsville, Maryland, Monthly Vital Statistics Report, Vol 33, No 13

76. National Incidence Study on Child Abuse Neglect. Washington, D.C., National Center on Child Abuse and Neglect, 1981

77. National Center for Health Statistics: Advance Report of Final Natality Statistics, 1982. Hyattsville, Maryland, Monthly Vital Statistics Report. Vol 33, No 6(Suppl)

78. National Center for Health Statistics: Advance Report of Final Natality Statistics, 1983. Hyattsville, Maryland, Monthly Vital Statistics Report. Vol 34, No 6(Suppl)

79. National Center for Health Statistics: Advance Report of Final Divorce Statistics, 1983. Hyattsville, Maryland, Monthly Vital Statistics Report. Vol 34, No 9(Suppl)

80. Nersesian WS, Petit MR, Shaper R, et al: Childhood death and poverty: A study of all childhood deaths in Maine, 1976–1980. Pediatrics 75:41, 1985

81. Norton AJ, Glick BC: One-parent families: A social and economic profile. Fam Relat 35:9, 1986

82. O'Hare WP: Poverty in America: Trends and new patterns. Popul Bull 40:1, 1985

83. Ooms T: The necessity of a family perspective. J Fam Issues 5:160–181, 1984

84. Oschman HP, Manosevitz M: Father absence: Effects of stepfathers upon psychosocial development in males. Dev Psych 12:479–480, 1976

85. Patton RD, Harvill LM, Michal ML: Attitudes of single parents toward health issues. J Am Med Wom Assoc 36:340, 1981

86. Poznanski E, Maxey A, Marsden G: Parental adaptations to maternal employment. J Am Acad Child Psychiatry 13:31, 1974

87. Pratt WF, Mosher WD, Bacharach CA et al: Understanding U.S. fertility: Findings on the national survey of family growth, Cycle III. Popul Bull 39:1, 1984

88. Pratt WM, Horn MC: Wanted and Unwanted Childbearing, U.S., 1973–1982. Advanced Data from Vital and Health Statistics. No 108. DHHS. Pub No (PHS) 8F 1215. Hyattsville, Maryland, Public Health Service, 1985

89. Prosen S, Farmer J: Understanding stepfamilies: Issues and implications for counselors. The Personnel and Guidance J 60:393–397, 1982

90. Raschke HJ, Raschke VJ: Family conflict and children's self-concepts: A comparison of intact and single-parent families. J Marriage Fam 41:367–374, 1979

91. Rosenbaum J, Rosenbaum V: Step-parenting. New York, E.P. Dutton, 1977

92. Rothenberg PB, Varga PE: The relationship between age of mother and child health and development. Am J Public Health 71:810, 1981

93. Rubenstein J, Howes C: Caregiving and infant behavior in day care and in homes. Dev Psych 15:1–24, 1979

94. Rutter M: Social-emotional consequences of day-care for preschool children. Am J Orthopsychiatry 51:4–28, 1981

95. Sack WH et al: The single-parent family and abusive child punishment. Am J Orthopsychiatry 55:252, 1985

96. Sanick MM, Maudlin T: Single vs. two-parent families: A comparison of mothers' time. Fam Relat 35:53, 1986

97. Santrock JW, Warshak R, Lindbergh C et al.: Children's and parent's observed social behavior in stepfather families. Child Dev 53:472–480, 1982

98. Schwartz P: Length of day care attendance and attachment behavior in 18-month-old infants. Child Dev 54:1073–1078, 1983

99. Sharma RK: Maternal employment and adverse pregnancy outcome: An exploratory study. Paper presented at the American Statistical Association meeting in Las Vegas, Nevada, August, 1985

100. Spence JT (ed): Achievement and Achievement Motives. San Francisco, WH Freeman & Co, 1983

101. Spivak H, Weitzman M: Social barriers faced by adolescent parents and their children. JAMA 258:1500–1504, 1987

102. Taylor B, Wadsworth J, Butler NR: Teen-age mothering, admission to hospital, and accidents during the first five years. Arch Dis Child 58:6, 1983

103. U.S. Bureau of the Census, Statistical Abstract of the United States: 1986, 106th edition. Washington, D.C., 1985

104. U.S. House of Representatives, Select Committee on Children, Youth, and Families: Teen Pregnancy: What Is Being Done? A State-by-State Look. Washington, D.C., U.S. Government Printing Office, 1986

105. U.S. Bureau of the Census, Current Population Reports, Series P-60, No 146, Money Income of Households, Families, and Persons in the United States: 1983. Washington, D.C., U.S. Government Printing Office, 1985

106. U.S. Bureau of the Census, Current Population Reports, Series P-20, No 398, Household and Family Characteristics: March 1984. Washington, D.C., U.S. Government Printing Office, 1985

107. Vaughn B, Gove F, Egeland B: The relationship between out-of-home care and the quality of infant-mother attachment in an economically deprived population. Child Dev 51:1203–1214, 1980

108. Wallerstein JS, Kelly JB: Surviving the Break-up: How Children Actually Cope with Divorce. New York, Basic Books, 1980
109. Wallerstein JS, Kelly JB: Surviving the Breakup: How Children and Parents Cope with Divorce. New York, Basic Books, 1980
110. Wallerstein, JS, Kelly JB: The effects of parental divorce: Experiences of the child in later latency. Am J Orthopsychiatry 46:256, 1976
111. Wilson M, Daly M, Weghorst SJ: Household composition and the risk of child abuse and neglect. J Biosoc Science 12:333–340, 1980
112. Wise PH, Kotelchuck M, Wilson ML et al: Racial and socioeconomic disparities in childhood mortality in Boston. N Engl J Med 313:360–366, 1985
113. Zambrana RE, Hurst M, Hite RL: The working mother in contemporary perspective: A review of the literature. Pediatrics 64:862–870, 1979
114. Zimmerman IL, Bernstein N: Parental work patterns in alternative families: Influence on child development. Am J Orthopsychiatry 53:418–425, 1983
115. Zuckerman BS, Frank DA, Hingson R et al: Impact of maternal work outside the home during pregnancy on neonatal outcome. Pediatrics 77:459–464, 1986

Division of Pediatric Medicine
700 W. Lombard Street
Baltimore, Maryland 21201

Divorce and Children

Michael Weitzman, MD,* and Robin Adair, MD†

Divorce, or the legal dissolution of a marriage, is a common event in the United States today. The divorce rate for the United States is currently the highest in the world.[4, 5] In 1985 there was one divorce for every two marriages, as compared to one divorce for every four marriages 25 years ago.[1, 2, 30] In 1983, approximately 1 million children, or slightly less than 2 per cent of all American children, experienced their parents' divorce, doubling from 20 years ago.[9, 30] An estimated 45 per cent of all American children born in 1983 will have the same experience sometime during the course of their lifetimes.[27]

Although designed as a social remedy for an unhappy marriage, research over the past 20 years reveals that divorcing parents and most of their children of all ages tend to experience divorce as an extremely stressful experience.[24, 27] For adults, divorce is second only to the death of a spouse or a parent in terms of its intensity as a stressor and the length of time required to adjust to it.[24] Divorce also differs from other common stresses experienced by children in at least two important ways: it is a process rather than a discrete event, and it is always the result of a voluntary decision on the part of at least one parent.[3, 24] Children frequently realize the latter fact and blame their parents for their unhappiness. Understanding, accepting, and relinquishing their anger and sense of blame is often a central and long-term theme for many of these children.[24]

Divorce often produces anger and a sense of failure for parents, conflicted loyalties, guilt, grief, and anxiety for children, and concern on the part of all about whether the children will suffer long-term harm.[7, 21] Divorce has also created new family patterns for which few norms or guidelines are available.[3]

The pediatrician is in a strategic position to help many of these children and families, particularly when the family is well known to the practice. He or she can provide developmentally appropriate counseling to the family on an anticipatory basis, as well as during or after the divorce when behavioral and emotional problems are quite frequent.[5] Parents also may approach the pediatrician to request testimony on their behalf in a custody battle. Thus, the pediatrician can play a number of different and significant roles for the divorcing family.

This article reviews the current knowledge about the effects of divorce on children and the roles of the pediatrician in caring for such children and families.

---

*Associate Professor of Pediatrics and Public Health, Boston City Hospital and the Boston University, School of Medicine and Public Health, Boston, Massachusetts
†Fellow in Behavioral Pediatrics, Boston City Hospital and the Boston University, School of Medicine, Boston, Massachusetts

FAMILY CHANGES BROUGHT ON BY DIVORCE

In over 90 per cent of cases mothers are awarded custody of the children.[3, 5] These mothers tend to become less available to their children both emotionally and physically due to their new responsibilities, as well as the emotional stress of the divorce.[17] Family finances are almost always negatively affected by divorce. This can bring with it a loss of social status as housing, schools, and activities are surrendered because of expense. A significant number of custodial mothers subsequently take on new employment outside the home. This may result in new day care arrangements for younger children while older children are often expected to take care of themselves for greater parts of the day, very often in an empty home. An affordable activity for a child may have to be dropped because of lack of transportation. Thus, at least transiently, children may "lose" both parents and their routines and regular activities.

Not infrequently the family relocates as a result of the divorce.[6] Mothers may choose to move in with their parents as a cost-saving measure, to acquire the services of grandparents for daycare, or to obtain emotional support. Loss of income or new maternal employment may require the family to move to an entirely new setting. Changing residence requires the child to leave familiar neighborhoods, schools, and friends, and may also be associated with adjustment problems.

During the early divorce process the children are often exposed to new and disturbing parental behaviors.[5, 8, 24] This is often a result of decreased parenting skills in the face of overwhelming depression or anger but may be part of coercive efforts by one parent to injure the other. The divorced mother with custodial responsibilities must raise and discipline the children, face economic hardships and decisions, and arrange for child care all by herself.[17] Some mothers resent their children for the increased child care responsibilities that often result in greatly limiting their freedom.[8] Children also often take out their angry feelings on the custodial mother rather than the physically and emotionally unavailable father.[22] Moreover, in the acute stage, a mother often experiences an overwhelming sense of personal loss, regardless of whether the divorce was initiated by her or was mutually agreed on.[8] She still must contend with a sense of loss, and this is often more than she anticipated. Divorce is also frequently a terrible insult to one's self-image and in many cases, both spouses feel rejected and inadequate.[8]

The divorced mother also must often contend with loneliness. Increased childcare responsibilities may limit her ability to socialize outside the family. Many old friends become unavailable following a divorce.[8] Some people have difficulty maintaining a friendship with both estranged individuals and choose one or the other. Other friends may feel burdened by the newly divorced individual's unhappiness, preoccupation with her life circumstances or perceived "neediness," and may not wish to spend time with her. Married friends often cannot respond to divorced individual's problems, either because they are alien to them or because their own marriages are troubled and it is threatening for them to discuss marital difficulties, especially those that end in divorce. The married women with whom the divorced mother used to socialize may now find her a threat. There still exists a stereotype that divorced women are easy sexual prey and, not infrequently, divorced women receive sexual advances from the male partners of female friends.

Virtually all elements of predivorce friendships may be altered by a divorce. Married couples, for example, frequently socialize with other couples and spend a great deal of time discussing their children and respective families, and divorced women are often deprived of this type of informal social support. Even more than parents in an intact family, divorced mothers need to make arrangements for regular time away from the children, and they frequently must accommodate to the loss of some friends and the need to seek new ones.[8]

In most divorces, the fathers are turned into noncustodial parents.[3] For these fathers, problems range from what to do with the children on visiting days (and these are not trivial concerns since many fathers have had little previous experience in caring for and interacting with their children over a sustained 24- to 48-hour period), to profound concern about the emotional consequences of the divorce on their children. Every noncustodial father must adjust to his new and complicated role. This is especially difficult for the father who has been intimately involved in the care of the children. Some fathers fear that their children will abandon them. Some have unrealistic expectations about the kind of relationship they will have with the children and some believe divorce deprives them of the right to exercise authority and discipline the children. In addition, like divorced mothers, divorced fathers are often deprived of old friends and family. He also frequently must deal with the stereotype that he caused the divorce.[3]

STAGES OF DIVORCE: CHANGES IN THE FAMILY UNIT

While marriages are failing, parenting is often adequate and the children do not experience a crisis related to the parents' interpersonal problems until the time of parental separation.[29] The period immediately following the separation is referred to as the *acute stage* of divorce. This stage is characterized by maximal turmoil and generally lasts up to 2 years. The family then moves into the *transitional stage*, which is characterized by more controlled changes. The third and final stage is the *postdivorce stage*, which is reached when major family restructuring ceases, often following remarriage.

Acute Stage

This stage lasts, in general, from the time at which the family acknowledges the inevitability of a divorce to 2 years after the divorce actually occurs. During this time, all family members are confronted with disruptions of their expectations, relationships, and support systems.[24] Children, during this stage, are often faced with new and disturbing behavior by their parents. Parents are often depressed, irritable, preoccupied with personal concerns, and evidence diminished parenting abilities as well as fear of rejection by the children.

Studies have shown the first year after divorce to be the year of maximal negative behavior by children and the poorest parenting by parents.[5] Initially, many parents make fewer demands on the children, communicate less effectively, are less affectionate, and have difficulty disciplining children.[5, 8] Many parents are victimized by their children's angry and regressive behavior and many children side with their father and oppose their mother.[5] In almost one third of divorces, the troubled relationship between parents continues indefinitely and is still present at least five years after the divorce. Studies demonstrate that these are the cases in which children exhibit the greatest incidence of postdivorce maladjustment.[7, 24]

During this stage, two events appear to be most stressful to most children: learning about the divorce and the actual departure of a parent.[27, 29] The apparent intensity of a child's reaction to this stage does not predict longterm adjustment or maladjustment, or even necessarily reflect the intensity of the stress these children are experiencing.[29] The child's previous level of psychological adjustment, the availability of environmental support, and the length of time this stress continues all appear to influence the degree and length of psychosocial dysfunction.

Transitional Stage

The *transitional stage* is marked by new undertakings for the single-parent household. Change continues to be a part of the childrens' lives, but often in a more predictable and controlled manner. Children find they are involved more in decision making than during the acute phase when parental behavior was more autonomous and erratic. Despite the improvements, this stage is sometimes more unstable than the predivorce situation.[27] The children must accommodate to their parents' new relationship with each other, to new friends, and often to their parents' new sexual partners. Maternal work patterns and child care arrangements may also be altered.

During this stage children are often concerned about the well-being of the noncustodial parent and their relationship with him or her, particularly if a remarriage has taken place. Visitation patterns tend to have become more stable, whether or not they are acceptable to all parties.

The major exception to the general pattern of increased stability is the family in which the parents are still locked in battle, either informally through the children, or formally through the legal system.

Postdivorce Stage

The final stage is the *postdivorce stage,* when relative stability is achieved. The family may still be headed by one parent or a step-parent may now be present. Three out of four divorced women and four out of five divorced men eventually remarry.[27] Remarriage does not convey automatic stability but requires new adjustments due to the reawakening of unresolved issues and conflicts.[16, 27]

EFFECTS OF DIVORCE ON CHILDREN

Much of the understanding about the effects of divorce on children is based on the work of Wallerstein and colleagues who have prospectively studied 131 children of divorce from 60 largely white, middle-class families since 1971.[25, 26, 28, 29] These children, aged 2 to 18 years at the time of marital separation, were selected because they lacked preexisting emotional or behavioral problems.

Initial Effects

Wallerstein identified characteristic initial responses in children that are largely influenced by the developmental level of the child. Preschool children, aged 2 to 5 years at the time of the divorce, initially tend to manifest regressive behavior. Sleep disturbances, temper tantrums, separation anxiety, loss of bowel and bladder control, and increased need for parental attention and nurturance are common. Children of this age often demonstrate evidence of feeling responsible for the marital breakup and appear to fear abandonment by both parents. Their cognitive and linguistic limitations often interfere not only with their ability to articulate their fears and concerns but also with their parents' ability to assuage their anxiety. Their regressive behavior can also be highly stressful for depressed and preoccupied parents going through the turmoil of the early stages of divorce. Depression or hostility in the parents can heighten the child's fear of abandonment by both parents.

Early school age children, aged 5½ to 8 years, tend to become depressed and openly grieve. They fear replacement and rejection by the absent parent. School performance and peer relationships may suffer and phobias may emerge as channels for expressing anger that they cannot openly direct at their parents.

Later school-aged children, aged 9 to 12 years, demonstrate intense anger at one or both parents. Their anger is fueled by their developmental need to see things as "good" or "bad." They tend to feel wronged by the parent who first seeks the divorce and may feel anger toward the custodial parent for allowing the other to leave. At this age, the usual confusion regarding issues of sexuality may be compounded by new parental behaviors associated with divorce. Parents, for example, may express hostility and deprecation of former loved ones and demonstrate new, sexually solicitous behavior toward new partners. Children of this age frequently become preoccupied with these events with resultant deterioration of their school performance and peer relationships. Teachers find some of these children converted into daydreamers, whereas others throw themselves into vigorous activity. In addition, children at this age may still blame themselves for the divorce. Kalter and Plunkett have shown that as many as one third of children of this age actually believe that children may have caused their parents' divorce.[19] This sense of guilt may contribute further to children's behavioral functioning.

The adolescent of divorcing parents finds himself without the expected home base from which to move away. This often results in insecurity, loneliness, and depression, which may be overtly or covertly expressed in exaggerated "acting out" through school failure, truancy, criminal behavior, substance use, or sexual promiscuity. Additionally, adolescents may be distressed as they perceive their parents as sexual beings because of dating. This can be accentuated if the parents choose new sexual partners who are close in age to the adolescent. Although there is considerable potential for problems between adolescents and parents during this stage, there is also potential for more understanding and support for the parents from a child of this age.

As the child matures, like the family unit, he or she goes through stages of adjustment. In general, boys adjust less well, demonstrating more behavior and school problems than girls.[11, 14, 16] However, once becoming adolescents, or in the event of remarriage, girls tend to manifest more problems than do boys.[13, 20]

Long-term Effects

Recent studies reveal long-lasting effects of parental divorce.[16, 25, 26, 28] Hetherington et al. found that in the 6 years following divorce, the children of divorce had experienced more negative life changes than children in intact families and that this was associated with increased behavior problems after 6 years.[16]

In a followup study 10 years after the parental divorce, Wallerstein found that the youngest children seemed least disturbed by the divorce, recalling fewer distressing memories and being least fearful about their future marriage or possible divorce.[25] In contrast, children who were 6 to 8 years of age at the time of the divorce later expressed fear and apprehension about love relationships, as well as a sense of helplessness.[28] The oldest group expressed sadness as a result of their parents' divorce. They express anxiety about their love relationships and often nearparalyzing fear of entering into a bad marriage. Most are determined not to divorce if they should have children.[26]

TASKS FOR THE CHILDREN OF DIVORCE

Several specific tasks for the children of divorce have been identified.[24] These tasks often are worked on simultaneously and to varying degrees of success. While the developmental level and the sex of the child are important, mastery of these tasks is facilitated by support and cooperation by both parents.

Acknowledging the Divorce and Relinquishing Longings for the Restoration of the Predivorced Family

This task requires the child to separate out the reality of the divorce from strong tendencies to deny that the family unit is dissolving and fearful fantasies of abandonment. Preschoolers may persist in believing the departed parent will magically return. Although older children are better able to accept the separation intellectually, they too have strong tendencies to deny the divorce, and they may persistently and desperately try to persuade the parents to reconcile. Even in the face of remarriage, children have been known to harbor hopes of parental reconciliation. As thoughts of the divorce stir up fewer feelings of acute anxiety, the child moves closer to accepting its permanence.

Regaining a Sense of Direction and Freedom to Pursue Customary Activities

During the acute stage, children of all ages tend to become quite focused on the events at home, sacrificing age-appropriate activities. Immediately following a divorce, many children experience emotional and behavioral difficulties, and many seem to lose interest in school, friends, and leisure time activities. Generally, the return to more typical activities for the child takes about a year. If this has not occurred within this period, then referral of the child or family for psychotherapy may be indicated. Children who are better adjusted prior to the marital breakup, those who are not enmeshed in a prolonged battle between the parents, and those who are supported in their efforts to understand their feelings are better able to accomplish this task.[24]

Dealing with Loss and Feelings of Rejection

Departure of a parent through divorce is experienced by children of all ages as a major assault on their self esteem and sense of security. Ideas of "If he loved me he wouldn't have left" often translates into "If I was lovable he wouldn't have left."[3] Young children may fantasize that they are responsible for the loss, therefore must be "bad," and consequently believe that they are at risk for further abandonment. Older children, appreciating that the departing parent is exercising a choice to leave, often feel anger as well as grief. This results in a complex interplay of negative emotions that is often directed at the custodial parent. Visitation in some cases prolongs the time needed to master this task because the loss of the noncustodial parent is incomplete and the child is faced recurrently with chances to "prove" that he is worth loving. Alternatively, infrequent or absent visitation may reinforce the negative impression. Regardless of the visitation experience, long-term followup by Wallerstein[26, 28] indicates that this important task may never be accomplished in a significant number of children of divorce.

Forgiving the Parents

This is most often a task for older children. It requires the ability to appreciate the parents' need to separate as more important than any reason to stay together, including the desires of the children. The child must overcome grief over the loss of the intact family, as well as the anger and resentment generated by the resulting changes in his or her life. This is especially difficult because the people responsible for the problems are the very ones who can help the child to master this task.

Resolving Issues of Relationship

Divorce often leaves children fearful and unable ". . . to reach, sustain, and support the personal vision that love, mutual understanding, and constancy are expectable components of human relationships. Perhaps the major developmental task posed by divorce is this: To achieve realistic hope regarding future relationships and the enduring ability to love and be loved."[24] This has been shown to be a difficult task that has not been resolved in a significant number of Wallerstein's original subjects who are now of adult age.[26]

CUSTODY

Traditionally, legal custody of the children has been awarded to one parent—the mother in 90 per cent of sole-parent custody cases.[4, 5, 27] The father, in these situations, usually is given visitation rights, most often alternate weekends. Often this results in the father spending more time overall with the children than prior to the divorce and spending it in more stimulating ways. Discipline and economy are often sacrificed due to this "Santa Claus father" syndrome. If the parental relationship has been acrimonious or child support inadequate, custodial mothers may find this phenomenon particularly distressing.[15] Historically, 10 per cent of these cases go on to litigation;[27] parents in this group have a significantly higher rate of psychological disorder and their children are often profoundly stressed.[18, 27]

During the 1970s, a shift away from this arrangement occurred, with sole custody being awarded in 70 to 90 per cent of cases.[23] The alternative, joint custody, usually takes the form of joint *legal* custody, in which children reside with one parent but both parents participate in child-related decisions. In approximately 2 per cent of all custody cases, joint *physical* custody is arranged, in which the children alternate residence frequently between both parents' households. The rationale of joint custody is "(1) parents cooperate and share authority and responsibility for their children after divorce, (2) mothers and fathers are viewed as equally important to their children, and (3) the children alternate living in both parental homes."[23]

While sole custody is well recognized as problematic, preliminary research on joint custody shows mixed results. Steinman and colleagues, for example, reported their results after 1 year of a 3-year longitudinal study of 51 joint custody families.[23] These families, from a cross-section of social and racial groups, were in the initial stages of arranging joint custody. Twenty-seven per cent of families were classified as successful, 40 per cent as stressed, and 31 per cent as failed in their custody arrangements. Parents from the successful group demonstrated respect for the parent–child bond involving former spouses, could view the former spouse as both ex-spouse and current parent, and were generally more psychologically flexible. Failure was associated with the opposite characteristics as well as inability to separate their own psychological needs from those of the child(ren), increased history of physical abuse, and increased substance use by the parents. The stressed group fell in between on many characteristics. It remains to be seen if intervention can improve outcome in this group or if the rates of successful joint custody arrangements will change over longer periods.

REMARRIAGE

One of the most common outcomes of divorce is remarriage, and this can have positive or negative effects on children.[8] In many cases, it restores a secure, two-parent environment and it may provide children with a model of a loving, caring relationship that a single parent family cannot provide. It also has the potential of creating new tensions and stresses.

When one parent remarries, the other may fear that the children will abandon him or her for the new step-parent and may consequently overindulge the children or fail to discipline them. Many children feel as if they are betraying one parent if they form a close relationship with the other parent's new spouse. Children often experience a great deal of ambivalence, and many continue to wish for a parental reunion. Many children have a complicated set of irrational and contradictory feelings toward the step-parent, and he or she is often the target of hostility.[8] If the new spouse has children from a previous marriage or if new children are born, there is the potential for jealousy and competition between the children.

THE PEDIATRICIAN'S ROLE

The pediatrician is often in a position to act as the child's advocate and to help the family anticipate, prevent, or address some of the many problems that frequently accompany divorce.[5] Divorce inevitably raises numerous questions about potential effects on children and the differential impact of various arrangements. The pediatrician can help families with many of these questions, provide anticipatory guidance, provide counseling for problems as they arise, and assess and refer children and family members for more extensive or detailed psychosocial intervention when needed. There are also a number of books for parents and children with useful advice and information that pediatricians may wish to recommend.[3, 8, 10, 17, 22, 29] What follows is a brief list and discussion of some of the more common issues and areas of concern that pediatricians can help divorcing families address.

Effects on Children

Parents should be informed of the short-term and long-term effects of divorce on children, as described earlier. The first year after the divorce is likely to be the year of maximal negative child behavior, in part a consequence of altered parenting styles.[5] Parents should be informed that a conflict-ridden intact family may be more harmful to children than divorce and that the presence of two parents in a home does not guarantee a child's happiness or optimal development.[5] What evidence exists suggests that divorce need not be more than a transient stress on children, but if the turbulent relationship between the parents persists, and especially if the children become enmeshed in their parents' difficulties, then the likelihood of long-term negative effects on the children is greatly increased.[7] Thus, if parents want to help their children cope with the divorce, they need to be encouraged to work together. If the parents are not in counseling, the pediatrician may offer to meet with both of them to facilitate cooperation regarding childcare.

How to Inform Children About Divorce

Many parents feel guilty, are afraid of hurting their children, and are consequently uncomfortable informing them about the divorce.[8, 22] Many parents do not realize that children often can face an unpleasant truth much better than the pervasive sense that something is wrong and being hidden.[8, 10] As to just what to say, it is likely to be difficult and different in every case. One approach is to explain that when people marry they hope that they will be happy together and live together always, but it sometimes does not work out that way and when it doesn't, it is better to live apart.[17] The child needs to be reassured that every attempt has been made to work out problems so that he does not cling to vain hopes of reunion. He must be reassured that he is still loved and that he did not cause the divorce; the parents are getting divorced, not the parent and child.[10, 22]

Although difficult, parents should try to protect the integrity of each other so the child is not confronted with divided loyalties.[22] It is probably best if both parents inform the children together, or at least agree on what to tell them.[8] Parents should try to avoid placing the child in the difficult position of which parent to believe and how to interpret his perceptions when the two most significant adults in his life have such differing views.[7]

Parents should realize that behind many of their questions, children are asking "Do you still love me and can I trust you?"[3] They should also be concrete about the children's future—where they will live, who will care for them, where the noncustodial parent will live, and how often he or she will visit.[17] Although all children react differently, many feel both devastated and betrayed, and so it may be difficult to assure them of their parents' love. Children need reassurance that they are not unique in having the feelings they are having and that there is nothing wrong with feeling this way.[10] They also should be encouraged to ask questions and express feelings, and they should be brought to see that it is useless to use up a great amount of energy hoping their parents will be reunited.[10]

Discussing the Noncustodial and Abandoning Parent

The custodial parent should attempt to protect the integrity of the noncustodial parent, but she should not defend him if he were abusing, rejecting, or irresponsible.[22] If the father has abandoned the children or does not show interest in them, this should be regularly and openly discussed so that the children can come to terms with this. Children should not be encouraged to seek love from those who do not return it. If the mother insists that the father loves the children despite evidence to the contrary, the children will not trust her and may become confused about what constitutes love.[10] The best approach is to give children an accurate picture of the parent's assets and liabilities. If the father is rejecting, it should be explained to the child that he did not cause this and that the father needs to be by himself. If the noncustodial parent has not abandoned the family and wants to remain involved with the children, it is essential that the custodial parent not attempt to sabotage this relationship.

Encouraging Visitation with the Noncustodial Parent

If the noncustodial parent wants to maintain a relationship with the children, which is most often the case, a number of concrete suggestions can be offered. Contact during the acute stage should be often, even every day in the form of telephone contact.[3, 8] The children should be encouraged to call. Initially, visitation should be often, for short periods, and structured so that all involved are comfortable. New noncustodial fathers are often uncomfortable entertaining their children and therefore they should do things that are fun for the children.[3, 8] When the children visit the noncustodial parent at his new home, they should stay overnight and in their own space if possible so that they are given the message that they are an intimate and permanent part of the noncustodial parent's life.[8] The noncustodial parent should attempt to encourage the children to speak about themselves, not just what they are doing, but what they are feeling, even if this is painful.[3]

If there is more than one child, the question may arise about whether the father should visit each alone or both together. There is no simple answer to this question. It is often easiest if most visits are with all children together, but occasionally time should be spent with each alone.[8] If a child does not wish to visit, he should be treated with love and respect. In such a situation, the child should not be made to feel guilty and the offer to visit soon should be extended; the child should be informed that he can initiate the contact. Persistent refusals to visit the noncustodial parent may suggest that the child is enmeshed in the parental difficulties, siding with the custodial parent, or that the custodial parent may be using the child to hurt the noncustodial parent.

Should Families Be Encouraged to Move After a Divorce?

If possible, most families probably should attempt to remain in the same house so as to minimize disruptions of environment, friends, and school.[6] In many cases, families find this emotionally or economically difficult. Some custodial mothers may ask about the wisdom of moving in with their parents. This obviously relieves some of the financial burden, loneliness, and fatigue associated with single parenthood, but the decision should be viewed in the context of the quality of the relationships between mother, children, and grandparents, and the implications such a move has on the children's relationship with their father and friends.

Decisions About Parental Dating and Remarriage

Parents should be encouraged to establish and nurture adult relationships after the divorce. Until the divorced parents are relatively certain that a new relationship is going to be long-term, children probably should not be encouraged to become intensely involved with new social contacts.[8] Many children are very eager for their mothers to remarry, if not to their father, then to someone else. Other children do not want their mothers to remarry, are intimidated by the mother's dating, and many actually try to prevent mothers from going out. Some are jealous and resent new parental friends. New parental friends may evoke anxiety because the child yearns for the return of the biologic father, but also may wish for someone to fulfill everyday needs. This may make the child feel as if he is betraying the biologic parent. If a parent decides to remarry, he or she should not request the child's permission, but rather inform the child and help him work through his conflicted emotions. Similarly, children should be invited to their parent's wedding, but if their choice is not to attend, this should be honored.

SUMMARY

The divorce rate in the United States is currently half the rate of marriages. Whether this rate will continue is not known. Millions of American children have already experienced their parents' divorce and millions more are likely to share the experience in the future. This makes divorce a problem that frequently appears in a pediatrician's patient population.

Most children of divorce will experience it at the least as a potent transient stress that disrupts virtually all aspects of their lives. Many will accommodate to their new life circumstances successfully, but a substantial percentage will suffer long-term negative effects. Many of the problems of these children and their families can be anticipated, prevented, or alleviated by thoughtful and timely intervention. The pediatrician can be helpful by serving as the child's advocate, offering anticipatory guidance, helping the family weather the turmoil of the acute stage, screening for maladjustment or maladaptive behavior of children and parents, providing counseling, and referring the children and family for more specialized mental health input when indicated.

ACKNOWLEDGMENT

Support for this work was provided in part (R.A.) from a grant entitled Academic Training Program in Behavioral Pediatrics, funded by the Bureau of Health Care Delivery and Assistance, Maternal and Child Health Branch (Grant # MCJ-009094).

REFERENCES

1. Annual summary of births, deaths, marriages and divorces, United States, 1960: Monthly Vital Statistics Report, National Center for Health Statistics, 9(13), May 31, 1961
2. Annual summary of births, deaths, marriages and divorces, United States, 1985: Monthly Vital Statistics Report, National Center for Health Statistics, 34(13), Sept 19, 1986
3. Atkins E, Rubin E: Part time father. New York, Signet Books, 1977

4. Better health for our children: A national strategy. Vol III: A statistical profile. The report of the select panel for the promotion of child health. Public Health Service, DHHS (PHS) Publication No. 79–55071, pp 5–6
5. Brown RH: Marital discord and divorce. In Friedman SB, Hockelman RA (eds): Behavioral Pediatrics: Psychosocial Aspects of Child Health Care. New York, McGraw-Hill, 1980, pp 255–258
6. Chapman AH: Management of Emotional Problems of Children and Adolescents. Philadelphia, JB Lippincott, 1974, pp 89–94
7. Chess S, Hassidi M: Principles and Practice of Child Psychiatry. New York, Plenum Press, 1972, pp 105–106
8. Dodson F: How to Discipline with Love. New York, The New American Library, 1987, pp 141–169
9. Final divorce statistics, 1983, advance report: Monthly Vital Statistics Report, National Center for Health Statistics, 34(9 Suppl), Dec 26, 1985
10. Gardner RA: The Boys' and Girls' Book about Divorce. New York, Bantam Books, 1970
11. Guidubaldi J, Perry JD: Divorce, socioeconomic status and children's cognitive-social competence at school entry. Am J Orthopsychiatry 54:459–468, 1984
12. Guidubaldi J, Perry JD: Divorce and mental health sequelae for children: a two-year follow-up of a nationwide sample. J Am Acad Child Psychiatry 24:531–537, 1985
13. Hetherington EM: Effects of father absence on personality development in adolescent daughters. Dev Psychol 7:313–326, 1972
14. Hetherington EM, Cox M, Cox R: The aftermath of divorce. In Stevens JH, Matthews M (eds): Mother–Child, Father–Child Relations. Washington, D.C., National Association for the Education of Small Children, 1978
15. Hetherington EM, Cox M, Cox R: Effects of divorce on parents and children. In Lamb ME (ed): Nontraditional Families. Hillsdale, New Jersey, Erlbaum, 1982
16. Hetherington EM, Cox M, Cox R: Long-term effects of divorce and remarriage on the adjustment of children. J Am Acad Child Psychiatry 24:518–530, 1985
17. Ilg FL, Ames LB: The Gessell institute's child behavior from birth to 10. New York, Harper & Row, 1955, pp 331–337
18. Johnston J, Campbell LEG, Mayes SS: Latency children in post-separation and divorce disputes. J Am Acad Child Psychiatry 24:563–574, 1985
19. Kalter N, Plunkett JW: Children's perceptions of the causes and consequences of divorce. J Am Acad Child Psychiatry 23:326–334, 1984
20. Kalter N, Reimer B, Brickman A, Chen JW: Implications of parental divorce for female development. J Am Acad Child Psychiatry 24:538–544, 1985
21. Kenniston K: All Our Children: The American Family Under Pressure. New York, Harcourt, Brace, Jovanovich, 1977, pp 21–22
22. Salk L: What Every Child Would Like His Parents to Know. New York, Warner Books, 1972, pp 173–175
23. Steinman SB, Zemmelman SE, Knoblauch TM: A study of parents who sought joint custody following divorce: Who reaches agreement and sustains joint custody and who returns to court. J Am Acad Child Psychiatry 24:554–562, 1985
24. Wallerstein JS: Children of divorce: Stress and developmental tasks. In Garmezy N, Rutter M (eds): Stress, Coping and Development in Children. New York, McGraw-Hill, 1983, pp 265–302
25. Wallerstein JS: Children of divorce: preliminary report of a ten-year follow-up of young children. Am J Orthopsychiatry 54:444–458, 1984
26. Wallerstein JS: Children of divorce: Preliminary report of a ten-year follow-up of older children and adolescents. J Am Acad Child Psychiatry 24:545–553, 1985
27. Wallerstein JS: Children of divorce. Emerging trends. Psychiatr Clin North Amer 8:837–55, Dec 1985
28. Wallerstein JS: Children of divorce: report of a ten-year follow-up of early latency-age children. Am J Orthopsychiatry 57:199–211, 1987
29. Wallerstein JS, Kelly JB: Surviving the breakup. New York, Basic Books, 1980
30. Wegman ME: Annual summary of vital statistics—1985. Pediatrics 78:983–994, 1986

HOB 421
Boston City Hospital
818 Harrison Ave
Boston, Massachusetts 02118

0031-3955/88 $0.00 + .20

Children with Chronic Illness

The Prevention of Dysfunction

James M. Perrin, MD,* and William E. MacLean, Jr., PhD†

Conservative estimates are that 10 to 20 per cent of children in America experience some long-term illness.[50] For most children, the illness is mild, interfering in only limited ways with the sorts of daily activities that most children participate in. About 10 per cent of children with long-term illnesses have severe disease, at least by physiologic criteria. Other children, whose disease may be physiologically less severe, may nonetheless face major limitations from illness. Thus, perhaps 2 to 4 per cent of children have severe health conditions that affect their daily activities on a regular basis. The goal of services for these children and their families is to diminish the impact of the illness and to prevent dysfunction where possible.

Dysfunction may be manifest in several ways. Important distinctions may be made among disease, disability, and handicap.[15] All chronically ill children have some disease. For some children, the disease causes disability, such as a knee that functions poorly. The disability can become a handicap, preventing the child from participating in certain school activities or playground efforts, because the interaction between the malfunctioning knee and the environment creates barriers to the child's effective participation. Handicap therefore usually represents an interaction between a disability and the child's physical and social environment. The prevention of handicap may require different interventions from those needed to prevent disability.

Intuitively, one might expect that the more severe the illness or disability, the more severe the handicap. Although there is some truth to that statement, many children with moderately severe disability face little handicap, and similarly, some children with very limited disability are severely handicapped.[51] Handicap may appear at all levels of illness severity, and preventive efforts should be directed not

*Associate Professor of Pediatrics, Harvard Medical School, Boston, Massachusetts

†Assistant Professor of Psychology, George Peabody College, Vanderbilt University, Nashville, Tennessee

From the Children's Service, Massachusetts General Hospital, Boston, Massachusetts, and the Department of Psychology and Human Development, George Peabody College, Vanderbilt University, Nashville, Tennessee.

only to those children with severe disease but also to children with milder disease who are still at risk of handicap.

The consideration of long-term illness in childhood often neglects concepts of prevention. It is typically assumed that the issues are all treatment ones. Prevention has primary, secondary, and tertiary components.[25] The etiologies of the many chronic illnesses that affect children are varied; some are genetic, some environmental, many unknown. Primary prevention means the prevention of the conception of a fetus affected by a genetic disease or preventing the onset of an illness by diminishing environmental exposure, such as ridding the environment of lead or preventing exposure to potential carcinogens. For many genetic diseases, the only form of primary prevention currently available is that of foregoing conception of a potentially affected infant. Secondary prevention refers to preventing the expression of an illness once it has already developed in the organism. The many recent advances in *in utero* determination of genetic illnesses have allowed many families at risk for genetic diseases to know whether their fetus is affected. For most families, secondary prevention at this point is the termination of a pregnancy of an affected fetus. Efforts in genetic engineering over the next decade may bring new forms of secondary prevention, with genetic or surgical manipulation of an affected fetus to eradicate the biochemical or anatomic elements of the disease.

Tertiary prevention attempts to limit the effects of the disease, diminishing the disability and handicap the disease may engender. Tertiary prevention is what clinicians typically do in the management of long-term illness in children. Even at this tertiary level, however, an important distinction may be made between prevention and treatment. Treatments often are directed toward what can be done to improve the physiological or anatomic aspects of the illness: maintenance of adequate blood sugar level in diabetes or the proper surgical management of meningomyelocele. A preventive approach changes the focus from only maintaining optimal blood sugar to determining ways to achieve good control in the context of diminishing interference of diabetes with the functioning of the child and family. Preventing handicap or dysfunction necessarily entails a series of health status outcomes broader than traditional physiologic ones. Additional realms include functional status (e.g., school attendance, performance of household chores, time with friends), psychological status of children and families, and the economic impact of illness on the family. Greater clinical and consumer awareness of the importance of measuring health outcomes in ways broader than physiologic status has led to new conceptualizations of health status and new ways to measure functioning for children and families.[54]

CHILDHOOD CHRONIC ILLNESS: DEFINITIONS AND EPIDEMIOLOGY

Chronic illnesses in childhood encompass a wide variety of diseases, such as juvenile arthritis, immunodeficiency syndromes, asthma, sickle cell anemia, hemophilia, cystic fibrosis, malignancies, and congenital heart disease. The epidemiology of childhood chronic illnesses differs from that of adult chronic illness. Children face a large number of rare diseases; adults face a much smaller number of common diseases (e.g., degenerative arthritis, coronary artery disease, diabetes, and other vascular diseases). Estimates from several epidemiologic studies vary from a low of about 15 per cent to a high of about 35 or 40 per cent of children having some chronic health condition.[7, 21, 40] The larger percentages likely reflect conditions that, although they may last for some months, are still transient in nature and are not persistent, long-term health conditions. Most long-term illnesses are mild by most considerations: intermittent hay fever, mild acne, milder forms of asthma, minimal limp, and the like. Among the severe chronic illnesses, only asthma is fairly common, occurring in about 3 per cent of children. Most asthma, however, is mild, with only about 5 per cent of children with asthma having severe disease.[57]

Gortmaker[20] has examined the more common varieties of severe chronic illnesses, finding that on average 80 per cent of children with long-term severe illnesses currently survive to young adulthood. In other words, much (but not all) of the achievable improvement in mortality already has occurred. The clinical corollary is that greater attention must now go to the morbidity of long-term illness. Further, assuming no change in the incidence of chronic illness, the population of children with long-term illnesses is likely to be stable over the next two or three decades. This finding is in contrast to the past two or three decades, during which the percentage of children with severe long-term illnesses and disabilities appears to have increased,[36] likely because of real improvements in mortality rates for many health conditions, including leukemia, some congenital heart anomalies, and end-stage renal disease. Even for diseases like cystic fibrosis, for which the average life span is still severely curtailed, survival rates allow most children to live into the third decade. Continued improvement in mortality rates is likely, but even a rise from the current 80 per cent survival to 100 per cent survival would increase the percentage of children with severe long-term illness only from 2 to 2½ per cent. These data assume no change in the *incidence* of severe long-term illness and should therefore be interpreted with caution. New health conditions such as childhood AIDS and severe respiratory disease in survivors of neonatal intensive care units may change the incidence of childhood chronic illness.

THE FUNCTIONING OF CHILDREN AND FAMILIES

Long-term illness affects the functioning of both children and families. The impact on children may be reflected in their psychological well-being, their involvement with peers, and in their school performance. The impact on family may affect the psychological status of parents, their work activities and performance, the economic status of the family, the structure and functioning of the family directly, the extent of their community involvement, and the psychological status and school performance of siblings.

PSYCHOLOGICAL STATUS OF CHILDREN WITH LONG-TERM ILLNESS

Children with long-term illnesses appear to be at greater risk than their able-bodied colleagues for having significant behavioral problems. Interest in the relationship between behavior and illness goes back many years, at least to the psychiatric investigations of Alexander and others of disease-specific personalities.[2] Although little research supports the idea of condition-specific behavioral problems, it is clear that the presence of long-term illness creates special tasks and problems that may interfere with the normal growth and behavioral development of children.[12]

Most studies with a firm epidemiologic base indicate that the risk of behavioral consequences is about twice that of the able-bodied population. These studies include the Isle of Wight studies from England,[45, 46] the Rochester Child Health Studies,[46] recent examination of the National Health Interview Survey, and the Ontario Child Health Studies.[7] Of interest is the fact that studies that are based on populations seen in tertiary care referral centers do not bear out the findings of studies of unselected populations. Tavormina et al.,[55] for example, found little evidence of overt psychopathology among chronically ill children. Why this disparity exists is unclear, but it may represent both issues in sample selection and the fact that children in most of the studied sites receive high-quality services that address directly the risk of psychological problems. In other words, the provision of high-quality services in these comprehensive centers may prevent the development of psychological problems.

In the clinical approach to patients and families, it is important to recognize that, even though the risk may be doubled, most children with severe long-term illnesses have no apparent problems with psychological adjustment. We have only limited understanding of how most families who cope well do so. Better understanding of this effective work on the part of families would help other families who are coping less well.

School represents the major workplace of children. School attendance is one of the better predictors of long-term effective functioning of children, and maximizing regular school attendance is therefore a responsible goal. Children with chronic illnesses miss a good deal more school on the average than do their able-bodied classmates. Data from the National Health Interview Survey in 1981, for example, indicate that children with chronic health conditions missed about 6½ days compared to 4 days for children without chronic health conditions.[53] Other studies have come up with approximately the same rate of increase among chronically ill children, although for teenagers, school absence rates are higher for both healthy and chronically ill adolescents.[16, 56, 58a]

Children with chronic illnesses miss school for a variety of reasons.[57] Sometimes, the illness or its treatment interferes with the child's stamina or diminishes his or her mobility. At other times, physician visits or other health service visits take place during regular school hours, interfering with the child's school attendance. Services to remedy results of school absence are limited in most jurisdictions. Home-bound teaching is typically available only after children have missed 2 or more consecutive weeks of school; yet, most children with long-term illnesses have frequent short absences that accumulate over a year. Even when home-bound teaching is available, it may be limited to a few hours per week during which time the full range of a youngster's academic subjects must be covered. Most school systems lack effective emergency procedure policies and medication or treatment policies to allow children with illness to receive treatments that otherwise require them to be away from school grounds during regular school hours.

IMPACT OF CHRONIC ILLNESS ON THE FAMILY

Chronic illness in the child affects the labor force participation of parents and therefore the economic status of the family.[47] The illness typically creates a great deal more in-home work for families, with the brunt of this additional work being carried by mothers.[3] Increased family work may include the physical burdens of lifting children with mobility impairments, in-home therapy such as respiratory care for a child with cystic fibrosis, or additional transportation time to carry a child to needed services, medical and other. Many families respond to this additional work by limiting parents' (primarily mothers') participation in work outside the home. Among middle class families, the presence of a long-term illness in a child significantly reduces the likelihood that mothers will have out-of-home jobs. For poor families, especially in single parent households, the effect is less pronounced. Here, mothers have about the equal likelihood of having jobs outside the home, regardless of whether their child has a long-term illness.[4] In addition to diminishing the direct earning power of many families, chronic illness increases the economic demands on the family by sizably increasing the out-of-pocket costs families must endure as a result of a long-term illness. Furthermore, the potential loss of benefits, especially health insurance, limits the job mobility of many families, for whom a several thousand dollar raise may be offset by the lack of insurance coverage for a child with hemophilia or cystic fibrosis.[55]

Families cope with long-term illness in their child in a variety of ways. Illness may affect how they raise their child and how they spend their leisure time, and the inter-relationship among family members. A common concern of families with children with long-term illnesses is the lack of any form of respite care. Babysitters are harder to find than for able-bodied children. Other family members are reluctant to take on the care of children, even for brief periods. For some families, the increased strain leads to family breakup and divorce, although with the relatively high background rate of divorce in American society currently, the marginal impact of chronic illness is slight. Here again, although families may be at somewhat higher risk of divorce as a result of childhood long-term illness, most families do not respond to illness through this means. Clinicians should be aware of the increased strain on families brought about by long-term illness in their children and seek ways to foster better parental coping.

Impact of Chronic Illness on Siblings

Relatively little work has been done to examine carefully the impact of childhood long-term illness on healthy siblings. Just as for parents, such illness typically causes increased demands on growing siblings. For some, the issues relate to less attention from parents, who are concerned about the health status and illness issues in a frequently ill sibling. For others, there are additional opportunities as well as burdens in direct care of a sick brother or sister. Just as for parents, these burdens can be viewed as an obstacle that interferes with the normal growth and development of children or as an opportunity for stimulating the effective development of mature capacities and strengths. We understand little about the means by which some siblings respond well and effectively to these challenges and others face great impediments to their best growth. Although processes are not clearly understood, there appear to be both birth order and sex differences in childhood coping in general. Younger sisters and older brothers of chronically ill children seem to cope better than do older sisters and younger brothers.[5]

FACTORS THAT MAY INCREASE RISK OF DYSFUNCTION

Several research groups, most notably those of Pless and Stein, have noted the large number of similarities among the variety of childhood chronic illnesses, in distinction to the very different specific medical treatments that may be available to them.[39, 49] These differences relate apparently to the chronicity of the illness itself rather than to the specific nature of the disease. Some of the common issues that parents frequently discuss are the high cost of illness, the tremendous amount of daily care provided by parents and other family members, problems with conflicting multiple providers and treatments, the unpredictability of long-term courses of many conditions, the pain and embarrassment suffered by their children, and the isolation engendered by the relative rarity of most childhood chronic illnesses.[24] Stein and Jessop[50] examined a large number of parameters of child performance and psychological adjustment, maternal psychiatric symptoms and functioning, and family functioning among children with asthma, hemoglobinopathies, myelomeningocele, and multiple handicaps. For essentially all measures, Stein and Jessop found more within-disease variation than between-disease variation. In other words, at least for this large group of measures of child and family functioning, what dysfunction was found seemed not to follow from a specific disease but rather from chronicity itself.

If risk of dysfunction seems not to follow from specific diseases, how else might

Table 1. *Characteristics of Childhood Chronic Illness*

TYPOLOGY OF CHRONIC ILLNESS
Age of onset
Course (progressive, stable, exacerbating)
Prognosis (improvement, fatal, persistent)
Impact on mobility
Impact on cognitive abilities
Predictability
Visibility

risk be categorized? Some characteristics of disease or even more how it is manifest in an individual child may play some role in determining risk of psychological or developmental or family dysfunction. Some of these characteristics are listed in Table 1. The natural history or course of the disease probably is important; whether the course is uniformly fatal with a persistently downhill course, whether it seems stable, and whether it is likely to remit after a few years are aspects that likely affect children in different ways. Different ages of onset present different tasks for children.[35] The child born with a missing limb faces a different set of developmental and adaptive tasks than those of a teenager who loses a limb in a major accident. Whether the condition is stable or exacerbating prevents different challenges. The degree of mobility impairment and the degree of interference with normal intellectual capacities and cognitive development both may be important predictors of risk. These concepts may lead to a new typology of chronic illness, although careful research that examines the role of these characteristics and others, such as the visibility of the disease, is typically lacking at this point.

Poverty interacts with long-term illness in several ways. Although the total rate of chronic illness appears only slightly increased among poor families, there is some evidence that severity is much greater in lower class children than among middle class ones.[45] Asthma, for example, seems to have little class difference in incidence[19a]; on the other hand, severe asthma seems skewed to poor populations. Whether this finding reflects a real difference in innate severity or differential access to adequately comprehensive services is unclear.

Differential access to treatment services could account for some differences in dysfunction. Despite the presence of private and public health insurance programs, a large number of American children still lack any adequate form of health care coverage.[6] Only about 50 per cent of poor children in America are currently enrolled in Medicaid. For poor children with long-term illness, the likelihood of not being on Medicaid is about twice that of poor children without any evident illness. Thus, chronic illness and poverty provide a form of double jeopardy. The work of Davis[11] and Starfield[48] among others suggests that Medicaid has positively affected the availability of services for many poor children in America. Conversely, they note that the presence of more severe long-term illness in poor populations indicates a need for more services than required by a relatively able-bodied middle class population and that Medicaid has not fully closed that gap.

MECHANISMS OF DYSFUNCTION

It should be clear from the data presented that the morbidity associated with chronic childhood illness, as expressed in conventional terms such as psychopathology or divorce, is relatively low. There is an increased risk of dysfunction among children with chronic illness and their families, however. The difference between outright morbidity and dysfunction is obviously arbitrary, especially if chronic illness is viewed as having a continuum of effects. However, these effects may divert children and families from normal developmental pathways.

There is nothing really different about children with chronic illness. They are best understood as normal children in an abnormal situation.[44] We favor this view for two reasons. First, it casts children with chronic illness and their families in a normalizing framework. Such a view allows the use of theories of development in conceptualizing and predicting the difficulties that will be encountered by these families. Second, the illness becomes an atypical situation in which a conventional stress and coping paradigm may be used to delineate a set of coping tasks brought about by the illness. This coping process determines whether a child adjusts adequately to the illness or exhibits dysfunction. Interventions aimed at enhancing the coping of all children with chronic illness are a crucial aspect of any preventive effort.

HOW DOES CHRONIC ILLNESS HAVE AN EFFECT ON CHILDREN?

The most obvious mechanism is the disruption of normal ongoing processes of development. These processes have been outlined in a developmental task model by Cerreto and Travis.[10] Their model emphasizes physical, personal–social, and cognitive and moral development, and the development of children's understanding of health and illness. These processes proceed in a specific sequence and pace unless affected by extraordinary external influences such as disease. Disease may make these tasks more difficult to achieve or limit progress altogether.

Similarly, the effects may be mediated by parents. Children with chronic illness are subject to the same processes of disequilibrium as healthy children. The degree to which their developmental experience is characterized by disordered parenting (perhaps related to parental psychopathology), disturbed rearing conditions (such as those associated with extreme marital discord), or disadvantaged environments affects their risk for dysfunction.[17-19]

STRESS AND COPING WITH ILLNESS

Coping is a complex process that can best be defined as "constantly changing cognitive and behavioral efforts to manage specific external and/or internal demands that are appraised as taxing or exceeding the resources of the person."[27] The first step in coping is cognitive appraisal. The appraisal process is critical to determining the ways in which the disease will impact on a particular child. Whereas some have argued in support of a noncategorical approach to conceptualizing childhood chronic illness,[49] at this level of analysis there are disease-specific tasks that must be coped with for adequate adjustment to occur. The day-to-day management of juvenile diabetes mellitus is different from that required for epilepsy. The degree to which the child can meet these daily obligations and still participate in regular activities is a function of coping.

In summary, chronic illness presents children and families with a tremendous coping burden. The risk for dysfunction is high, although psychological morbidity for chronically ill children is only twice that of healthy children. The best way of conceptualizing the effects of disease on children and families is through the disruption of normal processes of child development and family functioning. A stress and coping model facilitates understanding the disruption and suggests intervention approaches.

INTERVENTIONS

Just as chronically ill children are susceptible to the same risk factors as healthy children, so are they affected by the same protective factors as healthy children.

That is, there are identifiable, enduring qualities of children, parents, and families that mitigate against untoward influences. These protective factors may include "positive parent and child temperaments that provide a good fit, a benign family environment marked by cohesion, warmth, positive parental values and aspirations, parental reinforcement of the child's self-help activities, external supports to assist family with a handicapped child, and the presence of supportive teachers, school administrators, and peer group."[15]

One approach to preventive intervention is to provide whatever necessary to strengthen the family unit. Such an approach has been endorsed generally by Hobbs et al.[23] Those recommendations hold as well for chronically ill children. A number of intervention studies, however, have demonstrated enhanced coping abilities of children with chronic illness and their families. A comprehensive review of these studies is beyond the scope and purpose of this article. Examples will be presented as they illustrate the various approaches that have been taken. Each approach affects the coping process in some readily identifiable way.

Education About Disease

Perhaps the most common preventive intervention method has been through education about disease. The assumption is that children will cope more adequately if they have a greater understanding of their disease and its treatment. Certainly for conditions characterized by frequent exacerbations, such as asthma, there would be advantage in teaching children to avoid circumstances in which their disease becomes active or how to minimize the severity of an attack by early intervention. One may expect that changes in knowledge will be associated with less frequent asthma attacks, fewer emergency department visits and hospitalizations, and less medication use. With regard to functional outcomes, such intervention may be associated with decreased school absenteeism and increased participation in usual childhood activities. It is further assumed that increased knowledge, and its attendant effects on disease management, lead to more optimal psychological adjustment. Unfortunately, interventions have not always included measures at each level of outcome. For example, some studies demonstrate increased knowledge as a result of intervention with no assessment of health status or adjustment.[22, 25, 56] A few recent studies have examined disease-related outcomes of educational interventions. Parcel and colleagues reported decreased medical care utilization among children with asthma through the use of educational groups in a school setting.[37] A controlled trial of a nurse-educator in an allergy practice led to decreased hospitalizations, emergency department use, and school absenteeism.[14] Rubin et al.[43] reported a randomized clinical trial of a computerized teaching game for children with asthma. The experimental group demonstrated a significant increase in children's knowledge of asthma and parent report of more appropriate responses on an asthma behavior questionnaire. They found no changes in psychological measures, including the Child Behavior Checklist and the Piers-Harris self-concept scale, and no significant impact on morbidity (acute visits due to asthma, hospital days due to asthma, or school days absent). The researchers did find changes in parents' reports of asthma-related behaviors, although they had no direct assessment of behavior change as a result of the intervention. Increased knowledge may affect psychological adjustment by providing the child with a repertoire of illness management skills that may serve to minimize the impact of disease on daily functioning.

A variant of the educational approach is the systematic training of self-care strategies to children with chronic illness and their families. Examples of this approach can be found in the asthma and diabetes literatures. McNabb and colleagues developed a self-management program for children with asthma (AIR WISE).[34] AIR WISE is integrated with the medical management of asthma and has been shown to decrease emergency department use, improve knowledge of asthma, and lead to changes in self-management behavior. Similar findings were reported by Lewis et al. for a self-management curriculum called Asthma Care Training.[31] Johnson and colleagues have developed self-management programs matched to the child's developmental level and have applied these mainly in teaching management skills to adolescents with diabetes.[26, 27]

Although many interventions are carried out in clinical settings, other forums have been studied. There has been considerable interest in summer camps for chronically ill children. Camps provide an opportunity to separate children from parents, promote independence in aspects of daily functioning, facilitate acquisition of illness knowledge, promote personal growth through the formation of friendships with children who have similar health difficulties, and enhance disease management skills through systematic instruction and increased internal locus of control. Examples are available for diabetes[35] and chronic renal failure.[45] Drotar and Bush[12] maintain that peer socialization to the "illness experience" through participation in camps or contacts in clinic or inpatient settings may serve an important preventive intervention function.

Social and Family Support

Another approach is stress management training. Here the focus may be illness specific, in the sense of contingency coping exercises ("What do you do if?") or relaxation skill training where children are taught how to apply relaxation in strategies to prevent or diminish the effects of illness exacerbations. Most studies have demonstrated at least improvement in pulmonary function with these techniques.[1, 60] In a recent study conducted by the authors, a combined education and stress management curriculum had an effect on the subjects' resistance to negative life events. That is, children with asthma who received the training were less likely to respond to stressful life events with internalizing symptomatology than a group of control subjects. Furthermore, their psychological status improved, as did other functional status, as indicated by time playing with age-mates and their performance of daily household chores.[38a]

An area that should receive greater attention is the social experience of children with chronic illness. These children find themselves isolated from the typical childhood milieu and deficient in age-appropriate social skills. Social skill training is an area of growing interest and sophistication and offers a clear intervention approach.

Participating in a support group related to a child's illness may have a number of therapeutic effects. First, parents may benefit from increased knowledge by promoting a sense of mastery. Second, there is a cathartic experience of sharing impressions of being a parent of a child with chronic illness. Although such meetings need not be construed as group psychotherapy, there are similar elements in that parents' perceptions may be challenged by group members and acceptance may result. As an example, Mattson and Agle reported on group therapy with parents of children with hemophilia.[33] The group meetings had two objectives: to facilitate understanding of the parents' emotional reactions to hemophilia and to learn methods of coping used by other parents in raising a child with chronic illness. While there was no formal objective empiric analysis of the intervention, the authors reported therapeutic gains that could be assessed objectively in future investigations.

A family counselor intervention program described by Pless and Satterwhite demonstrated improved psychological status among a group of chronically ill children as compared with a group of controls.[41] The family counselors visited families routinely over a 1-year period. Their activities clustered in two broad categories: counseling and service provision. The specific activities included listening to parents discuss stresses related to the rearing of their ill children, educating about medical conditions, providing child rearing advice, tutoring, transporting families to clinic, coordinating various agencies involved with the child, advocacy for the family, and facilitation of social relations in the family. There was no standard package; rather there was a matching of family needs with available skills and resources of the family counselor.

A similar finding has been reported by Stein and Jessop (1982) from their Pediatric Ambulatory Care Treatment Study (PACTS).[52] In contrast to Pless and Satterwhite, this was a comprehensive program of medical, psychological, and social services that included close monitoring of the child, delivery of direct care, coordination of services, advocacy, health education, and social support. Instead of a family counselor, an interdisciplinary team was responsible for each family. Clearly, the assistance provided by such a program would decrease the stressors associated with health care provision, enhance parent–child relations, and reduce the uncertainty of how to care for a child with chronic illness. Although a program of this type seems best fit for a disadvantaged minority population, the elements of the program should be available to all families with chronically ill children.

Prevention in the Schools

Success in school is an important focus for preventive efforts. Failure in school quickly limits a child's future. The lack of educational success limits future employment opportunities and is a frequent concomitant of later psychological dysfunction.[46] Children need to participate regularly in an educational program appropriate for their abilities, in the least restrictive physical setting possible. Homebound instruction is necessary for children unable to attend school. A hospital-based educational specialist can ensure transfer of the child's curriculum from school, for children hospitalized for long periods. Tutoring, resource assistance, or special education may be necessary for children to maintain optimal performance. Unfortunately no current systematic set of procedures ensures that children with chronic illness receive needed educational opportunities. P.L. 94–142 has helped many children, mainly those with the most severe learning difficulties (e.g., learning disability, mental retardation, or perceptual handicap). What is needed is a comprehensive approach for children with chronic illness. One program described by Case and Matthews may serve as a model.[9] The Chronic Health Impaired Project (CHIP) is a federally funded program that provides responsive in-home teaching when needed and integrates chronically ill children back into school as soon as possible. Although the efficacy of this program may not have been studied empirically, the services provided are appropriate for chronically ill children and their families and should reduce the impact of the disease on normal child and family processes.

The appropriateness of an educational curriculum for a child with chronic illness should be considered by professionals who assume responsibility for long-term followup. Many diseases, as well as their treatments, can affect cognitive functioning and make academic tasks difficult.[30] For example, many children treated with cranial irradiation for acute lymphoblastic leukemia appear to have learning difficulties that warrant special consideration by school personnel.

SUMMARY

Children with long-term illnesses are at risk of developing problems in psychological adjustment and in functioning in activities of daily life. Their families face increased risks of marital and economic dysfunction, and siblings too face special tasks living with a chronically ill child. A variety of interventions can help children and families to cope effectively with the tasks of chronic illness.

Pediatricians should be alert to effects on the family. Children respond to family stress in very predictable ways. Inasmuch as the stress of chronic illness may affect the marital relationship, there is a likelihood of concurrent behavioral and school problems. Relatively sudden changes in behavior may signal family issues that require professional attention.

Drotar et al. maintain that professionals should serve as guides or advocates for children with chronic illness and their families.[13] The relationship that develops between families and professionals is based on trust. They believe that "trust appears to evolve from the following principles: (1) continuity of relationship, (2) active participation by professional caregivers, (3) mutual participation of child and family, (4) advocacy, (5) a focus on coping and competence, (6) a developmental perspective, and (7) a family-centered focus." Cadman et al. identified a similar set of elements that characterizes an efficacious preventive intervention approach.[7] In addition, they propose specific programmatic efforts that are associated with less morbidity. These include ongoing education and counseling for the child, family, and community regarding chronic illness and its management, use of stress management techniques to promote mastery and reduce the impact of stressful life events, and facilitation of social support mechanisms for families with chronically ill children. We have added consideration of the child's performance in school.

ACKNOWLEDGMENT

The preparation of this paper was supported in part by a grant from the William T. Grant Foundation (#82–0836–00) and by Maternal and Child Health Grant MCJ–250537 awarded by the Division of Maternal and Child Health, Bureau of Health Care Delivery and Assistance, HRSA, PHS, DHHS.

REFERENCES

1. Alexander AB, Cropp GJA, Chai H: Effects of relaxation training on pulmonary mechanics in children with asthma. J Applied Behav Anal 12:27–35, 1979
2. Alexander F: Psychosomatic Medicine. New York, W.W. Norton, 1950
3. Breslau N: Care of disabled children and women's time use. Medical Care 21:620–629, 1983
4. Breslau N, Salkever D, Staruch KS: Women's labor force activity and responsibility for disabled dependents. J Health Soc Behav 23:169–183, 1982
5. Breslau N, Weitzman M, Messenger K: Psychological functioning of siblings of disabled children. Pediatrics 67:344–353, 1981
6. Butler JA, Budetti P, McManus MA et al: Health care expenditures for children with chronic illness. In Hobbs N, Perrin JM (eds): Issues in the Care of Children with Chronic Illness. San Francisco, Jossey-Bass, 1985, pp 827–863
7. Cadman D, Boyle M, Szatmari P, Offord DR: Chronic illness, disability, and mental and social well-being: Findings of the Ontario Child Health Study. Pediatrics 79:805–813, 1987
8. Cadman D, Rosenbaum P, Pettingill P: J Prevent Psychiatry 3:147–165, 1987
9. Case J, Matthews S: CHIP: The Chronic Health Impaired Program of the Baltimore City Public School System. Children's Health Care 12:97–99, 1983
10. Cerreto MC, Travis LB: Implications of psychological and family factors in the treatment of diabetes. Pediatr Clin North Am 31:689–710, 1984
11. Davis K: Medicaid payments and utilization of medical services by the poor. Inquiry 13:127–135, 1976
12. Drotar D, Bush M: Mental health issues and services. In Hobbs N, Perrin JM (eds): Issues in the Care of Children with Chronic Illness. San Francisco, Jossey-Bass, 1985, pp 827–863
13. Drotar D, Crawford P, Ganofsky MA: Prevention with chronically ill children. In Roberts MC, Peterson L (eds): Prevention of Problems in Childhood. New York, John Wiley & Sons, 1984

14. Fireman P, Friday GA, Gira C et al: Teaching self-management skills to asthmatic children and parents in an ambulatory care setting. Pediatrics 68:341–348, 1981

15. Fit for the Future: Report of the Committee on Child Health Services. London, H.M.S.O., 1976

16. Fowler MG, Johnson MP, Atkinson SS: School achievement and absence in children with chronic health conditions. J Pediatrics 106:683–687, 1985

17. Garmezy N: Children under stress: Perspectives on antecedents and correlates of vulnerability and resistance to psychopathology. In Rabin AI, Aronoff J, Barclay AM et al (eds): Further Explorations in Personality. New York, John Wiley & Sons, 1981

18. Garmezy N: Broadening research on developmental risk: Implications from studies of vulnerable and stress-resistant children. In Frankenburg WK, Emde RN, Sullivan JW (eds): Early Identification of Children at Risk. New York, Plenum Press, 1985

19. Garmezy N, Masten AS, Tellegen A: The study of stress and competence in children: A building block for developmental psychopathology. Child Development 55:97–111, 1984

19a. Gergen PJ, Mullaly DI, Evans R: National survey of prevalence of asthma among children in the United States, 1976 to 1980. Pediatrics 81:1–7, 1988

20. Gortmaker SL: Demography of chronic childhood diseases. In Hobbs N, Perrin JM (eds): Issues in the Care of Children with Chronic Illness. San Francisco, Jossey-Bass, 1985, pp 827–863

21. Gortmaker SL, Sappenfield W: Chronic childhood disorders: Prevalence and impact. Pediatr Clin North Am 31:3–18, 1984

22. Hindi-Alexander MC, Cropp GJA: Evaluation of a family asthma program. J Allergy Clin Immunol 74:505–510, 1984

23. Hobbs N, Dokecki PR, Hoover-Dempsey KV et al: Strengthening Families. San Francisco, Jossey-Bass, 1984

24. Hobbs N, Perrin JM, Ireys HT: Chronically Ill Children and Their Families. San Francisco, Jossey-Bass, 1985

25. Holtzman NA, Richmond JB: Genetic strategies for preventing chronic illnesses. In Hobbs N, Perrin JM (eds): Issues in the Care of Children with Chronic Illness. San Francisco, Jossey-Bass, 1985, pp 827–863

26. Johnson SB: Knowledge, attitudes, and behavior: Correlates of health in childhood diabetes. Clin Psychol Rev 4:503–524, 1984

27. Johnson SB, Rosenbloom AL: Behavioral aspects of diabetes mellitus in childhood and adolescence. Psychiatr Clin North Am 5:357–369, 1982

28. Kaye RL, Hammond AH: Understanding rheumatoid arthritis: Evaluation of a patient education program. JAMA 239:2466–2467, 1978

29. Lazarus RS, Folkman S: Stress, Appraisal, and Coping. New York, Springer–Verlag, 1984

30. Lehr E: Cognitive effects of acute and chronic pediatric medical conditions. In Magrab PR (ed): Psychological and Behavioral Assessment. New York, Plenum Press, 1984

31. Lewis CE, Rachelefsky G, Lewis MA et al: A randomized trial of A.C.T. (Asthma Care Training) for kids. Pediatrics 74:478–486, 1984

32. Masters JC, Cerreto MC, Mendlowitz DR: The role of the family in coping with childhood chronic illness. In Burish TG, Bradley LA (eds): Coping With Chronic Disease. New York, Academic Press, 1983

33. Mattson A, Agle DP: Group therapy with parents of hemophiliacs. J Am Acad Child Psychiatry 11:558–571, 1972

34. McNabb WL, Wilson-Pessano SR, Hughes GW et al: Self-management education of children with asthma: AIR WISE. Am J Public Health 75:1219–1220, 1985

35. Moffatt MEK, Pless IB: Locus of control in juvenile diabetic campers: Changes during camp, and relationship to camp staff assessments. J Pediatr 103:146–150, 1983

36. Newacheck PW, Budetti PP, McManus P: Trends in childhood disability. Am J Public Health 74:232–236, 1984

37. Parcel GS, Nader PR, Tiernan K: Impact of a health education program for children with asthma. Paper presented at the Ambulatory Pediatric Association Meeting, San Antonio, April, 1980

38. Perrin EC, Gerrity S: There's a demon in your belly: Children's understanding of illness. Pediatrics 67:841–849, 1981

38a. Perrin JM, MacLean EW: Education and Stress Management in Childhood Chronic Illness. Final report to William T. Grant Foundation, Grant No. 82–0836–00, 1987

39. Pless IB, Pinkerton P: Chronic Childhood Disorder: Promoting Patterns of Adjustment. London, Henry Kimpton Publishers, 1975
40. Pless IB, Roghmann KJ: Chronic illness and its consequences: Observations based on three epidemiologic surveys. J Pediatr 79:351–359, 1971
41. Pless IB, Satterwhite B: Chronic illness in childhood: Selection, activities, and evaluation of non-professional family counselors. Clin Pediatr 11:403–410, 1972
42. Primack WA, Greifer I: Summer camp hemodialysis for children with chronic renal failure. Pediatrics 60:46–50, 1977
43. Rubin DH, Leventhal JM, Sadock RT et al: Educational intervention by computer in childhood asthma: A randomized clinical trial testing the use of a new teaching intervention in childhood asthma. Pediatrics 77:1–10, 1986
44. Russo DC, Varni JW: Behavioral pediatrics. In Russo DC, Varni JW (eds): Behavioral Pediatrics, Research and Practice. New York, Plenum Press, 1982
45. Rutter M, Graham P, Yule W et al: A Neuropsychiatric Study in Childhood. London, Spastics International Medical Publications, 1970
46. Rutter M, Tizard J, Whitmore K: Education, Health and Behavior. London, Longmans, 1970
46a. Sabbeth BF, Leventhal JM: Marital adjustment to chronic childhood illness. Pediatrics 73:762–768, 1984
47. Salkever DS: Parental opportunity costs and other economic costs of children's disabling conditions. In Hobbs N, Perrin JM (eds): Issues in the Care of Children with Chronic Illness. San Francisco, Jossey-Bass, 1985, pp 827–863
48. Starfield B: Family income, ill health and medical care of U.S. children. J Public Health Policy 3:244–259, 1982
49. Stein REK, Jessop DJ: A non-categorical approach to chronic childhood illness. Public Health Reports 97:354–362, 1982
50. Stein REK, Jessop DJ: What diagnosis does not tell. Paper presented at annual meeting of Society for Pediatric Research, Washington, D.C., May 1982
51. Stein REK, Jessop DJ: Relationship between health status and psychological adjustment among children with chronic conditions. Pediatrics 73:169–174, 1984
52. Stein REK, Jessop DK: Does pediatric home care make a difference for children with chronic illness? Pediatrics 73:845–853, 1984
53. Stein REK: Personal communication, 1987
54. Stein REK, Gortmaker SL, Perrin EC et al: Severity of Illness: Definitions and Issues. Lancet (in press)
55. Tavormina JB et al: Chronically ill children—a psychologically and emotionally deviant population? J Abnormal Child Psychol 4:99–110, 1976
56. Vignos PJ, Parker WT, Thompson HM: Evaluation of a clinical education program for patients with rheumatoid arthritis. J Rheumatol 3:155–165, 1976
57. Walker DK, Jacobs FH: Public school programs for chronically ill children. In Hobbs N, Perrin JM (eds): Issues in the Care of Children with Chronic Illness. San Francisco, Jossey-Bass, 1985, pp 827–863
58. Weeks KH: Private health insurance and chronically ill children. In Hobbs N, Perrin JM (eds): Issues in the Care of Children with Chronic Illness. San Francisco, Jossey-Bass, 1985, pp 880–911
58a. Weitzman M, Klerman LV, Lamb G et al: School absence: A problem for the pediatrician. Pediatrics 69:739–746, 1982
59. Williams NE, McNicol KN: The spectrum of asthma in children. Pediatr Clin North America 22:43–52, 1975
60. Zeltzer L, LeBaron S, Barbour J et al: Self-hypnosis for poorly controlled adolescent asthmatics. Presented at the Meeting of the Southern Society for Pediatric Research, New Orleans, 1981

WACC 615
Massachusetts General Hospital
15 Parkman Street
Boston, Massachusetts 02114

0031-3955/88 $0.00 + .20

Dying Is No Accident

Adolescents, Violence, and Intentional Injury

Howard Spivak, MD,* Deborah Prothrow-Stith, MD,† and
Alice J. Hausman, PhD, MPH‡

Violence and its consequences of injury and death represent a major health problem in this country. The United States has one of the highest homicide rates in the industrialized world, 10 times higher than that of England and 25 times higher than that of Spain.[27] In 1980, homicide and assault were responsible for over 23,000 deaths, 700,000 potential years of life lost, 350,000 hospitalizations, 1½ million hospital days, and $640 million in health care costs.[15] Fatalities from violence represent only the tip of the iceberg; nonfatal intentional injuries occur as much as 100 times more frequently.[3] Assault and intentional injuries identified in medical settings can be four times that reported to the police, suggesting that medical institutions are a primary site for identification of individuals with violence-related problems.[3] Violence must be perceived by the medical and public health communities as a serious and large scale problem they need to address.

Violence is a major cause of death among adolescents and young adults. Homicide has risen over the past several decades to become the second leading cause of death for all 15 to 24 year olds in the United States.[7] Young black men are at the greatest risk for death and injury from violence. Their rate of death from homicide is from six (for 15–24 year olds) to twelve (for 25–44 year olds) times higher than the national rates.[8]

These statistics have generated a growing concern within the health care community about the need to address the problem of violence more aggressively. Indicative of this attention, the U.S. Department of Health and Human Services has made the reduction of homicide in the 15 to 24-year-old age group a major objective to be met by 1990.[24] This article describes the epidemiology and characteristics of violence and intentional injury among adolescents and discusses the various ways in which clinicians and the public health community can help to reduce the extent of this problem. (Although abuse and suicide contribute to

─────────────

*Assistant Professor of Pediatrics, Boston University School of Medicine; Director, Adolescent
  Services, Boston Department of Health and Hospitals, Boston, Massachusetts
†Assistant Professor, Boston University School of Medicine; Commissioner, Department of
  Public Health, The Commonwealth of Massachusetts, Boston, Massachusetts
‡Assistant Professor, Boston University School of Public Health, Boston, Massachusetts

adolescent intentional injuries, their prevention and intervention differ from assaultive violence and are not discussed in this article.)

CHARACTERISTICS AND CONTRIBUTING FACTORS

Although the media presents assaultive violence as either coldly premeditated
or randomly directed to innocent bystanders, statistics demonstrate that social and
cultural factors place certain persons at greater risk of violence. Individual factors,
such as family history of violence or low self-esteem, also increase the risk of
violence. Knowledge of these factors can help health care providers to identify and
intervene with individuals at special risk for intentional injury.

Most of our knowledge of the epidemiology of interpersonal violence comes
from the most extreme and rarest outcome, homicide. Information on nonfatal
intentional injuries is extremely limited because data on these events are not
routinely collected and evaluated. As a result, many assumptions about intentional
injury are extrapolated from what is known about homicide. Cases of intentional
injury are only identified by obvious evidence (i.e., gunshot wound) or physician
interest regarding the circumstances of the injury event. Even when asked,
information about circumstances of an injury is difficult to obtain from injured
persons, particularly when there is the possible threat of involvement by the
criminal justice system. Furthermore, an unknown number of episodes of interpersonal violence may not even reach the attention of any institution that could collect
data. Despite these difficulties, recent studies have confirmed that homicide and
nonfatal intentional injuries are associated with the same set of characteristics and
risk factors.

Societal and Cultural Factors

A number of factors related to the risk of intentional injury and homicide
reflect specific societal and cultural influences. These include racial issues, socioeconomic factors, gender expectations, age, and pressures associated with adolescence.

A common misconception about violence is that it is inter-racial. It is true that
blacks are over-represented in the homicide statistics: 44 per cent of homicide
victims are black, which is significantly higher than the proportion of blacks in the
general population.[7] This over-representation of blacks in homicide is corroborated
by the Northeastern Ohio Trauma Study of intentional injuries.[3] However, the
analysis of homicide statistics by the Violence Epidemiology Branch of the Centers
for Disease Control (CDC) has shown that 80 per cent of homicides occur between
members of the same race.[6] Although racism adds to the anger and stress that can
contribute to violence, little violence actually is racially instigated. Rather, it is
increasingly clear that socioeconomic status is a greater predictor of violence and
that the over-representation of blacks in violence statistics reflects their over-
representation in poverty.

The importance of the role of socioeconomic status is demonstrated in a recent
study from Atlanta.[10] Using the number of people per square foot in each housing
unit as a socioeconomic indicator, racial differences in homicide rates were eliminated when socioeconomic status was controlled. Lower socioeconomic status was
significantly associated with death by homicide. The Northeastern Ohio Trauma
Study also indicated that lower socioeconomic status and residence in urban areas
played a role in the likelihood of intentional injury.[3] The notion of economic stress
leading to increased risk of violence finds further support in a study of homicide in
Dayton, Ohio, where rises in unemployment rate were associated with an increased

homicide rate with a lag period of 1 to 2 years.[6] These findings are consistent with the Centers for Disease Control (CDC) analysis that shows homicides most often occur in urban areas characterized by low socioeconomic status, high population density, poor housing, and high unemployment rates.[8] Knowledge of these socio-economic factors helps to target special intervention efforts to specific high risk populations.

Whereas most homicide victims (77 per cent) are male,[7] female subjects are also subject to and involved in intentional violence.[13] Differences in weapon-carrying behavior and social expectations may contribute to their lower rates of more serious injuries and homicide. However, with increases in the number of media-portrayed female heroes who are as violent as their male counterparts, we can expect that the gap between male and female homicide and intentional injury rates may be reduced.

Adolescents are at high risk for violence because of the rapid psychological and physical changes that occur in the transition to adulthood. Teenagers face a number of major developmental tasks, including (1) individuation from family through a narcissistic period of self-development; (2) development of a sexual identity that includes a period of identification with sexual extremes, such as the macho image for males and extreme femininity for females; (3) development of a moral and personal value system through experimentation; and (4) preparation for future employment and responsibility.[12, 17]

Many of the behaviors associated with these developmental tasks predispose adolescents to violence. Narcissism has a strong component of self-consciousness, making a teenager extremely vulnerable to embarrassment. Adolescents' preoccupation with themselves, their appearance and their image, makes them particularly susceptible to over-reacting to even a mild insult. Linking this with identification with the extreme sex role stereotype often sets an individual up for the use of violence. Furthermore, peer pressure, important in facilitating success in many developmental tasks, also can enhance the likelihood of violent behavior. If fighting is expected by peers, then an adolescent will have considerable difficulty disregarding the pressures to fight.

The situation is exacerbated when poverty and racism are superimposed on adolescence. Anger associated with limited economic options and racism, understandable as it is, lowers the individual's threshold for violence.[12]

Individual Factors

It is the personal, behavioral, and spontaneous characteristics of violence that both raise the most concern and offer direction for intervention. Almost 60 per cent of victims and assailants know each other, and 20 per cent of victims and assailants are members of the same family. One half of homicides are precipitated by an argument as compared to only 15 per cent of homicides occurring in the course of committing another crime.[6] Alcohol use also contributes to violent behavior; approximately half of all homicide victims have elevated blood alcohol levels.[9, 25] These characteristics indicate that the key to prevention may lie in greater understanding of the behavioral components that contribute to violence.

Because a large number of homicides involve firearms, there is an important concern regarding the availability and the carrying of handguns even when there is no premeditated intent to actually use it. Knives follow handguns as the primary weapons related to homicide.[6] The availability of such weapons is particularly concerning given the evidence that a large number of youths carry weapons at least occasionally. A survey done in the Boston Public Schools by the Boston Commission on Safe Schools, for example, revealed that 37 per cent of males and 17 per cent of females carried a weapon in school at some time during the school year.[5] Fear for their own safety was a major reason given by students for this behavior. The carrying of a weapon, however, greatly increases the possibility for escalation of violence and the potential for its use for other than protective purposes.

Evidence is mounting that violence is a learned response to stress and conflict. Violence in the home has been associated with adolescent violent behavior.[1, 2] Violence observed on television also has been associated with violent behavior in children and youth.[13, 18, 28] This is particularly relevant given the extent of violence displayed in the media and the predominance of heroes in television and movies who use violent means to solve problems. The evidence strongly suggests that young people demonstrate violent behavior that they observe on television. On the other hand, several studies show children also can learn nonviolent behavioral strategies for dealing with conflict from television.[13, 20] When children observe nonviolent problem-solving strategies on television, they are found to mimic these behaviors in their play when conflicts arise or are presented.

Psychological and descriptive characteristics of victims of intentional injury and assailants provide additional insight into contributing individual factors associated with violence. One study demonstrated that early exposure to family violence, incomplete schooling, illiteracy, depression, chronic alcohol and drug use, and low self-esteem were risk factors for being a victim of homicide.[1] A second study, which further substantiates these characteristics, also found many similarities in behavior and psychological makeup between homicide assailants and victims of serious assaults. These two groups, when compared to a group of matched, randomly selected young men obtained from household sampling, appeared significantly similar and clearly distinct from the matched control group.[11] This study also reported a number of subjects having interchanged the role of victim and assailant during the study period. This suggests that individuals with high-risk characteristics can present either as a victim or an assailant initially, and are at risk for either in the future.

Despite the overwhelming evidence of the psychosocial context of violence, organic factors also may contribute to violent behavior. In a review of the literature on central nervous system impairment and the occurrence of violent behavior, Bell concluded that there were clear associations between biologic factors (i.e., history of severe head trauma) and violence, and calling for the identification of such impairments as one important component of prevention of violence.[4] This observation, however, needs to be balanced with the fact that in actual numbers, this group represents a relatively small portion of the larger population of individuals with violence-related problems.

Summary of Characteristics

A large number of contributing factors have been identified as being associated with violent behavior and intentional injury. Some of these factors, such as poverty, race and gender expectations, represent major societal issues that give little direction for a clinical role in prevention and treatment. However, some of the behavioral factors provide clearer indication for clinical and public health interventions through patient contact, outreach programs, and health education. Medical and public health settings have great potential for contributing to both the primary prevention of intentional injury and the avoidance of future problems related to violence.

INTERVENTION STRATEGIES

Addressing the problem of interpersonal violence involves the collaboration of a broad base of professionals and community organizations. Given the relatively recent focus on the problem, there are only a few programs to look to for assistance in developing interventions. Most efforts to date have focused on the role of the criminal justice system, which has for the most part provided after-the-fact, punitive responses to violent events. The fact that most intentional injuries are produced by known assailants, are not premeditated, and are associated with identifiable psychosocial and behavioral risk factors suggests that other avenues of response to the problem must be developed. Efforts to handle these characteristics can and should be implemented in the following ways: (1) primary prevention of violence as a response to anger and conflict; (2) screening for and early identification of high-risk individuals: (3) increased availability of secondary level services for the high-risk population; and (4) improved rehabilitative services. Within this context, the medical and public health communities can play an important role in collaboration with other appropriate human service, mental health, education, community, and criminal justice institutions.

Clinical and Health Strategies

Individual clinicians have many opportunities to incorporate violence prevention in their medical care. One such opportunity involves raising the issue of violence prevention as part of anticipatory guidance.[22] Because we know that violence is a learned behavior, parents can be enlisted to help to prevent violent behavior in their children. Parents have daily opportunities to teach their children how to handle anger, such as encouraging verbal rather than physical expression of angry feelings. With some guidance, parents can play an active, conscious role in teaching their children positive, nonviolent strategies in directing and resolving their anger. Pediatric health providers can facilitate this process. Issues, such as styles of discipline, regulating television viewing, and negotiating conflicts between siblings also can be addressed during pediatric encounters.

As children grow older and enter adolescence, pediatric providers have the opportunity to raise the subject of anger and violence directly with them. Raising awareness of the risks of fighting and the factors that lead to violent situations can open the opportunity to discuss the issue in more depth. As noted earlier, studies have indicated that many youths have concerns about risks of violence and some even carry weapons for a sense of self-protection. Discussing these fears and helping the adolescent to identify and develop alternative strategies for avoiding violent situations may assist young people to better understand their behavioral options. Anger must be legitimized as a normal emotion, but individuals must be offered options for the resolution of conflict.

Beyond the level of primary prevention, clinicians have the opportunity to play an important role in the early identification of youth at high risk for violent behavior. The work that has been done around identifying characteristics of persons who are victims or perpetrators of violence can be used to recognize potentially violent youth. Screening of children and youth for a history of family or peer violence, substance abuse, depression and low self-esteem, carrying of weapons, and history of central nervous system injury or pathology can lead to the identification of youth who may be able to be helped by referral to and earlier intervention from mental health and other related services.

This effort of primary care health providers must, of course, be linked to the increased development and availability of intervention services directed toward violent behavior. Merely identifying high-risk youth without appropriate referral resources would lead to considerable frustration on the part of clinicians. Educational, mental health, and support services for adolescents need to be enhanced, and intervention strategies addressing the underlying emotional and behavioral components of violent behavior must be developed.

Of equal importance is the need to modify the response of health care professionals to youth with intentional injuries. Health care institutions, particularly emergency departments, are the major site of contact with persons with violence-related problems. Diagnostic and intervention services for such events as rape, child and sexual abuse, and suicide attempts are well established in the medical setting, and the extent of support services for children and families displaying these symptoms is considerable. Many intentional injuries do not clearly fit these categories. These generally are managed from the perspective of treating the injury itself without investigating or responding to the circumstances of the injury or the underlying issues and behaviors that may have led to the injury. Suturing a superficial stab wound and sending a patient home will not reduce the risk for future injury. Such patients present a double risk in that some persons who present as victims may be assailants in the future. Intentional injury victims often explicitly express their intent to seek revenge.[11] In addition, there is evidence that victims are not necessarily passive in creating the violent encounter and may in fact display provocative behaviors that led to the injury-related event.[26] Routine and adequate assessment of intentional injury victims are of extreme importance. This assessment should minimally include investigation of the following factors:

1. Circumstances of the injury event
2. Victim's relationship to the assailant
3. Use of drugs or alcohol
4. Presence of underlying emotional or psychosocial risk factors (especially violence in the family)
5. History of intentional injuries or violent behaviors
6. Predisposing biologic risk factors
7. Intent to seek revenge

In many cases, this information can help to identify a need for referral to appropriate intervention and support services that may reduce the risk of further problems.

Increased awareness, understanding, and attention to violence by health care providers can contribute in a significant way to addressing this problem. Violence needs to be incorporated into the health care system agenda.

Public Health Strategies

Individual clinicians cannot address violence in isolation and the public health sector can play a role in establishing a broader context for violence prevention. Individual level interventions are unlikely to be successful without the supportive attitudes and values in the community. An increased level of awareness and understanding needs to be established at the community level. One such effort is currently in progress in the city of Boston.[19] This program is a large-scale initiative concerning violence prevention that includes community-based education through a wide range of existing community agencies, and mass media. The program is targeting two specific urban neighborhoods with high adolescent homicide rates in an effort to assess the impact of a Violence Prevention Project. The premise of this approach is based on the cognitive learning theory model where knowledge and understanding lead to changes in attitudes and behavior.[21] Although there is little experience with violence prevention in the public health arena, evidence to support this approach exists from programs using a community-based prevention model to deal with other behaviorally related health conditions such as heart disease and hypertension.[14, 23]

Another public health approach used in addressing health problems involves attempts to manipulate the environment to reduce risk. For example, the use of safety locks on firearms (analogous to safety caps on medication bottles) might be indicated. While this would not necessarily be expected to significantly reduce premeditated intentional injuries, it might reduce the extent of unintentional firearm injuries as well as providing a moment of second thought in unplanned violent events. It is important to keep in mind that this sort of environmental intervention is limited in its potential effect when the intent to hurt someone is a primary factor in a violent episode.

The public health system also can contribute to the establishment of improved secondary prevention and intervention services. The public health system has the responsibility for advocating for more extensive mental health services for youth and young adults to address problems of violent behavior. Furthermore, there is great need to increase the collaboration of the health care system with other institutions that deal with violent individuals such as the police and courts. The criminal justice system has the largest number of identified individuals at extremely high risk for violent behavior. Improving access to supportive services for these individuals is an important consideration for the human service system.

Societal Strategies

Clearly, there are also components related to violence that must be addressed at the broadest societal level. Poverty and racism are associated risk factors for homicide and intentional injury as they are with many other health problems. Stress related to economic survival, overcrowding, limited options for employment, and racial barriers play a significant role in emotional status and behavior. The observation that socioeconomic status and race are associated with homicide rates is just one additional reason why we, as a society, must increase efforts to reduce or resolve these problems. Such resolutions require long-term strategies and cannot be expected to have a shorter term impact on violence and its consequences. There are, however, a number of efforts that are potentially less complicated to pursue and may have more immediate impact.

Improved control of weapons is one short term intervention. The availability of lethal weapons plays a major role in the most serious consequences of violence. Reduced access to guns or more stringent regulation of firearm licensing may contribute to a reduction of the more serious injuries seen in this country. Gun control is an extremely controversial issue in the United States, with strong, well-financed lobbies in opposition. The medical and public health sectors can contribute greatly to counter this opposition and further increase awareness of the serious implications of easy access to weapons.

Increased efforts to reduce the level of substance abuse in this country, which have already begun to occur, also can potentially decrease the extent of violence. Even here, however, the broader focus is on controlled, illegal substances. The association between alcohol and violence is less well publicized and the medical community can help to educate the public about this important link.

Changing or modifying media messages with respect to violence is of equal importance. The pervasive image of the "violent hero" is a dangerous model for our children and adolescents. Violence is represented in all levels of television programming, including cartoons, as a major behavioral response to stress and conflict. Media heroes who display nonviolent strategies to resolve conflict are difficult to find. The sensationalism of the news media, who persist in maintaining inaccurate stereotypes of violence, make improved awareness and understanding of the problem all the more difficult.

Again, the medical and public health communities can play an important, visible role. It is essential that health care providers actively participate with others in advocating for a reduction in the potential display of violence to our youth as well as advocating for more accurate and responsible reporting on violence in the news media. Medical and public health professionals cannot influence these factors alone, but their contribution can greatly strengthen existing efforts to address these factors as they have around other problems such as diet and nutrition, smoking, toxic exposure, and automobile safety.

FUTURE NEEDS

While the effectiveness of the above interventions has not been demonstrated, they have sound basis in what is already known about violence, in what has previously been done for other behavior-related health problems, and in the experience of several existing violence-related interventions. The health care sector must increase its role but can only do so with certain key institutional changes.

At the clinical level, training about violence for primary care clinicians, mental health providers, and other human service professionals must be incorporated into both initial training and continuing education programs. Increased knowledge on the subject will help professionals feel more comfortable and competent when addressing the problem. Furthermore, the incorporation of violence in the routine health care and educational systems is an important mechanism for increasing general community level awareness and understanding. Research in this area is equally important for the development of screening instruments that can predict violent behavior and appropriate protocols for managing individuals who present with intentional injuries. Instruments such as these should not be difficult to develop, but they require adequate interest and funding to make them a reality.

From a public health perspective, further development and evaluation of primary prevention initiatives will contribute greatly to our understanding of the problem and its potential solution. As this is an issue that particularly affects the minority community, input and involvement of that community is of great importance to assure that inappropriate stereotypes are avoided and cultural perspectives are maintained in addressing the problem.

Research efforts also must be increased. Establishment of adequate data bases and surveillance systems for intentional injuries are essential to improve our knowledge of risk factors related to violent behavior as well as maintaining a close eye on changes in the magnitude and characteristics of the problem. We need better definition of the etiology of nonfatal intentional injuries and fighting behavior. Much also is to be learned from communities and countries that experience lower rates of violence indicators. Again, interest and funding need to be generated to allow such activities to occur.

SUMMARY

Violence and its consequences are a major issue to be addressed by the health care community. The magnitude and characteristics of the problem cry out for new, creative approaches and provide for some insight into the direction that needs to be taken. Some of the components related to violence are societal in scope and will require long-term strategies well beyond the immediate realm of the health care system. Others provide direction that more clearly present a role for health providers and public health planners. Although there will be no easy answers or solutions to this problem, it is essential that support be developed for experimental efforts. The health community cannot ignore this problem and can in fact make a real contribution to its resolution through prevention, treatment, and research.

REFERENCES

1. Allen NH: Homicide prevention and intervention. Suicide and Life Threatening Behavior 11:167, 1981

2. Bandura A, Ross D, Ross S: Vicarious reinforcement and imitative learning. J Abnorm Soc Psychol 63:601–607, 1963
3. Barancik J, Chatterjee B, Green Y et al: Northeastern Ohio Trauma Study. I. Magnitude of the problem. Am J Public Health 73:746–751, 1983
4. Bell CC: Coma and the etiology of violence, Part 2. J Nat Med Assoc 79:79–85, 1987
5. Boston Commission on Safe Public Schools: Making Our Schools Safe for Learning. Boston, Boston Public Schools, 1983
6. Centers for Disease Control: Homicide—United States. MMWR 31:599–602, 1982
7. Centers for Disease Control: Violent deaths among persons 15–24 years of age—United States, 1970–78. MMWR 32:453–457, 1982
8. Centers for Disease Control: Homicides among young black males—United States, 1978–82. MMWR 34:629–633, 1985
9. Centers for Disease Control: Homicide Surveillance: High-Risk Racial and Ethnic Groups—Blacks and Hispanics, 1970–83. Atlanta, Centers for Disease Control, 1986
10. Centerwall B: Race, socioeconomic status and domestic homicide, Atlanta 1971–2. Am J Public Health 74:1813–1815, 1984
11. Dennis RE: Homicide among black males: Social costs to families and communities. Public Health Reports 95:556, 1980
12. Erickson E: Identify, Youth and Crisis. New York, W. W. Norton, 1968
13. Eron L, Huesman LR: Television violence and aggressive behavior. In Lahey B, Kazdin A (eds): Advances in Clinical Child Psychology. New York, Plenum Press, 1984
14. Farguhar J: The community-based model of life style interventions. Am J Epidemiol 108:103–111, 1978
15. Federal Bureau of Investigation: Uniform Crime Report: Crime in the United States. Washington, D.C., U.S. Department of Justice, 1981
16. Heller A: Job loss and impact on health in Dayton, Ohio. American J Soc Psychiatry 3:47, 1983
17. Jessor R, Jessor S: Problem Behavior and Psychosocial Development: A Longitudinal Study of Youth. New York, Academic Press, 1977
18. Liebert R, Neale J, Davidson E: The Early Window: Effect of Television on Children and Youth. New York, Pergamon Press, 1973
19. Prothrow-Stith DB, Spivak HR, Hausman AJ: The Violence Prevention Project: A public health approach. Science, Technology and Human Values. (in press)
20. Slaby R, Quarfoth G: Effects of television on the developing child. Adv Behav Pediatr 1:225–266, 1980
21. Stokols D: The reduction of cardiovascular risk: An application of social learning perspectives. In Enlow A, Henderson J (eds): Applying Behavioral Science to Cardiovascular Risk. New York, American Heart Association, 1975
22. Stringham P, Weitzman M: Violence counseling in the routine health care of adolescents. J Adolesc Health Care (in press)
23. Tuomilehto J, Nissinen A, Salonen J et al: Community program for control of hypertension in North Karelia, Finland. Lancet ii:900–903, 1980
24. U.S. Public Health Service: Promoting Health/Preventing Disease: Public Health Service implementation plans for attaining the objectives for the nation. Public Health Reports (Suppl):3, 1983
25. University of California at Los Angeles, Centers for Disease Control: The Epidemiology of Homicide in the City of Los Angeles, 1970–79. Atlanta, Department of Health and Human Services, 1985
26. Wolfgang ME: Patterns in Criminal Homicide. New York, John Wiley & Sons, 1958
27. Wolfgang M: Homicide in other industrialized countries. Bull N Y Acad Med 62:400, 1986
28. Zuckerman D, Zuckerman B: Television's impact on children. Pediatrics 75:233–240, 1985

Deputy Commissioner
Massachusetts Department of Public Health
150 Tremont Street
Boston, Massachusetts 02111

0031–3955/88 $0.00 + .20

Drug Use, Depression, and Adolescents

Neela P. Joshi, MBBS, MPH, DCH,* and Marcia Scott, MD†

The twentieth century has witnessed a substantial decline in early childhood mortality. In the last 20 years, however, the death rate among teenagers has risen frighteningly, reinforcing assumptions that adolescence—with its increased expectations and independence—is a dangerous time.[48] Whether in the form of accidents, suicide, or homicide, violence is the leading cause of the rise in teenage mortality.[48] These high-risk behaviors often are associated with other disruptions of normal adolescent functioning.

Turmoil in adolescence is no longer perceived as part of a necessary, normal developmental process in adolescence. More than half the youngsters studied by Offer and Petersen[79] completed adolescence without significant upheavals in functioning or in interpersonal relationships. Another third had minor or intermittent difficulties. The rest of these youngsters, whose adolescence was characterized by disruptions, included half the teenagers with severe psychiatric problems. High-risk behaviors, disrupted relationships, and troubled functioning frequently are associated with teenage substance abuse. Drug abuse, therefore, often is seen as the primary cause of morbidity and mortality in adolescents. It has become the symbol of "what is wrong" with adolescents. In fact, however, drug use is usually a symptom of pervasive developmental disruption.

It is crucial for physicians to understand the pharmacologic effects of alcohol and other psychoactive substances, as well as the social patterns of drug use. Physicians can best interpret drug-using behaviors if they conceptualize them as deviant attempts at coping and remember that the drugs—beyond their characteristic toxicity—interfere with social and emotional functioning and with interpersonal relationships, thereby threatening normal development. The physician's ability to intervene appropriately with youngsters and their families depends on a knowledge of the genetic, constitutional (internal), and environmental (external) factors that predispose an adolescent to use drugs as a way to cope. Whereas many children and adolescents handle environmental stressors and developmental challenges well, others are more vulnerable. Their development and functioning are characterized by frustrations and helplessness that make them especially susceptible to continuing or intense drug use, deviant behavior, and developmental arrest.

Depression has long been recognized as a factor in drug use. For many years,

---

*Assistant Professor, Pediatrics, Boston University School of Medicine, Boston, Massachusetts
†Assistant Professor, Psychiatry, Boston University School of Medicine, Boston, Massachusetts

it was commonly assumed that adolescents and children did not get depressed. The work of Rutter,[93] Sroufe and Rutter,[111] and Poznanski[85] makes it clear that children and adolescents often express feelings like depression nonverbally, that is, through behavior substantiating that depression is a significant component underlying behavioral and developmental problems.

Thus, drug abuse can provide a depressed youngster with emotional expression and a way, albeit dysfunctional, of coping with overwhelming feelings. These behaviors mimic a semblance of culturally appropriate adolescent functioning and superficially engage youngsters socially, but may in fact isolate them from needed experiences and relationships in ways that are ultimately self-defeating.

This article reviews both drug use and depression in adolescents. Whenever possible, drug use and depression are integrated around the theme that they represent efforts to manage different and possibly overlapping constitutional and social risk factors. To begin with, what are definitions of depression and drug use?

DEFINITIONS OF DEPRESSION AND DRUG USE

Depression

The term *depression* implies three meanings: (1) depressed mood, or a feeling of discouragement or hopelessness, (2) depressive symptoms, and (3) a major depressive episode or syndrome.[117] Recently, Boyd and Weissman have grouped depressive mood and depressive symptoms into one category of "feelings of sadness and disappointment."[17] Hence, youngsters may describe themselves as depressed, sad, blue, hopeless, low, down in the dumps, or irritable. The Diagnostic and Statistical Manual of Mental Disorders (DSM-III-R) is widely used to diagnose depression. By DSM-III-R criteria, a major depressive episode is defined essentially as having a depressed mood, or loss of interest or pleasure in all, or almost all, activities. At least five of the following symptoms must be prominent, relatively persistent for a period of at least 2 weeks, and occur daily: poor appetite, insomnia or hypersomnia; psychomotor agitation or retardation; loss of interest or pleasure in usual activities; loss of energy or fatigue; feelings of worthlessness, self-reproach, or excessive or inappropriate guilt; diminished ability to think or concentrate; and recurrent thoughts of death or suicide.[4] A major depressive episode can recur, and a depressive syndrome can be chronic. Diagnosis encompasses self-reports regarding depressive symptoms that should be substantiated by reports from others, such as parents and teachers, and professional assessment of clinical states such as anhedonia, or psychomotor retardation or agitation.[86] In this review, we will exclude secondary depressions associated with medical disorders.

Drug Use

The term *drug use* in this review includes both drugs and alcohol. Many, even most youngsters use drugs or alcohol at some time. Typically, adolescents state they use drugs out of curiosity or as part of their association with peers and friends.[26] According to many authorities, any use of psychoactive drugs by adolescents, except under medical supervision, should be considered abuse.[74]

Problem drinking is defined as being drunk six or more times or experiencing negative consequences in two out of five life areas during the preceding 12 months: trouble with teachers, difficulties with friends, criticism from dates, trouble with the police, and driving under the influence of alcohol.[30] Chemical dependence is defined as continued use of drugs or alcohol despite adverse physical, emotional, or sociocultural outcomes.[78, 113] Continued and intense use of drugs and progression to dependency are usually associated with particular vulnerability to emotional conflict (low self-esteem) or environmental stress (family disruption).

INCIDENCE OF DEPRESSION AND DRUG USE

Depression

Depression is a significant health problem for adolescents. Usually depression in adolescents is a reaction to age-appropriate stresses or difficulties in their environment. Vulnerability to affective illness and mood disorders can be expected to emerge at this stressful time of life and manifest itself as behavioral problems representing underlying difficulty with coping.

In a sample of 384 junior high school students from a North Carolina school district, a major depressive syndrome was found in 2.9 per cent of the adolescents.[100] The measurements for depressive symptoms in this study were obtained by using the Center for Epidemiologic Studies Depression Scale (CES-D) and scored along the lines of the Research Diagnostic Criteria for major depressive disorders. When a short form of Beck Depression Inventory (BDI) was administered to 63 seventh and eighth grade students, 33 per cent were judged to be experiencing moderate to severe depression.[1]

In a community survey, Kandel and Davies focused exclusively on exhibited depressive moods in 14 to 18 year olds: 19.7% reported feeling "sad or depressed" in the year prior to the survey.[61] Using the BDI to measure a broad spectrum of depressive symptomatology in adolescents, Kaplan et al. reported a point prevalence (i.e., the proportion of individuals ill at any one point in time) of 8.6 per cent for major depressive disorders.[67] The total percentage was 22.1 per cent of adolescents with scores on the BDI that were indicative of depression. This finding is remarkably similar to results from Rutter's study where 22 per cent of the teens in a general population responded to self-reported substantial depressive symptomatology.[92]

In college or college-aged populations, approximately 30 per cent of the men and women were found to have had an affective disorder.[49, 72, 103] Female adolescents had higher rates of depression than males in many of these studies.[61, 67, 92] In addition, adolescents living in poverty appear to have higher rates of depression in comparison to more privileged teens.[61, 67, 100] Overall, the prevalence of depressive symptoms tends to be higher in adolescents than in adults.[61, 99]

Drug Use

Experimentation with drug use is extremely common among adolescents. The prevalence of drug use in adolescents differs markedly for various drugs: alcohol and cigarettes have a higher frequency of use than illegal drugs. In the 1985 national survey, Monitoring the Future Project on High School Seniors, the lifetime substance abuse prevalence was 92 per cent for alcohol, 69 per cent for cigarettes, 54 per cent for marijuana, 26 per cent for stimulants, 17 per cent for cocaine, 12 per cent each for sedatives, tranquilizers, and hallucinogens, 10 per cent for other opiates, and 1.2 per cent for heroin.[56] Six out of every ten seniors (61 per cent) have tried some illicit drug by the time they leave high school.[56] The 30-day prevalence of drug use was 66 per cent for alcohol, 30 per cent for cigarettes, 26 per cent for marijuana, and 7 per cent each for amphetamines and cocaine.[56] During this period, daily smoking was reported by 20 per cent and daily drinking by 5 per cent of all seniors in 1985.[56] Similar prevalence rates of drug use by adolescents are reported in the National Survey on Drug Abuse.[40]

Although reported use of all these substances increases with age during adolescence, the period of 15 to 17 years old has been identified as the time of highest risk for initiation into marijuana use.[62] After age 25, there is a sharp decline in the use of marijuana and other illegal drugs. It has been suggested that in some individuals this decrease is associated with assumption of adult social roles that are incompatible with drug use such as marriage and parenthood.[62]

Gender differences are definitely revealed in the studies of prevalence of drug use.[7, 55, 62–64] Girls generally report less drug use. Consumption of five or more alcoholic drinks in a row, at least once in 2 weeks prior to the survey, was reported by 30 per cent of high school seniors in 1985.[56] The prevalence of this behavior was considerably higher for male (45 per cent) than for female (28 per cent) subjects.[56] Gender differences in marijuana use are less frequently reported.[55] Drinking is common among youths from all major ethnic groups—whites, Hispanics, American Indians, and blacks—in the United States.[96] Findings regarding ethnic differences in marijuana use are inconclusive. No differences for marijuana use by blacks, whites, and British West Indian teens were reported by Brook et al.,[19] whereas Johnston's study revealed higher retrospective rates of use by high school blacks than whites,[54] and Brunswik found that whites were less likely to report having tried marijuana than were black or Hispanic adolescents in a New York sample.[21] It is of crucial importance that physicians and other professionals working with teenagers are knowledgeable of these gender and ethnic differences in use of alcohol and marijuana because this awareness has important implications for interventions as discussed later in this article.

Studies in Drug Use and Depression

A number of studies demonstrate an association between depression and drug use.[32, 33, 81, 82] Even though the relationship between mood disorders and alcohol is more commonly discerned than between mood disorders and drugs,[77] drug abuse also has been associated with both a major depressive disorder (MDD) and other psychiatric diagnoses, such as phobic, panic and obsessive/compulsive disorders, and schizophrenia.[29, 103] Increased depression certainly has been found to be connected with the heavy use of marijuana and other drugs.[18, 70, 73] Furthermore, in a longitudinal study of adolescent drug use, a depressive mood was found to be an important predictor of initiation into illegal drugs other than marijuana in teenagers who had already used marijuana.[81] In the same study, these depressed adolescents reported a decrease in their depressive mood over time with the continued use of illegal drugs. Based on these same data, Paton and Kandel have reported a relationship between drug use and depressive mood for white male, and white, black, and Puerto Rican female adolescents. Among black and Puerto Rican boys, there was no relationship discerned between drug use and depression.[82]

The evidence for a temporal or causal relationship between MDD and drug and alcohol abuse is contradictory. MDD always preceded drug abuse in the study by Deykin et al.,[29] whereas in Schuckit's study, 60 per cent of young men reported that alcohol or drug problems preceded depression.[103]

It seems clear, however, that the prevalence of drug use and depression in adolescents is high. The relationship between the use of drugs and depression in adolescents has been reported by many investigators.[29, 32, 33, 81, 82, 103] There is little systematic information to clarify the causal relationships between depression and drug use, or to explain the long-term effects of depressive mood on drug use, or of long-term drug use as it affects or exacerbates depressive mood, however.[62] Further research is needed to clarify long-term effects of depressive mood on drug use or of long-term drug use as it affects depressive mood.

THEORIES OF DEPRESSION AND DRUG ABUSE

A variety of causes have been explored over the years to explain why depression occurs, as well as to shed light on why people turn to drug use. Early formulations of depression were based on psychoanalytic models.[41] Recently, Sameroff's transactional model,[95] and Greenspan's[46] and Sroufe and Rutter's[111] developmental/adaptation models explain adolescent depression as an adaptive failure that results when underlying vulnerabilities and multiple social and individual risk factors impact too severely on the adolescent.

Earlier studies of drug and alcohol abuse relied on genetic theories[59, 101] or focused on disturbances in personality.[6, 38, 43, 69] Later sociocultural theories[15, 20, 35–37, 52, 112, 114] emphasized the effects of cultural experience, social context, and peer-oriented life-styles. More recent work encompasses developmental issues[45] and psychosocial theories.[53]

Drug use and depression, like all behaviors and moods, are attempts to master feelings to negotiate normal, age-related conflicts, painful life disruptions, or new life roles. Depression and self-destructive behaviors can emerge when underlying vulnerabilities, developmental deficits, or social risk factors distort these attempts at adaptation. Genetic, developmental, and social theories may all affect different stages of drug involvement, social factors playing a more important role in the early stages, psychological factors in later ones.[60]

To realize how these different models may apply to particular life stages or to individual children, it is helpful to understand the developmental process. Sameroff described development as an interaction or transaction of both internal and external resources. Internal resources include genetic, neuroendocrine, and biochemical factors; intelligence; temperament; and personality traits, such as ego strength, self-esteem, and likeability. External resources are environmental, involving socioeconomic status, and family and peer relationships. In a transactional model, internal and external factors operate together to produce certain outcomes at any given age or stage of development.[95] Thus Cicchetti and Schneider-Rosen have defined normal adolescent development as a series of interlocking social, emotional, cognitive, and constitutional competencies.[25]

In this context, competence—as pointed out by Beardslee[11] and Waters and Sroufe[115]—is the ability to use internal and external resources to accomplish major, developmentally appropriate behavioral tasks. Achievements in school and formation of relationships embody success in the cognitive and social spheres, for example. According to Sroufe and Rutter, competence at one period of development, which helps an individual broadly adapt to his or her environment, prepares the way for competent development at the next stage.[111] Important age- and stage-appropriate tasks are critical to a child's adaptation at any developmental stage.[46, 111] Some tasks decrease in salience as others emerge, whereas others are always prominent and necessary. According to Cicchetti and Schneider-Rosen,[25] attachment as a developmental task begins in the first year of life and continues throughout adolescence and adult life. It undergoes transformations and reintegrations, and during adolescence, accomplishments of increasing autonomy and entrance into the peer world become very important. Given a stable supportive environment in childhood, early competent adaptation is often predictive of later competence,[115] and it is hoped that protective factors or buffers against affective disorders such as depression have been created.

Pathologic development, on the other hand, may be conceived as a lack of integration of crucial social, emotional, cognitive, and constitutional factors, hence potentially precluding the achievement of competent adaptation.[24, 65, 110] This may occur at any particular developmental level. Since the early structures of styles of relating, intellectual competence and self-mastery are incorporated into later adaptations, early deviation may compromise later adaptation.

It is also true, however, that each stage of development can provide a new opportunity to rework these structures and restore the capacity to adapt. The teen years especially bring cognitive development, physical development, independence, and new social expectations. Hence adolescence represents both a stressor and an opportunity. Unfortunately, in an individual adolescent, long-standing patterns of maladaptation or of adverse social interaction may prove to be the significant risk factors that precipitate depression.

Psychodynamic theories and transactional developmental models explain drug abuse in terms of interacting genetic, psychological, and social factors that result in both adaptive and maladaptive behaviors.[50] For example, Hendin views the use of drugs as an attempt on the part of the individual person to handle conflicts that arise in relations with others and with society: Particular needs and pressures vary, as the person passes through various developmental stages.[50] Illustratively, early childhood experiences such as illness or parental marital discord may interfere with a youngster's competence in verbal or social expression in relationships or in self-esteem. Therefore it is critical to understand how these experiences are crucial and later may determine vulnerability to drug use. It becomes a way of experiencing and managing difficult feelings.

Children reared in chaotic or stressful environments may be less well equipped to negotiate critical developmental tasks successfully. These youngsters are at greater risk when they encounter problems with painful feelings, interpersonal conflicts, or social expectations. The emergence of depression or dependence on drugs that such stresses elicit can result in further withdrawal from developmental challenges and can begin a cycle that leads to social or emotional breakdown. Long and Valliant have pointed out that depression and alcohol dependence, rather than economic deprivation, may transmit social disadvantage.[71] Not all youngsters who use drugs are depressed or dysfunctional. Some become involved during a social or emotional crisis period. Drug and alcohol use represents ways of coping that seem culturally consistent for these adolescents and are often socially reinforced by peers or adults.

To summarize, for adolescent drug abuse or depression there are multiple vulnerabilities and risk factors, and different components play a critical role at different stages of development. Studies that have investigated these risk factors as they relate to adolescent depression and drug abuse are reviewed next.

EMPIRICAL EVIDENCE

Genetic and Neuroendocrine Factors and Psychobiological Markers

Based on a review of numerous twin and adoption studies of adults, Gershon et al. summarized explorations for the existence of genetic predisposition for bipolar and major depressive disorders.[42] However, biologic evidence of a genetic factor in these illnesses, such as genetic markers and linkages, is still inconclusive.[28] Little research has been done on children and adolescents in the area of genetic predisposition to mood disorders.

After puberty there is a change in sex ratio for mood disorders. A most striking rise in mood disorders occurs in female subjects.[94] This raises the possibility of change in the neuroendocrine system as a causative factor for depression. However, there is no existing evidence relating hormonal changes to the emergence of depression.[94] Some studies on depressive illness in prepubertal children and adolescents have investigated neuroendocrine markers. There is hypersecretion of cortisol (20 per cent) and growth hormone (GH), positive dexamethasone suppression (60 per cent), and diminished GH secretion in response to insulin tolerance[87–89] in depressed prepubertal children. Depressed adolescents, on the other hand, hypo-secrete GH,[91] indicating a strong effect of hormonal changes of puberty. The abnormalities of GH persist in prepubertal depressed children even after they recover from their depression.[90] This evidence is suggestive of a genetic trait marker, but data are not yet available regarding GH levels in normal siblings and in recovered adolescents.

Offspring of parents with a major mood disorder show a significantly high rate of mood disorders, in comparison to the children of controls.[27, 80, 116, 118] Whether the high incidence of depression in these children is due to familial transmission or to the effects of living with a depressed parent is not clear. Future quantitative research in genetics may help clarify these relationships.

Longitudinal followup studies[5, 84, 85] suggest that depression and related behavioral problems in childhood are often predictive of significant psychopathology in adolescence. Whether there is continuity between childhood and adult depression can be established only when good epidemiologic studies become available.

Alcohol and drug problems also may be genetically influenced.[102] Studies of alcoholism in twins raised in the same environment show that identical twins were much more likely to have similarities in alcohol abuse than fraternal twins.[57, 59] In a Swedish study of 2000 adoptees, a high incidence of alcoholism in parents was positively correlated with an incidence of alcohol abuse in adopted-away sons.[101] The transmission mechanism of genetic predisposition to alcoholism is still unclear, however.

Personality Structures

A significant relationship has been reported between self-esteem and depression,[8–10] and between alcohol-consumption patterns and self-esteem.[2, 12, 23, 77] Yanish and Battle have indicated that depression correlates significantly with almost all facets of self-esteem and also that a correlation exists between alcohol consumption and self-esteem.[119] Low self-esteem over time predicted initiation into various forms of drug use in a three-wave, longitudinal study of junior and senior high school adolescents.[66] Lack of mastery of social and intellectual skills, poor control in regard to various life tasks,[83, 106] and feelings of powerlessness or inadequacy[13] have been reported to be associated with increased alcohol and drug use. Other longitudinal studies have measured personality and other psychosocial variables prior to the onset of substance use in adolescence and have shown a dependable relationship between these variables and the likelihood and extent of later use of illegal drugs, such as marijuana, cocaine, and LSD.[104, 105, 107] Measures of socialization such as the ability to make friends were particularly efficient indicators of later use of illegal drugs. Socialization scores were highest among adolescents who remained nonusers of both legal and illegal drugs and lowest for those who became users of illegal drugs.[108]

Further longitudinal studies demonstrate evidence that patients who sought treatment for depression and other mood disorders, and who had alcohol or drug problems, were similar to individuals in the population who abuse drugs and alcohol, namely those who are young, male, unmarried, or from a lower socioeconomic background. Mood disorders were associated with high rates of alcohol and drug use in this analysis.[47]

Environmental and Social Risk Factors

Family disruptions associated with unemployment, poverty, and divorce contribute to stressors experienced by children.[14] The Ramsey Clinic in St. Paul, Minnesota, which provides substance abuse treatment to adolescents, maintains a database—the Chemical Abuse Treatment Outcome Registry (CATOR). From the initial assessment of these youngsters, grief and loss appeared as significant stressors: death of a family member, in 68 per cent; death of a friend, 45 per cent; separation of parents, 54 per cent; and divorce of parents, 46 per cent. Physical abuse was discovered in 32 per cent and sexual abuse in 7 per cent of the adolescents treated. Three quarters of them reported experiencing depression.[22] High rates of attempted suicide[68] and severe drug abuse[58] have been reported in children of alcoholic parents.

It is important to realize that a child's sense of helplessness in the face of these stressors is often the medium for acute emotional vulnerability and clears a path to depression or substance abuse. Implications of the theoretic frameworks presented need to be examined for clinical management and for public health interventions.

IMPLICATIONS FOR PUBLIC HEALTH INTERVENTIONS AND CLINICAL MANAGEMENT

Many current approaches to adolescent depression or drug use are simply applications of standard therapeutic techniques, designed to provide some structure and supportive relationship for teenagers, yet often these styles of treatment do not address specific determinants of the behavior or timely developmental issues. At other times, interventions are unfortunate responses to the feelings adults have, that is, anger about adolescent behavior and concern for their own or for the adolescent's safety. Although these feelings are understandable, interventions that arise from them do little to help and are often counterproductive. Often the failure of an intervention gives credibility to the notion that all adolescents are hopelessly self-destructive, that drug abuse is an intractable problem, and that psychological understanding is an ineffective approach that wastes time and money.

Understanding and evaluating depression and substance abuse demands widespread realization that all behaviors are expressions and that self-destructive adaptations have multiple constitutional, psychosocial, and sociocultural determinants both in the individual and in the culture. Treating depression and substance abuse requires a careful targeting of specific individual and social problems. Treatment also must accurately respond to a child's developmental level.

For example, many youngsters take drugs as part of peer group experiences. Having friends who are involved in obtaining and using drugs has been reported to be the strongest predictor at all levels of drug use in adolescents, but only a few youngsters go on to heavy or continuous substance use.[26] Physicians need to be able to distinguish these groups since the former often are reacting transiently to stressors with behaviors consistent with their culture. These particular youngsters may respond well to pressures within the culture that diminish the status of self-destructive behavior while assisting them with positive educational and adaptive strategies: For example, public health measures can stimulate a negative attitude toward drugs in the community and reinforce positive ways of coping with stress through self-help groups, economic opportunities, religious participation, and positive forms of emotional expression in work, play, and relationships. Caregivers also need to recognize that youngsters with serious internal pathology, such as depression, or with several external stressors, such as extreme poverty or abuse, often are unable to make use of such educational assistance or positive reinforcement. These adolescents require individual assessment and treatment to enhance motivation and skills, so that positive cultural norms, as well as individual and public health interventions, become accessible.

CLINICAL MANAGEMENT

An adolescent's drug abuse or depression may surface in a variety of ways: Trouble with the law may uncover problems; disciplinary issues in school or at home may point toward drug abuse; it may arise in counseling for depression or other mental disorders, or for family or school problems; or social isolation may bring a youngster's problems to the attention of family or friends. Often the substance-abusing adolescent is found to have multiple problems, such as conduct or attention disorders, complicated by deficits in learning or social skills.[51] These diagnoses often are associated with depression in youngsters.

It is possible to miss the early signs of drug abuse or depression if one is looking for needle tracks or a history of suicidal attempts or ideation. Adolescents rarely walk into a physician's office complaining of drug dependence or depression. Sometimes they express their frustrations and feelings verbally by describing problems with school, or unhappiness with job or family. More often, their emotional expression has been translated into behaviors: excessive smoking, trouble with the law, sleeplessness, sleepiness, deteriorating appearance or work habits, or weight problems. The symptoms of drug use, endocrine diseases such as hypothyroidism or diabetes, infectious diseases, or nutritional disorders often mimic and are confused with psychiatric illness.[44]

Drugs and alcohol are powerful mood-altering substances, and when youngsters use them to deal with emotional problems, more layers of behavioral problems often emerge. The physiologic effects of drugs and of drug withdrawal often interfere with normal patterns of sleep, appetite, energy, and sexual functioning. Disruption of these functions is also symptomatic of depression.

It is incumbent on a physician to make a comprehensive assessment of an adolescent with this constellation of symptoms. The youngster must be evaluated in terms of inherent vulnerability, developmental achievement, and social risk factors, using the developmental models outlined earlier. Early diagnosis and management are the most likely approaches to be successful.

Diagnostic Assessment

A thorough history needs to be gotten during the initial clinical interview(s), which includes: overall health and specific complaints; family's usual health patterns, including the family's possible psychiatric or substance abuse history; school and job performance; social activities and relationships with friends; sexual functioning and understanding; and interpersonal relationships within the family.

Inquiries about alcohol and drug use must be a routine, nonthreatening part of initial clinical interviews. Caregivers should ask about specific drug(s) used by the patient, including quantity and frequency of each drug as well as the possibility of sharing drug paraphernalia. Use of a simple checklist, for example, the Adolescent Drug Use History Checklist by Farrow and Deisher,[34] provides considerable information regarding the pattern and extent of drug use in a teenager.

In addition, specific information should be obtained about sleep patterns, changes in appetite and weight, level of energy, school performance, and sexual activity.

A complete physical examination should be performed to see whether there are signs of particular illness, such as infectious mononucleosis, hypothyroidism, or nutritional disorders. Laboratory screens should include tests to rule out infections (mononucleosis), anemia, hypothyroidism, or diabetes. Judicious use of blood and urine tests to detect drugs (marijuana, cocaine) will aid diagnosing some adolescents.

At this stage of assessment, in addition to indicating the presence of drug abuse or depression, the primary care physician needs also to determine the extent of depression and stage of drug involvement. The intensity of substance use can be appraised by observing irritability, mood swings, argumentative behavior, difficulty being a patient, trouble with explaining symptoms or feelings, or denial of wrong doing and blaming others. Severity of depression can be assessed further from a possibly poor appearance or reported deteriorating work habits and relationships.

Advanced stages of both drug use and depression are more easily recognizable: A youngster may have violated the law by shoplifting or vandalism, may be isolated from friends, may be involved in unusual sexual behaviors, or might be brought into the emergency ward with razor slashes on the wrist. Drug use is often associated with these troubling behaviors.

The next important step is to identify youngsters' understanding of their drug use to aid the formulation of its meaning in psychological and social terms. The management of these young people is not helped by simply labeling them as "delinquent" or "antisocial." A useful way to preceive them, however, is to recognize they are developmentally and socially thwarted[73] and that they are using aggressive adult behaviors in the service of likely unbearable childlike frustrations and helplessness. It will provide little or no help to focus intervention on the negative behavior because the youngster often lacks the skills or supports to initiate alternative ways of coping. Simple detoxification or threats leave them more isolated and feeling more helpless. Rarely can they engage in individual outpatient counseling, and such referrals are likely to fail. An integrated approach encompasses detoxification with psychiatric, family, and social assessment, and with counseling, much of which should take place within the youngsters' social and familial networks.

Treatment

The choice of a treatment setting for seriously drug-involved or depressed adolescents, whether inpatient, residential, or outpatient, depends on the severity of drug involvement, the coexistence of depression or other psychiatric disorders, the youngster's personal and environmental assets, and available community resources. Resources for adolescents with disruptive behavior are in short supply and often are directed primarily at controlling behavior, and hence do little to affect underlying emotional or social problems. For this reason, treatment of and in the family, even in the presence of serious deficits, is often the best way to provide a safe, effective milieu for the treatment of an adolescent drug user. In addition, family involvement may uncover drug use or depressive disorders in the family, engage other family members in needed treatment, provide support for the adolescent within the family, and prevent drug use or other problems in younger siblings. Ideal treatment involves attention to family, social, vocational, and psychological rehabilitation,[51] as well as striving for total abstinence. Appropriate referrals to organizations and groups for adolescents, which help to sustain abstinence while providing ongoing support for them and their families, also are needed.

If depression exists without drug involvement, a primary care physician may decide to treat the youngsters him- or herself. This is less feasible if there are indications of strong suicidal ideation or signs of psychosis. Alternately, primary care physicians—internists, pediatricians, family practitioners—can integrate mental health clinicians in their practices to provide early assessment as well as intervention for youngsters with mood and other psychiatric disorders. All adolescents expressing serious suicidal ideation or psychosis must be referred to a child psychiatrist for further evaluation and treatment.

PREVENTION

Prevention in conventional public health terms means preventing the problem before it begins, that is, *primary prevention*. Stopping the progression once it has begun is *secondary prevention* and stopping the worst consequences of the problem is *tertiary prevention*.[31] Public policy decisions and public health education efforts to prevent substance abuse should be aimed at preadolescent patients, parents, primary caregivers, and routine health maintenance clinic staffs, as well as the culture itself.

If physicians accept the opinion of McDonald[74] that any use of psychoactive substance, except under medical supervision, is drug abuse, then their efforts will be directed toward abstinence from alcohol and drug use. Pediatricians are in a unique position to participate in these efforts because they are trained in offering age-appropriate anticipatory guidance. Although an individual physician may define drug use as a totally moral problem, he or she has a special opportunity to treat the medical, social, and emotional factors that support drug use. This approach can enable youngsters and their families to make moral decisions and commitments that without intervention may be impossible to achieve given the social, emotional, and medical problems they may have.

Physicians are needed in community-wide prevention efforts working with parent and student groups such as MADD/SADD, with police and juvenile court officials, and with the media. Schools, where children and adolescents spend so many of their waking hours, are also fertile ground for vigorous prevention efforts. Physicians also can get involved with policy and legislative efforts directed toward containing substance abuse and helping to develop effective approaches to the treatment of youthful offenders.[74] Prevention in the 1960s at the federal level used the mass media to inform the public regarding the dangers of drug use; in the 1970s positive values were promoted in The Brand New Language (Health Educational Publication)[109] and with educational efforts to provide information about drugs. Evaluation of these varied efforts showed that teenagers did increase their knowledge about drugs, but there was no reduction in actual drug use.[97]

Using similar didactic sessions, counseling, and skills training used to prevent smoking in the schools have had only short-term effects in stopping smoking.[76, 98] In one study, combining information with skills training and peer support proved quite effective in reducing cigarette smoking.[16] Since most young people have their initial experience with smoking prior to high school, the American Academy of Pediatrics has suggested initiating educational endeavors in the prevention of smoking at early grade levels.[3]

To summarize, in DuPont's words: "The future of drug abuse prevention programs will be found less in any specific prevention effort than in the social environment in which individuals, families and communities are able to say 'no' to drugs in meaningful ways."[31] DuPont feels a society-wide prevention effort will succeed if there is a commitment to zero tolerance to drug use, testing to identify drug use, prevention programs for at-risk youth, and proliferation of programs—such as MADD, SADD, and Parents Peer Movement—that provide parental and peer encouragement of prevention.[31] These efforts must include interventions directed at the psychosocial factors that make children more vulnerable to drug abuse and depression.

Prevention and treatment of depression depend on early identification of the impact of stressors or losses experienced by a given adolescent. The physician should learn to use social support systems, extended family, peers, school teachers and counselors, clergy, and welfare departments staffs—in helping an adolescent cope with the impact of burdensome stressors. Such collaboration is one key to prevention of further pathology. These support systems are particularly important in inner-city or other areas where mental health services are limited.[75] Teachers, counselors, and peers can also be an especially valuable resource for early identification of depression. They can provide clues such as deteriorating school performance or work habits, alienation from friends and teachers, and absenteeism. Youngsters identified through schools can be assessed further by their primary care physicians and managed in their practices by using the social support systems mentioned above. Early and extensive use of mental health clinicians in primary care offices and clinics can meaningfully prevent serious pathology and lower costs of caring for at-risk adolescents.

CONCLUSION

Drug abuse and depression are leading causes for teenage mortality and morbidity. For adolescents, they are likely deviant attempts at coping and are many times the result of frustrated efforts to handle different or overlapping internal and external risk factors. Substantial work remains to be done in the field of genetic epidemiology and neuroendocrine chemistry to identify genetic markers in the transmission of depression and alcoholism. However, it is useful for physicians and professionals working with adolescents to understand how various factors predispose a youngster to use drugs as a way of coping. It is also critical to recognize that drug abuse and depression may coexist in an adolescent. Drug use, in fact, may be used to provide a dysfunctional adolescent with a way of temporarily coping with her or his depression. Comprehensive assessment is needed to evaluate accurately the specific intrapsychic, developmental, and environmental risk factors troubled youngsters are living with so that primary care providers can marshall appropriate prevention and intervention strategies.

REFERENCES

1. Albert N, Beck AT: Incidence of depression in early adolescence: A preliminary study. Adolescence 4:301–308, 1975
2. Allen LR: Self-esteem of male alcoholics. Psycholog Rec 381–389, 1969
3. AAP Committee on Adolescents: Tobacco use by children and adolescents. Pediatrics 79(3):479–481, March 1987
4. American Psychiatric Association: Committee on Nomenclature and Statistic: Diagnostic and Statistical Manual of Mental Disorders, Ed 3. Washington D.C., American Psychiatric Association, 1987, pp 222–223
5. Apter A, Borengasser MA, Hamovit J et al: A four year follow-up of depressed children. J Prevent Psychiatry 1:331–335, 1982
6. Ausubel DP: Drug addiction: Physiological, psychological and sociological aspect. New York, Random House, 1958
7. Bachman JG, Johnston LD, O'Malley PM: Smoking, drinking and drug use among American high school students: Correlates and trends, 1975–1979. Am J Public Health 71:59–69, 1981
8. Battle J: The relationship between self-esteem and depression. Psychol Rep 42:745–746, 1978
9. Battle J: The relationship between self-esteem and depression among high school students. Perceptual and motor skills 51:157–158, 1980
10. Battle J: The relationship between self-esteem and depression among children. Bureau of child study, Edmonton Public Schools. Edmonton, Alberta, Canada, 1984
11. Beardslee WR: The need for the study of adaptation in the children of parents with affective disorders. In Rutter M, Izard CE, Read PB (eds): Depression in young people, developmental and clinical perspectives. New York, Guilford Press, 1986, p 197
12. Beckman LJ: Self-esteem of women alcoholics. J Stud Alcohol 39:491–498, 1978
13. Beckman L: Perceived antecedents and effects of alcohol consumption in women. J Stud Alcohol 41:518–530, 1980
14. Bernard J: Needs of families: An overview. Paper presented at MacArthur Foundation Conference: Child care: Growth fostering environments for young children, Chicago, Dec 1982
15. Blumer H, Sutter AG, Ahmed S et al: The World of Youthful Drug Use. School of Criminology, University of California, Berkeley, 1967
16. Botrin G: Prevention of adolescent substance abuse through the development of personal and social competence. In Glyn T, Leukeveld C (eds): Preventing Adolescent Drug Abuse: DMHS Publication No. (ADM) 83–128. Washington D.C., U.S. Government Printing Office, 1983

17. Boyd JH, Weissman MM: Epidemiology of Affective Disorders, Ed 3. Washington, D.C., American Psychiatric Association, 1980
18. Brill NQ, Crumpton E, Grayson HM: Personality factors in marijuana use. Arch Gen Psychiatr 24:163–165, 1971
19. Brook JS, Luckoff IF, Whiteman M: Correlates of marijuana use as related to age, sex, ethnicity. Yale J Biol Med 50:383–390, 1977
20. Brown C: Manchild in the Promised Land. New York, Signet, 1965
21. Brunswik AF: Health needs of adolescents: How the adolescent sees them. Am J Public Health 59:1730–1745, 1969
22. CATOR Data, Ramsey clinics, St. Paul, Minnesota, 1985. In Zarek D, Hawkin DJ, Roger PD: Risk factors for adolescent substance abuse. Pediatr Clin North Am 34(2):481–493, 1987
23. Charlampous KD, Ford BK, Skinner TJ: Self-esteem in alcoholics and nonalcoholics. J Stud Alcohol 37:990–994, 1976
24. Cicchetti D, Schnider-Rosen K: Theoretical and empirical considerations in the investigation of the relationship between affect and cognition in atypical populations of infants: Contributions to the formulation of an integrative theory of development. In Izard C, Kagan J, Zajon C (eds): Emotions, Cognition and Behavior, London, Cambridge University Press, 1984
25. Cicchetti D, Schneider-Rosen K: An organizational approach to childhood depression. In Rutter M, Izard CE, Read PB (eds): Depression in Young People—Developmental and Clinical Perspectives. New York, Guilford Press, 1986, p 76
26. Clayton RR, Ritter C: The epidemiology of alcohol and drug abuse among adolescents. Adv Alcohol Substance Abuse 4:69, 1985
27. Cytryn L, McKnew DH, Bartho JJ et al: Offspring of patients with affective disorders II. J Am Acad Child Psychiatr 21:389–391, 1982
28. Cytryn L, McKnew DH, Waxler-Zahn C et al: Developmental issues in risk research: The offspring of affectively ill parents. In Rutter M, Izard CE, Read PB (eds): Depression in Young People—Developmental and Clinical Perspectives. New York. Guilford Press, 1986, pp 163–168
29. Deykin EY, Levy JC, Wells VW: Adolescent depression, alcohol and drug abuse. Am J Public Health 77(2):178–182, 1987
30. Donovan JE, Jessor R: Adolescent problem drinking. J Stud Alcohol 39:1506–1524, 1978
31. DuPont RL: Prevention of adolescent chemical dependency. Pediatr Clin North Am 34(2):495–505, 1987
32. El-Gueblay N: Manic-depressive psychosis and drug abuse. Psychiatr Assoc J 20:595–598, 1975
33. Famularo R, Stone K, Popper C: Preadolescent alcohol abuse and dependence. J Am Psychiatr Assoc 142:1187–1189, October 1985
34. Farrow JA, Deisher R: A practical guide to the office assessment of adolescent substance abuse. Pediatr Ann 15(10):675–684, 1986
35. Feldman HW: American way of drugging. Society: 32–38, May/June, 1973
36. Feldman HW: Street status and the drug researcher: Issues in participant-observation. Washington D.C., Drug Abuse Council, 1974
37. Feldman HW: A neighborhood history of drug switching in street ethnography. In Weppner RS (ed): Beverly Hills, California, Sage, 1977
38. Felix RH: An appraisal of the personality types of the addict. Am J Psychiatry 100:462–467, 1944
39. Finestone H: Cats, kicks, and color. Soc Probl 5:3–13, 1957
40. Fishburne P, Abelson H, Cisin I: The national survey on drug abuse: Main findings 1979. N.I.D.A. DHHS Pub. No. (Adm) 80–976. Washington, D.C., U.S. Government Printing Office, 1980
41. Freud A: Normality and Pathology in Childhood. London, Hogarth Press, 1966
42. Gershon ES, Nurnberger J, Nadi NS et al: The Origins of Depression: Current concepts and approaches, Berlin, Dahlem, Konfeserzen. New York, Springer-Verlag, 1982
43. Glover E: Psychoanalysis. London, Staples, 1949
44. Gold MS: When depression isn't. In The Good News About Depression: Cures and Treatments in the New Age of Psychiatry. New York, Villard Book, 1987, pp 74–88
45. Greenspan S: Substance abuse: An understanding from psychoanalytic, developmental and learning perspectives. In Blain J, Twins D (eds): Psychodynamics of Drug

Dependence. NIDA Research Monograph 12 DHEW Publ. No. (ADM) 77–470. Washington D.C., U.S. Government Printing Office, 1977

46. Greenspan S: Psychopathology and adaptation in infancy and early childhood. New York, International Universities Press, 1981
47. Hasin D, Endicott J, Lewis C: Alcohol and drug abuse in patients with affective syndromes. Comprehen Psychiatry 26(3):282–295, 1985
48. Healthy people: The surgeon general's report on health promotion and disease prevention. Washington, D.C., U.S. Dept. of Health and Human Services, Publication (PHS), 1979
49. Helzer JE, Robins LN, Davis DH: Depressive disorders in Vietnam returnees. J Nerv Ment Dis 163:177–185, 1976
50. Hendin H: Psychosocial theory of drug abuse—a psychodynamic approach. N.I.D.A. Research Monograph Series 30:195–200, 1980
51. Hoffman NG, Sonis WA, Halikas JA: Issues in the evaluation of chemical dependency treatment programs for adolescents. Pediatr Clin North Am 34(2):449–459, 1987
52. Hunt LG, Chambers CD: The heroin epidemics: A Study of Heroin Use in the United States, 1965–1975. New York, Spectrum, 1976
53. Jessor R: A psychosocial perspective on adolescent substance use. In Report of the Fourteenth Ross Round Table Conference, pp 21–28, 1983
54. Johnston LD: Drug use during and after high school: Results of a national longitudinal study. Am J Public Health (Suppl) 69:29–37, 1974
55. Johnston LD, Bachman JG, O'Malley PM: Highlights from student drug use in America, 1975–1981. Rockville, Maryland, N.I.D.A., 1981
56. Johnston LD, O'Malley PM, Bachman JG: Psychotherapeutic, licit and illicit use of drugs among adolescents, An epidemiological perspective. J Adolesc Health Care 68:36–51, 1987
57. Jonsson E, Nilsson T: Alkoholkonsumption hos monozygota och dizygota tvilligan. Nord Hyg Tidskr 49:21–25, 1968
58. Judd L, Mandell A: A "free-clinic" population and drug use patterns. Am J Psychiatry 128:1298–1302, 1972
59. Kaij L: Alcoholism in twins: Studies on the etiology and sequels of abuse of alcohol. Sweden, University of Lund, 1960
60. Kandel DB: Developmental stages in adolescent drug involvement. In Lettieri D (ed): Drug Theories. Washington D.C., U.S. Government Printing Office, 1980, pp 120–127
61. Kandel DB, Davies M: Epidemiology of depressive mood in adolescents—An empirical study. Arch Gen Psychiatry 39:1205–1212, 1982
62. Kandel DB: Epidemiological and psychosocial perspectives on adolescent drug use. J Acad Child Psychiatry 21(4):328–347, 1982
63. Kandel DB: Marijuana users in young adulthood. Arch Gen Psychiatry 41:200–209, 1984
64. Kandel DB, Logan JA: Periods of risk for initiation, stabilization and decline in drug use from adolescence to early adulthood. Am J Public Health 74:660–666, 1984
65. Kaplan B: The study of language in psychiatry: The comparative developmental approach and its application to symbolization and language in psychopathology. In Arieti S (ed): American Handbook of Psychiatry. New York, Basic Books, 1966
66. Kaplan HB: Antecedents of deviant responses: Predicting from a general theory of deviant behavior. J Youth Adolesc 6:86–101, 1977
67. Kaplan SL, Hong GK, Weinhold C: Epidemiology of depressive symptomatology in adolescents. J Am Acad Child Psychiatr 23(1):91–98, 1984
68. Kearny TR, Taylor C: Emotionally disturbed adolescents with alcoholic parents. Acta Paedopsychiatr 36:215–221, 1969
69. Kolb L: Types and characteristics of drug addicts. Ment Hyg 9:300–313, 1925
70. Kupfer DJ, Detre T, Doral J et al: A comment on the amotivational syndrome in marijuana smokers. Am J Psychiatry 130:1319–1322, 1973
71. Long JVF, Valliant GE: Natural history of male psychological health, XI: Escape from the underclass. Am J Psychiatry 141:341–346, 1984
72. Malikas JA, Goodwin DW, Guez SB: Marijuana use and psychiatric illness. Arch Gen Psychiatry 27:162–165, 1972
73. McAree CP, Steffenhagen RA, Zheutlin LS: Personality factors and pattern of drug use in college students. Am J Psychiatry 128:890–893, 1972

74. McDonald DI: Drugs, drinking and adolescence. Am J Dis Child 138:117–125, 1984
75. Mental Health Services in Primary Care Settings: Report of a Conference, April 2–3, 1979. Washington D.C., U.S. Department of HHS. ADAMHA Series DN#2, 1979
76. Midanik LT, Polen MR, Hunkeller EM et al: Methodologic issues in evaluating stop-smoking programs. Am J Public Health 75:634, 1985
77. Mitic W: Alcohol use and self-esteem. J Drug Educ 10:197–208, 1980
78. Morrison MA, Smith QT: Psychiatric issues of adolescent chemical dependence. Pediatr Clin North Am 34(2):461–480, 1987
79. Offer D, Petersen AC: Child psychiatry perspectives. J Am Acad Psychiatry 21:86–87, 1982
80. Orvaschel H, Weissman MM, Padian N et al: Assessing psychopathology in children of psychiatrically disturbed parents: A pilot study. J Am Acad Child Psychiatr 20:112–122, 1981
81. Paton SM, Kessler R, Kandel DB: Depressive mood and adolescent illegal drug use: A longitudinal analysis. J Genet Psychol 31:267–289, 1977
82. Paton SM, Kandel DB: Psychological factors and adolescent illicit drug use: Ethnicity and sex differences. Adolescence 13(50):595–598, 1978
83. Pearlin LT, Radabaugh CW: The sociological study of a social problem: A reply to Roman. Am J Sociology 83:991–994, 1978
84. Poznanski EO, Krahenbuhl V, Zrull JP: Childhood depression: A longitudinal perspective. J Am Acad Child Psychiatr 15:491–501, 1976
85. Poznanski EO: Childhood depression: The outcome. Acta Paedopsychiatrica 46:297–304, 1980–1981
86. Poznanski EO: The clinical phenomenology of childhood depression. Am J Orthopsychiatry 52(2):308–313, 1982
87. Puig-Antich J, Chambers W, Halpern F et al: Cortisol hypersecretion in prepubertal depressive illness: A preliminary report. Psychoneuroendocrinology 4:191–197, 1979
88. Puig-Antich J, Tabrizi MA, Davies M et al: Prepubertal endogenous major depressives hyposecrete growth hormone in response to insulin-induced hypoglycemia. Biological Psychiatry 16:801–881, 1981
89. Puig-Antich J, Novacenko H, Davies M et al: Growth hormone secretion in prepubertal major depressive children in response to insulin-induced hypoglycemia. Paper presented at the Annual Meeting of the Academy of Child Psychiatry, October, 1982
90. Puig-Antich J, Goetz R, Davies M et al: Growth hormone secretion in prepubertal major depressive children. IV. Sleep-related plasma concentrations in a drug-free fully recovered clinical state. Arch Gen Psychiatry 41:479–483, 1984
91. Puig-Antich J: Psychobiological markers: Effects of age and puberty in depression in young people: In Rutter M, Izard CE, Read PB (eds): Developmental and clinical perspectives. New York, The Guilford Press, 1986
92. Rutter M, Graham P, Chadwick OFD et al: Adolescent turmoil: Fact or fiction? J Child Psychol Psychiatr 17:35–56, 1976
93. Rutter M: Stress, coping and development: Some issues and some questions. J Child Psychol Psychiatr 22:324–356, 1981
94. Rutter M, Garmezy N: Developmental Psychopathology. In Mussen PM (ed): Handbook of Child Psychology. New York, John Wiley & Sons, 1983, p 810
95. Sameroff A: Transactional model in early social relations. Hum Develop 18:65–79, 1975
96. Sanchez-Dirks R: Drinking practices among Hispanic youth. Alcohol, Health and Research World 3(2):21–27, 1978
97. Schaps E, Diertal R, Moskowitz J et al: A review of 127 drug abuse prevention programs' evaluation. J Drug Issues 11:17–43, 1981
98. Schinke SP, Gilchrist LD, Snow WM: Skills intervention to prevent cigarette smoking among adolescents. Am J Public Health 75:665–667, 1985
99. Schoenbach VJ, Kaplan BH, Wagner EH et al: Depressive symptoms in young adolescents (abstr). Am J Epidemiol: 112–440, 1980
100. Schoenbach VJ, Kaplan BH, Wagner EH et al: Prevalence of self-reported depressive symptoms in young adolescents. Am J Public Health 73(11):1281–1287, 1983
101. Schuckit MA, Goodwin DW, Winokur G: A study of alcoholism in half-siblings. Am J Psychiatry 128:1132–1136, 1972
102. Schuckit MA: Biological markers: Metabolism and acute reactions to alcohol in sons of alcoholics. Pharmacol Biochem Behav (Suppl) 1:9–16, 1980

103. Schuckit MA: Prevalence of affective disorders in a sample of young men. Am J Psychiatry 139(11):1431–1436, 1982

104. Smith GM: Antecedents of teenage drug use. Paper Presented at the 35th Annual Meeting of the Committee on Problems of Drug Dependence. National Academy of Sciences, National Research Council 1973, pp 312–317

105. Smith GM, Fogg CP: Teenage drug use: A search for causes and consequences. In Lettier DJ (ed): Predicting Adolescent Drug Abuse: A Review of Issues, Methods and Correlates. N.I.D.A. Research Issues Series, II: 277–282. Washington, D.C., DHEW Pub. No. (ADM), 1975, pp 76–299

106. Smith GM, Fogg CP: Psychological predictors of early use, late use and nonuse of marijuana among teenage students. In Kandel DB (ed): Longitudinal research on drug use: Empirical findings and methodological issues. Washington, D.C., Hemisphere, 1978, pp 101–114

107. Smith GM, Fogg CP: Psychological antecedents of teenage drug use. In Simmons RG (ed): Research in Community and Mental Health: An Annual Compilation of Research, Vol I. Greenwich, Connecticut, JAI Press, 1979

108. Smith GM, Schwerin FT, Stubblefield FS et al: Licit and illicit substance use by adolescents: Psychosocial predisposition and escalatory outcome. Contemp Drug Prob 11:75–100, 1982

109. Special Action Office for Drug Abuse Prevention (SAODAP): The media and drug abuse messages. Washington, D.C., 1974

110. Sroufe LA: The coherence of individual development. Am Psychologist 34:834–841, 1979

111. Sroufe LA, Rutter M: The domain of developmental psychopathology. Child Develop 55:17–29, 1984

112. Sutter AG: Worlds of drug use on the street scene. In Cressey CR, Wards DA (eds): Delinquency, Crime and Social Process. New York, Harper & Row, 1969

113. Talbot GD: Substance abuse and the professional provider. Ala J Med Sci 21:150–155, 1984

114. Thomas P: Down These Mean Streets. New York, Signet, 1967

115. Waters E, Srouf LA: Competence as a developmental construct. Develop Rev 3:79–97, 1983

116. Weissman MM, Siegel R: The depressed woman and her rebellious adolescent. Social Casework 53:563–570, 1972

117. Weissman M, Klerman G: Sex differences and epidemiology of depression. Arch Gen Psychiatry 34:98–111, 1977

118. Welner Z, Welner A, McCrary MD et al: Psychopathology in children of inpatients with depression: A controlled study. J Nerv Ment Dis 164:408–413, 1977

119. Yanish DL, Battle J: Relationship between self-esteem, depression and alcohol consumption among adolescents. Psychological Reports 57:331–334, 1985

Adolescent Center
ACC 5
Boston City Hospital
Boston, Massachusetts 02118

0031-3955/88 $0.00 + .20

Acquired Immunodeficiency Syndrome: A New Population of Children at Risk

Ellen R. Cooper, MD,* Stephen I. Pelton, MD,†
and Mireille LeMay, MD‡

The acquired immunodeficiency syndrome (AIDS) was first described in homosexual males and intravenous drug users. It was recognized subsequently in recipients of infected blood products and heterosexual partners of infected persons. More recently, AIDS has been described in the population of infants born to infected mothers. In 1982, the first descriptions of this illness in infants were reported. Retrospectively, however, children with clinical findings suggestive of HIV infection can be identified as early as 1979.[65] The total number of pediatric cases of AIDS reported to the Centers for Disease Control (CDC) was 908 as of March 21, 1988; however, by 1991 this number is expected to increase to over 3000, with an additional 2000 children manifesting symptomatic HIV infection but not yet fulfilling the strict case definition of AIDS.[24] Because of the unique mode of transmission as well as the different clinical spectrum of disease, pediatric AIDS is defined as occurring in children under 13 years of age. Children over age 13 have disease so strikingly similar to that of adults that they are included in those statistics.

Several factors initially prevented acceptance of the concept of pediatric AIDS as a specific disease entity. The difference in clinical manifestations between adults and children with AIDS encouraged skepticism regarding a common etiologic agent. Prior to the availability of specific serological tests, it was difficult to differentiate AIDS from other already described causes of congenital immunodeficiency syndromes. This differentiation required an elaborate combination of epidemiologic observations and pathologic studies in addition to the development of specific laboratory testing.

Two laboratories in the United States and France have identified the causative

*Assistant Professor of Pediatrics, Division of Infectious Diseases, Boston University School of Medicine; Clinical Director of Pediatric AIDS Program, Boston City Hospital, Boston, Massachusetts

†Associate Professor of Pediatrics, Vice Chairman of Department of Pediatrics, Division of Infectious Diseases, Boston University School of Medicine, Boston, Massachusetts

‡Research Fellow, Pediatric Infectious Diseases, Boston University School of Medicine, Boston, Massachusetts

agent for AIDS. Initially, two names, human T lymphotrophic virus III (HTLV-III) and lymphadenopathy-associated virus (LAV) were employed, depending primarily in which laboratory the scientists worked. More recently, human immunodeficiency virus (HIV) has been accepted universally as the common name for this retrovirus.

PATHOGENESIS

The acquired immunodeficiency syndrome is caused by a human T lymphotropic retrovirus. Evidence suggests that the monocyte or macrophage is the host cell, which is initially infected with HIV and subsequently serves as the vehicle of viral replication and persistent infection. Infection occurs in specific CD-4 receptor positive cells, and this may at least partially explain the occurrence of isolated brain or lung involvement in some patients.

HIV infection of previously immunocompetent cells may result in immunodeficiency by several mechanisms. Direct cell damage and subsequent death leads to T-cell depletion. Cytotoxic but uninfected T cells may destroy infected cells and result in a reduced number of T4 cells. There seems also to be a direct effect on immune function by HIV because abnormalities in function may be seen before the total numbers are depleted. These effects can lead to abnormal monocytic function as well as decreases in natural killer cell activity, antibody formation, and T-cell immunity. Deficiency in specific antibody response may result from chronic HIV antigenic stimulation or loss of suppressor T-cell regulation. There have been a variety of other immune defects demonstrated in patients with AIDS. These include abnormal neutrophil function and complement pathway derangements.[64]

SEROLOGIC TESTING

Although it is possible to culture the HIV virus from infected patients, the procedure is labor intensive and currently available only in research settings; therefore, indirect evidence by detection of antibody to major viral proteins remains the accepted diagnostic tool. Serologic testing for antibodies to HIV has become the standard test for documenting infection. A test that is both simple and sensitive is the enzyme-linked immunosorbent assay (ELISA), which currently measures antibodies to all viral proteins. When the ELISA is repeatedly positive it must be confirmed in a reputable reference laboratory by the more specific Western blot technique. This technique detects antibodies against specific HIV-associated antigens and confirms HIV seropositivity if antibodies to viral antigen p24 or gp41 are present. In infants, however, negative results of ELISA and Western blot techniques are increasing in number. Borkowsky and co-workers reported that in their group of 85 infants, as many as 10 per cent of children infected with HIV, and 25 per cent of those symptomatic with opportunistic infections were not identified by ELISA screening alone.[11] The sensitivity of the test may be insufficient to detect low levels of antibody. In children in whom the index of suspicion is high based on history or symptoms, it is worthwhile to request Western blot determination even when the ELISA is repeatedly negative. Similarly, both ELISA *and* Western blot may be negative in symptomatic patients when the decay in immune function has left them unable to mount the antibody response, or whose antibody titers are low.[29a] With the development of reliable and specific antigen detection methods, it will become possible to define HIV infection further.

EPIDEMIOLOGY AND MODES OF TRANSMISSION

Since HIV infection in infants and children in this country is a recently recognized entity, a clear understanding of the modes of transmission is still evolving. It is well known that in adults the major routes for HIV infection are through close sexual contact, the sharing of needles and syringes among intravenous drug users, or the receipt of blood or blood products.

In adolescents, HIV is associated with these same established routes of infection. Children also have been exposed to HIV during blood transfusions, and these cases currently represent 13 per cent of all cases of AIDS in childhood. Another 5 per cent of childhood AIDS cases can be attributed to blood products received as treatment for coagulation disorders. There also have been a few reports of HIV transmission to children occurring as the result of sexual abuse. [15, 23, 43]

Most children with AIDS are born to mothers who themselves carry the virus. Perinatal exposure accounts for approximately 80 per cent of the children with AIDS. This proportion is rapidly increasing as the number of new cases related to blood or blood products declines secondary to blood donor screening programs. [15] Mothers of high-risk children may have a history of intravenous drug use, prostitution, or multiple sexual partners. They may practice no "high-risk" behaviors but simply originate from particular geographic regions, such as Haiti and Central Africa, where heterosexual transmission is thought to play a major role. At the time of their pregnancy, the mothers may have AIDS or AIDS-related complex (ARC), or be totally asymptomatic. There is some suggestion that babies born to symptomatic women, or to women who seroconvert during their pregnancy, may have an increased risk of developing clinical symptoms. [49, 66]

The evidence for transplacental transmission of HIV includes the suggestion by some investigators that there are characteristic phenotypic facial features in HIV-infected infants. [42] This controversial claim would imply an embryopathy secondary to intrauterine infection. There has been isolation of the virus from the tissue of fetuses as early as 16 weeks' gestation that documents the presence of intrauterine viral transmission. Transmission has been documented in infants who have been born by cesarean section and so had no exposure to vaginal secretions during the birthing process. In addition, infants have been found to be seropositive and later symptomatic, even in instances in which there has been no postnatal contact with the biologic mother. [62, 67, 70, 75]

The incidence and the efficiency of HIV transmission *in utero* has not been well defined, nor have contributing cofactors been accurately identified. It does seem clear at this point, however, that transmission of the virus to the fetus, although common, is not inevitable. Cases of monozygotic twins have been reported in which only one infant was infected. By most conservative estimates, however, approximately 60 per cent of infants born to seropositive mothers are infected with HIV. [67] Other types of perinatal transmission of HIV must be considered, although they probably do not play as major a role as transplacental passage of virus. This includes passage via infected breast milk. In support of this as a potential risk, there has been a report of a child born by cesarean section to a mother who received blood contaminated with HIV after the delivery of the infant. This child seroconverted, with the only identifiable exposure being breast milk. [39a]

DIAGNOSIS OF HIV INFECTION IN CHILDHOOD

Two major problems have made it difficult to determine the full extent of HIV infection in children. Antibody to HIV is not reliably diagnostic of true infection in children less than 15 months of age. In addition, the definition of AIDS in children initially proposed by the Centers for Disease Control required rigid criteria that few children with HIV infection actually fulfilled.

HIV infection in children is identified by the actual presence of the virus in blood or tissues. This may be confirmed by direct viral culture or serologic antigen

Table 1. *Laboratory Abnormalities in Symptomatic Pediatric HIV Infection*

Hypergammaglobulinemia	Reversed T4:T8†
Hypogammaglobulinemia*	Neutropenia
Total lymphopenia	Anemia
T4 lymphopenia†	

*Unusual in comparison to *hyper*gammaglobulinemia.
†Often a late manifestation.

detection methods. As already mentioned, neither of these techniques is readily available. Physicians therefore must rely on the presence of antibody in serum as evidence of HIV exposure in neonates. This is a particularly confusing situation when the infant is born to an infected mother.

Antibody to HIV is passively transferred to the newborn in virtually all children born to seropositive women. However, many of these infants are not truly infected. Some have passively acquired only antibody to HIV from the mother, as they might acquire antibody to measles or varicella virus. In these uninfected children, the antibody decays over time. Longitudinal studies of antibody-positive newborns suggest a mean duration of seropositivity of 10 months with a maximal duration of 15 months in children who subsequently are proven to be uninfected. Seventy-five per cent of the children who become seronegative do so in the first year.[49, 50]

There have been a few reports of infants who have become seronegative but subsequently have developed symptoms of HIV infection.[11] In a few of these, virus has been isolated from blood or spinal fluid.[49] This underscores the difficulty in determining active infection given presently available serologic markers.

Other laboratory abnormalities may help to identify the seropositive infant who is at risk for progression of disease. We have found hypergammaglobulinemia a common finding, occurring in 93 per cent of symptomatic children. This elevation often precedes clinical manifestations. Immunologic abnormalities, as mentioned, are consistent with our present understanding of the pathogenesis of disease. A decreased number of T4 cells, which is a reliable marker of disease in adults, is often a very late finding in children (Table 1).

The second difficulty in identifying children with HIV infection has been the failure to recognize the spectrum of disease due to HIV in children. The CDC's initial criteria were extremely restrictive because of the concern for excluding children with congenital immunodeficiency and limited experience with the clinical disease in pediatric patients. With greater experience, sequential modification of the CDC criteria has been required. The current classification recognizes the difficulty in pediatric diagnosis prior to 15 months of age and also expands the clinical spectrum required to fulfill the case definition (Table 2).[15]

CLINICAL SPECTRUM OF DISEASE

Clinically, the incubation period seen in children born at risk has been variable, but seems to average between 4 and 6 months. Most cases of pediatric HIV infection are diagnosed early, with 50 per cent of cases diagnosed during the first year of life, and 82 per cent by the age of 3 years.

There are several profiles of the HIV-infected child that have been commonly identified and should serve as a warning sign to the pediatrician, especially when risk factors have been identified (Table 3).

Wasting Syndrome

Failure to thrive, with or without lymphadenopathy and hepatosplenomegaly, is seen in 20 to 50 per cent of symptomatic children.[8] This wasting syndrome was

Table 2. *Pediatric AIDS Classification: Summary of Current CDC Criteria*

P-0	Indeterminate infection (not tested or noninterpretable test results; includes infants born to HIV-positive mothers)
P-1	Asymptomatic infection
	A—Normal immune function
	B—Abnormal immune function
	C—Immune function not tested
P-2	Symptomatic infection
	A—Nonspecific findings (ARC)
	B—Progressive encephalopathy
	C—Lymphoid interstitial pneumonitis
	D—Secondary infectious diseases
	D–1 opportunistic infections (AIDS)
	D–2 recurrent bacterial infections
	D–3 recalcitrant infections, specifically candida and herpes
	E—Secondary malignancy

first recognized among infected adults in Kenya, where it was termed "slim disease." Height and weight often fall below the third percentile for age, but height can be appropriate for weight.

Wasting syndrome can be associated with chronic or recurrent diarrhea, either as a direct effect of HIV on the gastrointestinal tract or as a result of a secondary opportunistic infection.

Mucocutaneous candidiasis occurs in over 75 per cent of these patients. It is usually localized to the oral pharynx but can cause esophagitis in up to 20 per cent of children.[67] The candida can be resistant to all forms of therapy and even when responsive to treatment may reappear soon after therapy is withdrawn.

Lymphadenopathy/Parotitis

Lymphadenopathy and salivary gland enlargement may be seen together or as separate entities. Although they may remain the only manifestation of disease in an infected child, they are associated with later onset of pulmonary disease.

The parotitis may be mistaken for a swollen lymph node. It persists over months and years and usually is not associated with fever or elevation of amylase levels in the blood and urine.

Bacterial Infections

Bacterial infections seen in children with HIV infection can be recurrent and serious. They include sepsis, meningitis, pneumonia, cellulitis, focal abscesses, urinary tract infections, osteomyelitis, and otitis media.

The most common causative agents include *Streptococcus pneumonia*, *Hemophilus influenzae*, and *Salmonella*, although many cases of *E. coli* or *Staphylococcus aureus* also have been described, especially in the already hospitalized patient.[9]

As a general rule, the bacterial infections occurring in HIV-infected children are similar to those seen in children with hypogammaglobulinemia. This is not surprising in light of the shared abnormality in humoral immunity.[10]

Table 3. *Syndromes Associated with Pediatric HIV Infection*

Wasting syndrome	Lymphadenopathy syndrome
Interstitial pneumonitis	Cardiomyopathy
Recurrent bacterial infection	Hepatitis
Encephalopathy	Renal disease

Because these etiologic organisms do not easily differentiate those patients infected by HIV, it is up to the astute pediatrician to ascertain the appropriate history of risk factors in the child with recurrent infections if HIV infection is to be considered.

Pulmonary Syndromes

Pulmonary disease is the most common cause of morbidity and mortality in children with HIV infection, and it is often the first manifestation of HIV infection. In addition to bacterial and viral pneumonia, children, as do their adult counterparts, develop *Pneumocystis carinii* (PCP) infection.[73] However, another cause of chronic interstitial disease with progressive alveolocapillary block has been described. It has been termed *lymphoid interstitial pneumonitis* (LIP) but is also called *pulmonary lymphoid hyperplasia*. Its etiology remains unclear.

Although LIP is still considered uncommon in adults, it is being reported recently with greater frequency. It is associated with a progressive course that can result in dyspnea and hypoxia. The chest x-ray film demonstrates a diffuse nodular pattern, sometimes with widened superior mediastinum and hilum. Fever is distinctly uncommon and both auscultation and percussion are commonly normal. The laboratory findings may help differentiate LIP from PCP since the former often is associated with a marked hypergammaglobulinemia and lower lactate dehydrogenase than seen in PCP.[63] It must be emphasized, however, that these entities can indeed easily be confused and that an AIDS patient may have secondary infection that may alter the presentation of either.

Histologic examination of the lungs of patients with LIP can show peribronchial or parenchymal mononuclear cells forming nodules, or diffuse interstitial and peribronchiolar infiltration with lymphocytes and plasma cells.[38, 41]

Presently there is an unclear association of this lung disease with chronic Epstein-Barr virus (EBV) infection, since some children have persistently elevated antibodies to EBV nuclear antigen. EBV DNA as well as HIV DNA has been identified in lung tissue from children with LIP.[52, 63] Uncertainty, therefore, still exists as to the specific etiology. Some investigators feel that LIP may be a result of an interaction between the two viruses.

The clinical management of the HIV-infected child with pulmonary disease is a complex problem and discussed in more detail later in this article.

Neurologic Syndromes

Neurologic involvement occurs in 50 per cent of children with HIV infection. It is seen in 90 per cent of those who meet the case definition of AIDS and usually takes the form of a progressive encephalopathy.[25] More commonly, however, neurologic manifestations are characterized by developmental delay or loss of motor milestones. There is decreased brain growth, as evidenced by microcephaly and abnormal neurologic examination findings. Pathologic findings correlate with computed tomographic findings of cerebral atrophy, enlargement of the subarachnoid space and ventricles, and symmetrical calcification of basal ganglia and periventricular white matter. We have observed these calcifications in infants as young as 2 months of age. This further substantiates transmission *in utero* since the calcifications in the walls of small blood vessels are thought to develop over a prolonged time.

In addition to the progressive encephalopathy seen in children with HIV infection, there is also described a nonprogressive static encephalopathy in patients who have no other manifestations of disease. In a study of 20 children with progressive encephalopathy, the average time between onset of symptoms and death was 7.9 months, whereas all patients with static encephalopathy were still alive 19 months later.

Although children with HIV infection are at risk for secondary infections of the

Table 4. *Opportunistic Infections in Pediatric AIDS*

Pneumocystis carinii	Cryptosporidium
Candida sp.	*Toxoplasma gondii*
Mycobacterium avium intracellulare	*Cryptococcus neoformans*
Cytomegalovirus	*Histoplasma capsulatum*
Herpes simplex (disseminated)	

central nervous system, there is strong evidence to suggest that many of these neurologic findings result as a direct effect of HIV. Electron-microscopic demonstration of HIV in multinucleated giant cells and macrophages in the brain has helped resolve this issue.[25] In addition, antigen can be detected and virus isolated from CSF. This underscores the importance of demonstrating blood–brain barrier penetration of any antiviral agent that may be considered for testing in patients with AIDS.

Opportunistic and Viral Infections

Opportunistic infections are not as common a presentation of AIDS in children as in adults. It is often a late complication, and mean survival after first documentation of an opportunistic infection is 3 months, with 75 per cent mortality at 1 year.[2]

Pneumocystis carinii appears to be the most important opportunistic pathogen in children and has occurred in approximately 50 per cent of the childhood AIDS cases reported to the CDC.[67] Cytomegalovirus (CMV) infections also are increasingly reported and have caused a wide spectrum of disease. Retinitis, pneumonitis, hepatitis, and gastrointestinal ulcerations have all been observed. In children with perinatally acquired disease, CMV is often the first manifestation because initial exposure to the virus may be at the time of delivery. By strict definition, a CMV infection is considered truly opportunistic only if it occurs beyond the age of 6 months in an anatomic site other than the liver. However, the serious extent of CMV disease seen in the HIV-infected infant must be considered opportunistic since survival is substantially shortened in these patients. Children are less likely than adults to develop infection with *Toxoplasma gondii*. They have a smaller chance of harboring the organism because of lack of prior exposure.

Embryopathy

A characteristic dysmorphic syndrome in children with congenital HIV infection has been reported by one group of investigators.[42] From a group of 20 infected children born to drug-using mothers, they identified growth failure in 75 per cent and microcephaly in 70 per cent. The craniofacial features noted were ocular hypertelorism, prominent forehead, flat nasal bridge, mild obliquity of the eyes, long palpebral fissures, short nose, triangular philtrum, and patulous lips. If in fact this embryopathy can be proven to be causally associated with HIV, it is good evidence for early infection in vitro. Not all investigators have been able to confirm this observation, however.[57] Because of the variety of confounding variables, a more controlled survey needs to be undertaken before any conclusions can be made.

Other Manifestations

While secondary malignancies seem to be more common in adult AIDS patients, they have been reported to have occurred in children as well. Kaposi's sarcoma is rare in cases of pediatric AIDS, but lymphomas are being reported with increased frequency.[15]

Cardiac disease is common but is unusual as a presenting manifestation in children. Left ventricular dysfunction has been seen in 45 per cent of symptomatic children who have been echocardiographically studied. Eighteen per cent were shown to have pericardial effusions.[66, 68] Congestive heart failure unresponsive to digitalis therapy also is well described. Whether this cardiac abnormality is related to an opportunistic infection or to direct HIV damage remains unclear.

Hepatitis, as well as renal disease, may be presenting manifestations of AIDS.[8] Direct effect of HIV on the liver and kidneys has been postulated, and direct infection demonstrated by in situ hybridization techniques.

MANAGEMENT OF THE HIV-INFECTED CHILD

Immunizations

As in children with other immunodeficiencies, the concern about safety and immunogenicity of both live and killed vaccines has been raised in children with HIV infection.

In children with other immunodeficiency syndromes, live virus vaccines are considered contraindicated because of the potential for dissemination of the very infection they are meant to prevent. Limited clinical information is available regarding the safety or efficacy of measles and polio vaccines in HIV infected children however. Among 75 children with AIDS or ARC who received one dose of measles, mumps, and rubella vaccine, no adverse events were documented.[56] There have been no reports of adverse reactions to live oral polio vaccine (OPV) in small studies of HIV-infected children or their household contacts, in spite of the large theoretic risk. Limited studies have not demonstrated adverse effects from other live or inactivated vaccines including meningococcal, live adenoviral[4, 7] tetravalent influenza, 23-valent pneumococcal, and hepatitis B vaccines.[19, 73]

Inactivated vaccines usually are not considered a risk to the immunodeficient child, but questions regarding the potential of any immunization to accelerate the course of HIV infection have been raised.[20] It is possible that antigen-induced stimulation of CD4 positive T-lymphocytes (T-helper cells), which are the targets of HIV, could result in more rapid deterioration in infected persons. At this time no documentation of adverse effects has been published.

Efficacy of immunizations is uncertain and is another important area in need of further investigation. Limited studies suggest vaccine immunogenicity is significantly attenuated in the patient with symptomatic HIV disease.[12, 37] Even when the initial antibody response to immunization has been adequate, the titer may quickly decline to below protective levels with progression of the disease.

Presently, based on the limited information available, the Immunization Practices Advisory Committee (ACIP) guidelines recommend immunization for children with HIV infection.[4] Because polio virus may be excreted for several months in the stool of an immunized infant, all children residing in the household of an AIDS patient should receive inactivated polio virus vaccine (IPV). In addition, all children who are seropositive for HIV should receive IPV. It should be pointed out that these recommendations apply to children in developed countries, where the risk of disease is low. The World Health Organization (WHO) recommends administration of all regular immunizations to children in developing nations.[59]

In addition to routine immunizations, symptomatic children should receive pneumococcal and influenza vaccines. The pediatrician, however, must be aware that protective antibody levels may not be achieved in these patients. Significant exposure to infective agents such as pertussis, tetanus, or measles should be identified, and prophylaxis or passive antibody administered when possible.

Until recently, the administration of the measles–mumps–rubella (MMR)

Table 5. *CDC Recommendations for Routine Immunization of HIV-Infected Children (April, 1988)*

| | HIV INFECTION | |
VACCINE	Asymptomatic	Symptomatic
DTP	Yes	Yes
OPV	No	No
IPV	Yes	Yes
MMR	Yes	Yes
Hemophilus influenzae type B	Yes	Yes
Pneumococcal	No	Yes
Influenza	No	Yes

vaccine was not recommended in persons with symptomatic disease because of the risk of live virus exposure. However, in a recent issue of Morbidity and Mortality Weekly Reports (April, 1988) the CDC reports six cases of measles in HIV-infected children.[4] Two children died as a result of a nosocomial outbreak in New York City. Because of the scattered outbreak of measles in the United States, and the increased susceptibility of the immunocompromised child, it is now recommended that all patients receive MMR. (Table 5 contains a summary of the current recommendations.)

Approach to the Febrile Child with HIV Infection

Children with HIV infection are at risk for disease from a variety of opportunistic organisms as well as with the usual childhood pathogens. The child with HIV infection and fever requires a careful clinical evaluation and investigation for the possibility of pyogenic infection. Cultures of urine, blood and, when indicated, cerebrospinal fluid should be obtained. In most cases it is wise to initiate treatment with broad-spectrum antibiotics while awaiting culture results. If community-acquired disease is suspected therapy should be directed toward *Streptococcus pneumoniae*, *Hemophilus influenzae*, and *Salmonella* species. In cases of infection where an indwelling catheter is present, therapy to cover staphylococcal species should be instituted. In nosocomial infection, or infection following instrumentation, therapy to cover gram-negative organisms also should be included.

Approach to the Child with HIV Infection and Respiratory Symptoms

The major morbidity and mortality from acquired immunodeficiency syndrome in children is associated with pulmonary disease. Children with HIV infection are at risk for *Pneumocystis carinii* pneumonia (PCP) as well as the more common respiratory pathogens, which include respiratory syncytial virus (RSV), adenovirus, parainfluenza virus, pertussis, *Streptococcus pneumoniae*, and *Hemophilus influenzae*. Similarly, they are susceptible to infection with cytomegalovirus (CMV), *Mycobacterium avium intracellular* (MAI), and Candida sp.

When a previously well, seropositive infant less than 15 months of age presents with respiratory distress, the clinician is faced with a dilemma. This illness may be due to a common pathogen of childhood or may represent the first manifestation of the opportunistic infections associated with HIV disease.

An approach to this problem is shown in Table 6. In this algorithm, the seropositive child who is less than 15 months of age presents with an interstitial pattern on chest radiograph and undergoes an initial noninvasive evaluation. This includes bacterial and viral cultures, determination of arterial blood po$_2$, and serum lactate dehydrogenase levels. Age-appropriate antimicrobial therapy is started. In addition, trimethoprim-sulfamethoxazole (TMP-SMZ) is initiated as therapy for

Table 6. *Approach to the High-Risk Child with Respiratory Distress**

ACUTE RESPIRATORY DISTRESS WITH RADIOGRAPHIC FINDINGS

Initial work-up should include:

     Blood cultures, urine for *H. influenzae, S. pneumoniae* antigen.
     Nasopharyngeal aspirate for rapid detection of RSV; viral cultures.
     Nasopharyngeal swab for rapid diagnosis of chlamydia.
     Blood for EBV serology.
     Throat swab, urine for CMV culture.
     Ophthalmologic exam for presence of CMV retinitis.
     SGOT, SGPT, LDH.
     Arterial po$_2$ determination.

CHEST RADIOGRAPH

Diffuse Interstitial Pattern		*Noninterstitial Pattern*	
Deep tracheal suction (in intubated patients only) for bacterial and viral culture as well as silver stain for pneumocystis			
Start appropriate therapy for age plus Trimethoprim-sulfamethoxazole and		Start appropriate therapy for age.	
Arrange for bronchoscopy† within 24–48 hours.			
Diagnosis available from initial work-up. Postpone bronchoscopy. Individualize therapy.	No diagnosis, No change. Bronchoscopy.	Unchanged or worse at 48 hours Add Trimethoprim-sulfamethoxazole. Arrange for bronchoscopy.	Improved at 48 hours.

*Infants born to HIV Ab + mothers and/or infants known to be HIV Ab +.

†Bronchoalveolar lavage has been shown to be most useful. If this is not available, open lung biopsy may be necessary.

Pneumocystis carinii. If no etiology is found during the first 24 to 48 hours, and the child does not significantly improve, plans should be made to perform bronchoscopy or an open lung biopsy, depending on the availability of these procedures.[72]

     In the HIV-infected adult, bronchoalveolar lavage and transbronchial biopsy have yielded an etiologic agent in 95 per cent of patients with pulmonary infection.[69] In children, there is little published information. One group reported on the use of bronchoalveolar lavage in acute interstitial pneumonitis. Of eight children who underwent bronchoalveolar lavage, a diagnosis of *Pneumocystis carinii* pneumonia was made in four and of CMV in one. It remains unclear which procedure is the best, but in practice it largely depends on the available expertise in each institution. It would appear, however, that only bronchoalveolar lavage, in contrast to bronchiolar lavage, yields significant information about the etiology of pulmonary infection.

     After initial evaluation of the seropositive child who presents with a lobar infiltrate, one should initiate age-appropriate antibiotics and observe for 24 to 48 hours. At that time, if there is no improvement, bronchoscopy or open lung biopsy should be arranged. It is important to remember that in adult AIDS patients with respiratory symptoms, but with normal or nondiagnostic chest radiographs, 5 to 15 per cent ultimately have PCP documented at bronchoscopy.

     Once a diagnosis is made, therapy must be individualized. For the treatment of PCP, the drug of choice remains trimethoprim-sulfamethoxazole (TMP-SMZ). The drug is given intravenously in a total daily dosage of 15 to 20 mg per kg of trimethoprim, divided into three or four doses daily for 2 to 3 weeks.

     TMP-SMZ and pentamidine are equally effective for initial treatment of PCP

Table 7. *Treatment of* Pneumocystis carinii *in AIDS*

THERAPY	DOSE	INDICATION	ADVERSE EFFECTS
TMP-SMZ	20 mg/kg/day IV q6h, × 21 days	Drug of choice	Anorexia, nausea, vomiting, rash, neutropenia, thrombocytopenia, hepatitis, fever, nephritis, TEN
Pentamidine	4 mg/kg/day IV or IM once daily, × 21 days	Alternate choice	Painful, sterile abscess at IM site, azotemia, neutropenia, rash, hypoglycemia, hypotension, pancreatitis, ventricular arrhythmias
Aerosolized Pentamidine	300 mg/day (inhaled from nebulizer) 30 min/day, × 21 days	Experimental in adults	Few adverse effects Airway irritation and cough
Trimetrexate	30 mg/m²/day IV once daily, × 21 days. + Leucovorin 20 mg/m²/day IV or PO q6h, × 23 days	Experimental in adults (one uncontrolled study in 49 adult AIDS)	Neutropenia, thrombocytopenia, rash, elevated transaminases, peripheral myopathy
Dapsone-TMP	Dapsone: 100 mg/day TMP: 20 mg/kg/ day, × 21 days PO	Experimental (adults only)	Nausea, vomiting, rash, elevated transaminases, neutropenia

in AIDS, with survival rates of 75 per cent or higher.[33, 72] In adult patients, when pentamidine is substituted because the patient cannot tolerate TMP-SMZ, it is generally effective. When it is used because the patient has not responded to TMP-SMZ, however, it is often found also to be ineffective. Initial reports by Gordin et al. of adverse effects of TMP-SMZ in adult patients with AIDS suggested that 54 per cent of patients treated had serious adverse reactions that necessitated discontinuation of therapy.[48] Severe rash complicates the use of TMP-SMZ for both treatment and prophylaxis of PCP in adult AIDS patients. This is thought to be less of a problem in children, although there is limited information available. Newer therapies for PCP pneumonia are being studied in adults (Table 7), although at this time there is no reported experience in children.

Other causes of interstitial pneumonitis are more difficult to treat. There is limited experience in the treatment of CMV pneumonitis with the guanosine derivative 9-(2-hydroxy-1-[hydroxymethyl]ethoxymethyl)guanine (DHPG). Its efficacy in treating lung disease is questionable and one of its major side effects is bone-marrow suppression.[52] *Mycobacterium avium intracellulare* (MAI) is similarly difficult to treat. At the present time there is no effective therapy. Some of the drugs used have included clofazamine, ansamycin, ethionamide, cycloserine, and amikacin. The outcome is uniformly poor, and in most cases drug toxicity outweighs any potential benefit.

Lymphocytic interstitial pneumonitis (LIP) may present acutely, although it usually has an insidious onset. In established cases of LIP, clinical deterioration marked by tachypnea and decreased arterial pao₂ (< 65) has been used as the indication for treatment with immunoglobulins or steroids.[38] The dose used has

Table 8. *Differential Diagnosis of Enteritis in Children with HIV Infection*

CMV	Salmonella
Adenovirus	Shigella
Mycobacterium avium intracellulare	Campylobacter
C. difficile	*M. tuberculosis*
Giardia	*Isospora belli*
Cryptosporidium	Microsporidia
	E. histolytica

been 2 mg per kg per day of oral prednisone, which is tapered to alternate-day therapy when improvement has been documented.

Approach to the Child with Malnutrition or Other Gastrointestinal Symptoms

Failure to thrive is reported in over 90 per cent of cases of pediatric AIDS.[53] From early in life, children with AIDS are at risk for malnutrition because of frequent and severe infections. These prolonged periods of illness, especially pneumonia or esophagitis, result in poor intake. Poor growth may also be secondary to recurrent or chronic enteritis with malabsorption, a finding present in 10 to 50 per cent of children with AIDS.[47] Aggressive nutritional support is therefore of utmost importance and should be implemented as soon as HIV infection is identified. Nutritional status should be closely monitored, with anthropometric measurements as well as intake diaries. Screening laboratory determinations also may be used to document metabolic status. In selected cases, especially during periods of well-being, oral dietary supplementation may be useful. Overnight enteral feedings may be necessary to ensure sufficient caloric intake. During periods of illness and often during convalescence, it is necessary to institute long-term intravenous hyperalimentation. There are no published studies evaluating the risk of infection of central lines in patients with AIDS. It is a risk, and this must be weighed against the benefit of nutrition in each individual child.

Chronic or recurrent diarrhea is a common finding in children with HIV infection. The etiology may be common pathogens or numerous opportunistic organisms, including CMV, cryptosporidium, and *Isospora belli* (Table 8). In either instance, the infection tends to be more severe, more difficult to eradicate, and more likely to relapse in the HIV infected child as compared to the normal host.[58]

In addition, diarrhea has been reported in some cases, associated with intestinal mucosal damage as well as signs of malabsorption, in which no pathogen has been identified.[47] It has been hypothesized that this is due to the presence of HIV within the intestine or the host mucosal immune reaction to the virus.

It is important to attempt to find a cause for and treat the diarrhea since it may contribute significantly to the failure to thrive so prominent in HIV-infected children. Bacterial cultures may be obtained, but if these results are negative, a more aggressive search for an etiology should be attempted. Stool specimens looking for ova and parasites should be repeated, as well as viral cultures and rapid antigen detection. Because many of these children receive multiple courses of antimicrobial therapy, the possibility of pseudomembranous enterocolitis should be considered.

Documentation of malabsorption should also be sought and a 72-hour fecal fat determination may be helpful. Table 9 outlines a full evaluation of the child with gastrointestinal symptoms.

Oroesophageal Lesions

Oral candidiasis is the most common oral infection seen in children with HIV infection. It is difficult to eradicate and often is accompanied by extension into the esophagus.[47]

Table 9. *Evaluation of the Child with AIDS and Gastrointestinal Symptoms*

1. Nutritional Status	To set intake goals and monitor effect of nutritional therapy.
a) Anthropometrics	—Height, weight, head circumference
	—Triceps skin fold
	—Midarm circumference
b) Intake	—3-Day diary
c) Laboratory	—Serum albumin
	—Transferrin, prealbumin
	—Hemoglobin, RBC morphology
	—Serum iron, plasma zinc
2. Infections	Cultures and procedures determined by presenting symptoms.
a) Stool	—Culture and sensitivities (C + S)× 3, Ova + Parasites (O + P) × 3
	—*C. difficile* toxin
	—virology
	i. Rapid antigen (rotavirus)
	ii. Electron microscopy
	iii. Viral cultures
b) Endoscopy	—Esophageal brushings; biopsy
	—Duodenum aspirate for O + P, C + S; biopsy
	—Rectum C + S; biopsy

Endoscopic biopsies may be cultured and/or examined by light and electron microscopy for pathogens.

3. Malabsorption	Should be sought to help guide optimal nutritional therapy.
a) Fat	—Qualitative, 72 hr fecal fat
b) Carbohydrate	—Stool pH, reducing substance
	—Lactose breath hydrogen
	—D-Xylose 1 hour serum level
c) Protein	—Stool α-1-antitrypsin excretion
d) Biopsy	—Small intestine morphology

CMV and herpes also may cause esophagitis, sometimes coexisting with candida. Because all of these are potentially treatable, it is important to establish a diagnosis. Severe esophagitis can be seen on barium swallow. This method of detection is neither as sensitive nor as specific as endoscopy with biopsy, however.

Treatment for candida esophagitis has been successful with oral ketoconazole or with intravenous amphotericin. There also has been some success with clotrimazole troches in adults, but there has been little pediatric experience. No optimal pediatric formulation is available.[58]

Herpes esophagitis usually responds well to intravenous acyclovir. No adequate therapy for CMV esophagitis is currently available, although experimental antiviral agents have been attempted.[30]

Prophylaxis

Several investigators have advocated the use of intravenous immunoglobulin. Small groups of children with AIDS or ARC were given intravenous immunoglobulin and were reported to have both clinical and immunologic improvement.[13] The treated children had fewer episodes of fever and sepsis as well as stabilization of interstitial pneumonitis when present. Also described were an increase in T4-lymphocytes, increase in the lymphocyte proliferative response, and decreased circulating immune complexes.[31] The regimen used was 50 mg per kg intravenous immunoglobulin, increased by 50 mg per kg every 3 days, achieving a maximum of

200 to 350 mg per kg over 2 or 3 weeks. This was followed by a 200 to 250 mg per kg infusion every 2 to 4 weeks. To date, however, well-controlled studies documenting the efficacy of intravenous immunoglobulin have not been performed. Currently, a multicenter randomized and placebo-controlled trial is being conducted to answer this question. For now its use remains controversial.

The benefits of prophylactic TMP-SMZ for PCP pneumonia has been well established in those patients able to tolerate it. Without prophylactic treatment, PCP recurs within 6 months after initial therapy in about 25 per cent of adult patients with AIDS.[69] Therefore, after a documented episode of PCP, patients should receive prophylactic TMP-SMZ at a dosage of 10 mg per kg per day. In patients with leukemia, Hughes et al. showed that TMP-SMZ, one double-strength tablet b.i.d. given on three consecutive days each week was 100 per cent effective in preventing recurrence of PCP over a 2-year period.[34] It is not yet known whether this protocol will be effective in patients with HIV infection.[67]

Broader use of prophylactic therapy with TMP-SMZ has been advocated by some investigators. Whether all children with HIV infection should receive prophylaxis is an important question that has not been answered.

Therapy

The ultimate goal of therapy for HIV infection would be control or ablation of the infection altogether, coupled with an ability to reconstitute normal immune function in the individual.

Although there are many potential targets for antiviral drugs, most recent efforts have been aimed at attempts to inhibit the DNA polymerase that is unique to the retrovirus. Of the candidate antiviral agents for testing in children, the most publicized has been 3' azido-3'deoxythymidine (AZT).[30] Phase I trials already have begun in several centers so that optimal dosage regimens can be established. Although AZT has been shown to be efficacious in adults with AIDS and has been licensed for clinical use, it is not without problems. Most patients have developed anemia severe enough to necessitate blood transfusion. Other cell lines of the bone marrow also may be affected. In addition, there may be other side effects such as nausea, vomiting, and central nervous system disturbances. Although therapy with AZT decreases HIV antigenemia, this returns with cessation of treatment. Therefore, life-long therapy may be needed. It is not known how children will respond to this drug, however.

Many AIDS patients, both adult and pediatric, have received new therapies on experimental protocols after informed consent has been obtained. This has created a legal dilemma, especially with regard to the pediatric patient. Because of the social circumstances of many of these children they are often found in foster care families, with legal custody in the hands of the Department of Social Services. This raises many legal questions of risk and liability on the part of the governmental agency that grants permission for participation in experimental protocols.

This, of course, is a problem unique to pediatrics, since the patient is a minor and unable to give informed consent on his or her own behalf. Traditionally it has been difficult to obtain permission in circumstances such as these. However, as more protocols become available, and the number of children with devastating disease increases, these experimental therapies are likely to become standard of care. The legal questions regarding liability will need to be weighed against the ethical issue of withholding possibly effective therapy from children with otherwise fatal diseases.

PSYCHOSOCIAL ISSUES

In addition to all of the new and unusual questions that have been raised with regard to the medical management of HIV infection, there are new challenges to the health care system secondary to the psychosocial issues raised. Although most of these issues are familiar to pediatricians dealing with other problems of childhood, their special constellation and intensity are unparalleled in modern health care. The stigmatization of this disease has complicated the health and social care of the infected parties. Our ability to handle these concerns compassionately and intelligently will be very important to these families. School-aged children with HIV infection have become the focus of fears of teachers, other pupils, and neighbors. Ostracism and resultant low self-esteem often have been the consequences of the public's fear. Adolescents who have acquired this disease by engaging in "high-risk behaviors" must handle these admissions in addition to coping with the disease itself. Well-publicized incidents of discrimination, some with accompanying acts of violence, have created an environment in which the family, with the infected member, has chosen total anonymity instead of seeking help. This reduces the possibility of psychiatric, religious, or community support. The fear of contagion has made it difficult to find foster homes, and babies have remained hospitalized for up to a year awaiting placement. This thereby has influenced interventions on the part of social service.

In addition, misconceptions within different ethnic, cultural, or community groups has further increased the feeling of isolation on the part of the afflicted family. Some families have been forced out of housing, others turned away by their family or friends. In some cases, churches have hesitated to comfort families and have even refused to house funeral or memorial services.

Identification of a seropositive infant brings up other problems for the family. Many of these children are already the victims of drug-using families and low socioeconomic status. When a mother is told that her infant is seropositive, she must accept the likelihood that she also is infected with HIV. This message includes the serious, usually fatal illness in the infant, the likely infection and potential for illness and death in the parents, the need for changes in sexual expression to prevent further transmission, and the possibility of avoidance of future pregnancies. Fear, guilt, and sadness further confound an already difficult situation. Similarly, an older uninfected sibling must face the possible loss of several family members.

In addition to the obvious psychosocial burden on the family, this places a great responsibility on the medical community. Many patients and their families vent their frustration, anger, and sadness surrounding the diagnosis; because the medical team is considered safe, the staff often accept this burden alone. This can be an emotionally draining experience for the pediatricians, who usually see patients improve under their care. Even for physicians and other caretakers who care for chronically and terminally ill children, the social problems associated with this disease can be overwhelming and can lead to feelings of impotence on the part of the medical team. The large number of people required to care for a particular child stems from the multidisciplinary nature of the disease and can lead to miscommunications. Regularly scheduled discussion and support groups have been necessary to deal with this, especially when a particular child becomes more symptomatic, and hospitalizations become more frequent and prolonged. As the number of infected children and parents increase, we will have to look for other techniques to reduce burnout and depression among health care workers.

PUBLIC HEALTH CONTROVERSIES

Controversies Regarding Screening

It is mandatory that screening be only one part of a program of counseling, health care and support services if it is to be useful in the prevention of HIV disease. Maternal and fetal screening are widely utilized for diseases that are silent or have minimal symptomatology, but are regularly transmitted to the fetus and may be modified with appropriate therapy. Syphilis and toxoplasmosis are examples of this type of infection.

The same logic would apply to screening programs to detect HIV infection in the pregnant woman. The epidemiology of HIV infection in women and children suggests that silent infection may be detected in women if we focus our efforts on high-risk populations. To date, most children with infection have been black or Hispanic, with maternal intravenous drug use or history of an infected sexual partner the predominate risk factors.[22] The public health service has recommended that all high-risk women of childbearing age be offered testing for HIV antibody as part of their reproductive counseling.[21] They believe this offers women with risk-associated behaviors the opportunity to identify their HIV status and receive appropriate information and advice. If the woman tests seropositive, the risk to future pregnancies must be discussed and family planning can be stressed. If she is already pregnant, counseling should include alternatives to the continuation of the pregnancy.[22] In either case, risk of transmission to sexual or intravenous drug-using partners must be thoroughly discussed and modification of high-risk behaviors encouraged. In addition, planning for infant care may ensure early identification by the pediatrician and therefore optimal care for the affected newborn. Planning for delivery room precautions could reduce the risk to health care workers.

Objections to universal screening for HIV infection have centered on the potential impact of false-positive results, as well as the concern regarding confidentiality of results.[26] The specificity of the current ELISA test when used only in high-risk populations, however, is 99 per cent or greater when only repeatedly reactive test results are considered as positive. To further reduce any risk of a false-positive test result, confirmation by the Western blot techniques has become standard practice. The potential for this testing sequence resulting in a false-positive result appears to be low when utilized in high-risk groups only.

Newborn Screening. The documentation of IgG antibody in the serum of a newborn is neither diagnostic nor predictive of future disease. Identification of those infants at risk, however, could be useful so that optimal care could be provided. As already discussed in this article, current research is being conducted to evaluate other serologic markers that may be associated with true infection early in life.

Screening Other High Risk Pediatric Populations. Patients who received blood products potentially "contaminated" with HIV are at risk for being seropositive and developing subsequent infection. Children with hematologic illness (such as hemophilia or sickle cell disease) who are treated with blood fraction products or multiple transfusions of whole blood or red blood cells are at risk. Seropositivity has been reported in 33 to 92 per cent of patients with hemophilia A and 14 to 52 per cent of patients with hemophilia B.[32] Cases of AIDS have been recognized in both those populations. However, a surprisingly low frequency of progression of disease has suggested the contribution of cofactors to some investigators. Asymptomatic seropositive patients represent a risk to their sexual partners. A recent issue of the MMWR reported seroconversion among sexual partners of HIV seropositive hemophilia patients.[17] It seems appropriate that screening should be offered so that counseling regarding mechanisms of transmission and prevention be initiated. It may be advisable to encourage this population to seek voluntary and confidential serologic testing prior to initial sexual activity.

Children who received transfusions prior to universal screening of blood for HIV antibody (April, 1985) are also at some risk for infection. Only in cases in which a suspected source of blood has been identified is testing of asymptomatic individuals considered reasonable. However, physicians should routinely include exposure to blood or blood products as part of their medical history taking. Decisions regarding HIV testing should be individualized.

With the introduction of both donor interview/questionnaire and HIV serologic screening measures in April 1985, blood and blood products have no longer been a major contributor to the transmission of HIV infection. Indeed, this has been confirmed by an evaluation of the current epidemiology of HIV infection.[32] A recent review confirms the validity of screening techniques utilized in blood banks. Patients with presumed false-positive ELISA results for HIV antibody were screened for reactivity by Western blot. None of over 300 specimens were reactive. These studies suggest that ELISA testing for HIV essentially eliminates the use of plasma or blood from infected persons. However, problems with this approach still persist. Transmission from a seronegative donor who subsequently seroconverted has been documented in two cases. These reports confirm the existence of a "window of seronegativity" in the presence of viremia between exposure and seroconversion. This window may last from weeks to months and represents an ongoing, albeit markedly reduced, potential for transmission of HIV via blood and blood products. In addition, seroconversion has been observed in patients with hemophilia who received only heat treated factor concentrates. This suggests that heat treatment may not guarantee the safety of such products. Currently, only donor-screened heat-treated concentrates are recommended in the therapy of patients requiring factor replacement.[23]

Counseling Sexually Active Adolescents

Counseling and education of the sexually active adolescent requires special skill as well as knowledge of the current understanding of viral transmission. It should be incorporated into discussions including risk of pregnancy as well as the risk of other infectious agents. HIV status should be considered when planning the scope of one's sexual activities. However, HIV status remains largely unknown for most persons not involved in an ongoing monogamous relationship.

The most commonly asked questions involve the risks of kissing, hugging, or other intimate contacts not involving intercourse. The effectiveness of barrier methods for preventing transmission is also a major focus of concern. Exposure to semen, vaginal fluid, or blood is required for transmission of HIV. Skin and oral mucosa, if intact, are resistant to viral passage.[27, 36] The implications are that practices such as kissing and caressing will not result in viral transmission. Preliminary evidence suggests that transmission of HIV via vaginal or rectal intercourse can be reduced by the use of condoms.[21, 26] Latex condoms have been demonstrated to be effective barriers; however, failure rates as high as 17 per cent have been reported. Laboratory testing suggests "natural" lambskin condoms are considerably less effective for preventing both HIV and hepatitis B transmission.[16]

Counseling adolescents to abstain from sexual intercourse as the only reliable method to eliminate risk is necessary but may be ineffective.[29] Evidence that "say no" campaigns are effective is lacking. Use of condoms is a secondary strategy. Education must include information concerning the proper use of condoms as well as identification of high-risk sexual behaviors such as receptive anal intercourse. Techniques such as peer counseling and advertising campaigns need to be initiated and evaluated.

Education and Day Care

Education and day care for seropositive children is a difficult challenge for society. Although much about the transmission of HIV is known, unanswered questions persist. Although virus has been isolated from saliva, tears, and urine, no case of HIV infection has been identified in persons with contact to only limited these bodily fluids. The question of transmission by casual contact has been evaluated through the use of household studies. The only documented seroconversions among household contacts are limited to two persons who were involved in the care of terminally ill patients and had extensive contact with body secretions.[14] In studies of 137 household members who had contact with HIV-infected persons, no transmission was evident.[36] However, the number of household contact studies is relatively small, and extensive experience with day care and school settings is lacking.

Herein lies an emotionally charged dilemma. Transmission via the fecal–oral route, as well as droplet and urine contact, are important modes of transmission of common microbes in young children in day care centers. However, none of these secretions have been demonstrated to contribute to the transmission of HIV. It is because of the remote potential for transmission via urine or saliva that recommendations have been made to restrict HIV seropositive children from day care if they are (1) unable to control body secretions, (2) display biting or mouthing behaviors, or (3) have oozing skin lesions.[18] This is in keeping with the recommendations of the CDC and the American Academy of Pediatrics.[1, 53, 61] This is particularly relevant regarding early intervention programs for infants because HIV disease is often associated with developmental delay. Specific guidelines have been developed on the state and local level, and variations from locale to locale have been influenced by varying moral and political climates in addition to the basic scientific data.[45]

In the school-aged child with HIV infection, who is toilet trained and developmentally appropriate, concern for transmission of HIV has little scientific credibility. The report of the Surgeon General's Workshop on Children with HIV infection suggests the decision to attend school is best left to the individual child's physician. The report further states that under ideal circumstances an individual at the school should be aware of the diagnosis. The need for confidentiality in some instances gives the child the right to have the information withheld from the school, however. Other recommendations have included the formation of an advisory board to review the status of an HIV-infected child on a periodic basis and make recommendations regarding the school attendance of the individual student. In addition, schools must develop appropriate hygienic measures to deal with common events since not all seropositive students will be identified. By having policies to deal with children with epistaxis, gastroenteritis, or exposures to communicable diseases (i.e., varicella) potential risks to both healthy and infected students can be minimized. Programs which educate all children in an age appropriate manner must be developed and fear of HIV infection must be replaced with education regarding risk reduction.

The participation of the HIV-infected school-aged child as a full member of the school community is appropriate when behavioral risks are not present. However, we believe that placing the physician as the only decision maker regarding school attendance is inappropriate. The physician as advocate for all children may be conflicted if she/he also is given the role of advocate for an individual patient. Policies must be established in advance with the help of the local health department or school health team. Should a panel of experts be involved? Could such a panel exist and still maintain confidentiality? These critical questions must be addressed to provide credible leadership for the community.

Risk to Health Care Providers

Unfortunately, the risk to health care workers is not absolutely none. Apparent transmission of HIV has been reported following needle stick, ungloved contact with blood and secretions, and ocular contact with blood. Other potential routes of transmission include contact with amniotic fluid or cervical secretions during resuscitation of the newborn infant in the delivery room.

Although at least seven case reports of seroconversion following occupational exposure have been reported, the infrequency with which such infection has occurred supports the view that transmission is uncommon. The cause of most of the exposures is a needle stick event related to blood drawing or intravenous line placement (45 per cent), from collection boxes (12 per cent), events in the operating room (12 per cent), and skin contamination in an emergency department setting (12 per cent). Universal guidelines have been established by the CDC to minimize the risk of such events; however, complete elimination of occupational risk seems implausible.[28]

The risk to health care workers can be reduced by education concerning and application of infection control guidelines. Specific attention in the labor and delivery site should be given to the use of gloves in handling infants prior to bathing and proper equipment for suctioning infants with neonatal aspiration syndrome. In addition, gloves are indicated for procedures associated with blood drawing and line placement.

In the office, handwashing after each patient contact must be made routine. For care of high risk infants, gloves for handling secretions or excretions (i.e., diapers) should be added to routine practices. Although not all potential risks can be eliminated, one survey suggested 40 per cent of HIV-related exposures could "probably" have been prevented.[26]

Health care workers are at minimal risk for acquiring HIV in the workplace. Risk reduction can be further achieved through good infection control policies. This minimal risk cannot be exploited as a reason to avoid the physician's responsibility to children with HIV infection.

CONTROL OF THE EPIDEMIC

There are currently exhaustive attempts to develop a vaccine to prevent HIV infection in those individuals not yet exposed. Numerous problems exist, making the search for an effective vaccine a very difficult one. It is complicated by the diversity of subtypes of the virus, and the lack of knowledge regarding the actual role of antibodies and cell-mediated immunity in the defense against HIV.

The objective of most investigators working on candidate vaccines is to develop a vaccine that will induce neutralizing antibody. It has been shown, however, that most patients with HIV infection have antibody that is ineffective in preventing AIDS. Direct cell-to-cell spread of virus may exist in consort with viral latency to "protect" HIV from the immune system.[30] At the present time, it is not known how vaccination will affect either seronegative or seropositive donors. Animal testing is hampered by a shortage of chimpanzees, and so it will probably be necessary to test most vaccines in HIV seronegative human volunteers.[56] In short, we are a long way from being able to rely on a vaccine to control this epidemic, and other avenues must be explored.

Although universal screening of blood and blood products for HIV has not eliminated the risk of transfusion-associated acquisition of HIV, it was an important step in decreasing the number of new cases. Because of the long latency period of the virus, new transfusion-related cases will continue to be diagnosed for some time however.

Prevention of perinatally acquired disease will depend on the number of births to HIV infected women. Identification and education of infected women who can transmit HIV to their children must be aggressively attempted. Counseling high-risk women to be voluntarily screened must be done in conjunction with information regarding risk to their infants. Of course, education also must focus on behavioral change, with avoidance of high-risk sexual activities and intravenous drug use.

In addition to the counseling and education of already high-risk populations, the true spread of the AIDS epidemic will not be able to be controlled until the general public can be made aware of the risks. Containment of this disease will rest on our ability to effect changes in behavior and life-style so that the chain of transmission can be effectively broken. Mass media, which often emphasizes the sensational aspects of the AIDS epidemic, must educate the public so that fear does not spawn drastic policy measures that are unwarranted in terms of what is known about the actual risk. Significant portions of the population, including intravenous drug users, adolescents, and those with language barriers, are not being reached with the educational messages conveyed through traditional media. The techniques of marketing research should be used to identify the most effective means of communicating with all parts of the population. Alternative communication resources should be explored. It is only in this way that the stigmatization may be reduced, thus allowing affected persons to openly be counseled, tested, and receive care. Unless this occurs, the number of HIV-infected adults, children, and infants will continue to grow to even more tragic proportions.

ACKNOWLEDGMENTS

Thanks to Ms. Kelly Mills for excellent secretarial assistance and to P.F.L. for the inspiration needed to complete this article.

REFERENCES

1. American Academy of Pediatrics: School attendance of children and adolescents with human T lymphotropic virus III/lymphadenopathy associated virus infection. Pediatrics 77:430, 1986
2. Amman AJ: The acquired immunodeficiency syndrome in infants and children. Ann Intern Med 103(5):734–737, 1985
3. Amman AJ, Cowan MJ, Wara DW et al: Acquired immunodeficiency in an infant: possible transmission by means of blood products. Lancet 1:956, 1983
4. ACIP: Immunization of children infected with human immunodeficiency virus. MMWR 37:181–183, 1988
5. ACIP: Measles prevention. MMWR 31:217–224, 1982
6. ACIP: Mumps vaccine. MMWR 31:617–620, 1982
7. Allegra CJ, Chabner BA, Tuazon CU et al: Trimetrexate for the treatment of *Pneumocystis carinii* pneumonia in patients with the acquired immunodeficiency syndrome. N Engl J Med 317(16):978–985, 1987
8. Barbour SD: Acquired immunodeficiency syndrome of childhood. Pediatr Clin North Am 34:247–257, 1987
9. Bernstein LJ, Krieger BZ et al: Bacterial infection in the acquired immunodeficiency syndrome of children. Pediatr Infect Dis 4(5):472–475, 1985
10. Bernstein LJ, Ochs HD, Wedgewood RG et al: Defective humoral immunity in pediatric acquired immune deficiency syndrome. Pediatrics 107:352–357, 1985
11. Borkowsky W, Bebenroth D, Krasinski K et al: Human immunodeficiency-virus infections in infants negative for anti-HIV by enzyme-linked immunoassay. Lancet 1:1168–1171, 1987
12. Borkowsky W, Steele CJ, Grubman S et al: Antibody response to bacterial toxoids in children infected with the human immunodeficiency virus. J Pediatr 110(4):563–566, 1987
13. Calvelli FA, Rubinstein A: Intravenous gamma-globulin in infants with the acquired immunodeficiency syndrome. Pediatr Infect Dis 5(3):S207–S210, 1986
14. CDC: Apparent transmission of HTLV-III/LAV from a child to mother providing health care. MMWR 35:75, 1986
15. CDC: Classification system for human immunodefiency virus infection in children under 13 years of age. MMWR 36:593, 1987

16. CDC: Condoms for prevention of sexually transmitted diseases. MMWR 37:133–138, 1988
17. CDC: HIV infection and pregnancies in sexual partners of HIV-seropositive hemophiliac men. MMWR 36:225, 1987
18. CDC: Education and foster care of children infected with human T-lymphotropic virus type III/lymphadenopathy associated virus. MMWR 34:517, 1985
19. CDC: Immunization of children infected with human T-lymphotropic virus type III/lymphadenopathy-associated virus. Ann Intern Med 106:75–78, 1987
20. CDC: Immunization of children infected with human T-Lymphotropic virus type III/lymphadenopathy-associated virus. MMWR 35:595–606, 1986
21. CDC: Public health service guidelines for counseling and antibody testing to prevent HIV infection and AIDS. MMWR 36:509, 1987
22. CDC: Recommendations for assisting in the prevention of perinatal transmission of human T-lymphotropic virus type III/lymphadenopathy-associated virus and AIDS. MMWR 34:721–732, 1985
23. CDC: Survey of non-U.S. hemophilia treatment centers for HIV seroconversions following therapy with heat-treated factor concentrates. MMWR 36:121, 1987
24. Curran JW, Morgan WM et al: The Epidemiology of AIDS: Current status and future prospects. Science 229:1352–1357, 1985
25. Epstein LG, Sharer LR, Oleske JM: Neurologic Manifestations of Human Immunodeficiency Virus Infection in Children. Pediatrics 78:678–687, 1986
26. Francis DP, Chen J: The prevention of acquired immunodeficiency syndrome in the United States. JAMA 257:1357, 1987
27. Friedland GH, Saltzman BR: Lack of transmission of HTLV-III/LAV infection to household contacts of patients with AIDS or AIDS-related complex with oral candidiasis. N Engl J Med 314:344–349, 1986
28. Gerberding JL, Bryant-LeBlanc CE, Nelson K et al: Risk of transmitting the human immunodeficiency virus, cytomegalovirus, and hepatitis B to health care workers exposed to patients with AIDS and ARC. J Infect Dis 156:1–8, 1987
29. Goedert JJ: What is safe sex? N Engl J Med 316:1339, 1987
29a. Goetz DW, Hall SE, Harbison RW et al: Pediatric acquired immunodeficiency syndrome with negative human immunodeficiency virus antibody response by enzyme-linked immunosorbent assay and western blot. Pediatrics 81:356–359, 1988
30. Grierson HL, Purtilo DT: New Developments in AIDS. Infect Dis Clin North Am 1:547–558, 1987
31. Gupta A, Novick BE, Rubinstein A: Restoration of suppressor T-cell function in children with AIDS following intravenous gamma globulin treatment. Am J Dis Child 140:143–146, 1986
32. Hilgartner MW: AIDS in the transfused patient. Am J Dis Child 141:194, 1987
33. Hughes WT, Feldman S, Chauhary SC et al: Comparison of pentamidine isothionate and trimethoprim-sulfamethoxazole in the treatment of Pneumocystis carinii pneumonia. J Pediatr 92(2):285–291, 1978
34. Hughes WT, Rivera GK, Schell MJ et al: Successful intermittent chemoprophylaxis for Pneumocystis carinii pneumonitis. N Engl J Med 316:1627–1632, 1987
35. Isenberg HJ, Charytan M, Rubinstein A: Cardiac involvement in children with acquired immune deficiency. Am Heart J 110:710, 1985
36. Kaplan JE, Oleske JM et al: Evidence against transmission of human T-lymphotropic virus/lymphadenopathy. Associated virus (HTLV-III/LAV) in families of children with the acquired immunodeficiency syndrome. Ped Infect Dis 5:468–471, 1985
37. Krasinski K, Borkowski W: Response to polio vaccine in children infected with the human immunodeficiency virus. Albuquerque, New Mexico, Society for Pediatric Research, 925, 1987
38. Kornstein MJ, Pietra GG, Hoxie JA et al: The pathology and treatment of interstitial pneumonitis in two infants with AIDS. Am Rev Resp Dis 133:1196–1198, 1986
39. Leoung GH, Mills J, Philip C et al: Dapsone-trimethoprim for Pneumocystis carinii pneumonia in the acquired immunodeficiency syndrome. Ann Intern Med 105:45–48, 1986
39a. Lepage P, Van de Perre P, Carael M et al: Postnatal transmission of HIV from mother to child. Lancet 2:400, 1987
40. MacDonald KL, Dowla RN, Osterholm MT: Infection with human T-lymphotropic virus

type III/lymphadenopathy associated virus: consideration for transmission in the child day care setting. J Infect Dis 8:606, 1986

41. Marchevsky A, Rosen MJ, Chrystal G et al: Pulmonary complication of the acquired immunodeficiency syndrome. Hum Pathol 16(7):659–670, 1985

42. Marion RW, Wiznia AA et al: Human T-cell lymphotropic virus type III (HTLV-III) embryopathy: A new dysmorphic syndrome associated with intrauterine HTLV-III infection. Am J Dis Child 140:638–640, 1986

43. Martin K, Katz BZ, Miller G: AIDS and antibodies to HIV in children and their families. J Infect Dis 155:54–63, 1987

44. Marwick C: HIV antibody prevalence data derived from study of Massachusetts infants. JAMA 258(2):171–172, 1987

45. Massachusetts Department of Public Health: Governor's Task Force on AIDS. Policies and Recommendations, January, 1987

46. McCarthy VP, Charles DL, Unger JL: Transfusion associated HIV infection in a neonate from a seronegative donor. Am J Dis Child 141:1145, 1987

47. McLoughlin LC, Nord KS, Joshi VV et al: Severe gastrointestinal involvement in children with the acquired immunodeficiency syndrome. J Pediatr Gastroenterol Nutr 6:517–524, 1987

48. The Medical Letter on Drugs and Therapeutics: Treatment of *Pneumocystis carinii* 29:103–104, 1987

49. Mok JQ, DeRossi A, Ades AE et al: Infants born to mothers seropositive for human immunodeficiency virus. Lancet 1:1164, 1987

50. Mok JQ, Giaquinto C, Rossi A et al: Infants born to HIV-seropositive mothers: preliminary findings from a multicenter European study. Lancet 1:1165–1168, 1987

51. Montgomery AB, Luce JM, Turner J et al: Aerosolized pentamidine as sole therapy for *Pneumocystis carinii* pneumonia in patients with acquired immunodeficiency syndrome. Lancet 29:480–482, 1987

52. Murray JF, Felton CP, Garay SM et al: Pulmonary complication of the acquired immunodeficiency syndrome. N Engl J Med 310:1682–1688, 1984

53. Novick BE, Rubinstein A: AIDS-the pediatric perspective. AIDS 1:3, 1987

54. Ochs H: Intravenous immunoglobulin in the treatment and prevention of acute infection in pediatric acquired immunodeficiency syndrome patients. Pediatr Infect Dis 5:S207–S210, 1986

55. Oleske J, Minefor A, Cooper R et al: Immunodeficiency syndrome in children. JAMA 249:2345, 1983

56. Onorato I: Immunization, vaccine preventable diseases and HIV infection. 21st Immunization Conference, New Orleans, June 8–11, 1987

57. Qazi QH, Sheikh TM, Fikrig S et al: Lack of evidence for craniofacial dysmorphism in perinatal human immunodeficiency virus infection. J Pediatr 112:7–11, 1988

58. Quinn TC: Gastrointestinal manifestation of AIDS. Pract Gastroenterol 9:23–34, 1985

59. Reyn CF, Mann JM, Clements CJ: Human immunodeficiency virus infection and routine childhood immunization. Lancet 19:669–672, 1987

60. Rodgers VD: Gastrointestinal manifestation of AIDS. West Med J 146:57–67, 1987

61. Rogers MF: AIDS in children: A review of the clinical and public health aspects. Pediatr Infect Dis 4:230, 1985

62. Rubinstein A: Pediatric AIDS. Curr Probl Pediatr 16:362, 1986

63. Rubinstein A, Morecki R, Silverman B et al: Pulmonary disease in children with acquired immunodeficiency syndrome and AIDS-related complex. J Pediatr 108(4):498–503, 1986

64. Rubinstein A, Novick BE, Siclick MJ et al: Circulating thymulin and thymosin activity in pediatric acquired immunodeficiency syndrome: in vivo and in vitro studies. J Pediatr 109(3):422–427, 1986

65. Rubinstein A, Siclick M, Gupta A et al: Acquired immunodeficiency with reversed T4:T8 ratio in infants born to promiscuous and drug-addicted mothers. JAMA 249:2350, 1983

66. Sherran P, Pickoff AS, Ferrer PL et al: Echocardiographic evaluation of myocardial function in pediatric AIDS patients. Am Heart J 110:710, 1985

67. Silverman BK, Waddell A: Report of the Surgeon General's workshop on children with HIV infection and their families. U.S. Department of Health and Human Services, August 1987

68. Steinherz LJ, Brochstein JA, Robins J: Cardiac involvement in congenital acquired immunodeficiency syndrome. Am J D Child 140:1241–1244, 1986

69. Walzer PD: Diagnosis of *Pneumocystis carinii* pneumonia. J Infect Dis 154:629–632, 1988
70. Weinbreck P, Loustaud V, Denis F et al: Postnatal transmission of HIV Infection. Lancet 482, 1988
71. Weiss SH, Goedert JJ, Sarngadharan MG et al: Screening test for HTLV-III antibodies. JAMA 253:221, 1985
72. Wharton JM, Coleman DL, Wofsy CB et al: Trimethoprim-sulfamethoxazole or pentamidine for *Pneumocystis carinii* pneumonia in the acquired immunodeficiency syndrome. Ann Intern Med 105:37–44, 1986
73. Williford Pifer LL, Woods DR, Edwards CC: *Pneumocystis carinii* serologic study in pediatric acquired immunodeficiency syndrome. Am J Dis Child 142:36–39, 1988
74. Wood CC, McNamara JC, Schwarz F et al: Prevention of pneumococcal bacteremia in a child with acquired immunodeficiency syndrome related complex. Pediatr Infect Dis J 6(6):564–566, 1987
75. Ziegler JB, Johnson RO, Cooper DA et al: Postnatal transmission of AIDS-associated retrovirus from mother to infant. Lancet 1:896, 1985

Division of Infectious Diseases
Boston City Hospital
818 Harrison Avenue
Boston, Massachusetts 02118

0031–3955/88 $0.00 + .20

Children as Participants in Medical Research

Michael A. Grodin, MD,* and Joel J. Alpert, MD†

HISTORY OF THE USE OF CHILDREN AS RESEARCH SUBJECTS

While human experimentation dates back thousands of years, the planned use of human subjects for medical research is a phenomenon primarily of this century. The use of children as subjects for serious study in medical research has only occurred in the last 50 years.[32] The short history of children and research parallels the historical status of children.[20] Children were considered the chattels of their fathers until the mid-seventh century in England.[46] Physicians did not begin to care for children in earnest until the 17th century. Pediatric care was felt to be beneath the dignity of physicians, and the high infant mortality rate also discouraged medical science from focusing on childhood disease. The American Society for the Prevention of Cruelty to Children was established only in 1874.[17] As pediatrics and child welfare began to succeed in lowering mortality rates, medicine became increasingly interested in specialized therapies for children. Paralleling adult medicine, but lagging behind, medical scientists began to concern themselves with establishing the validity of pediatric care based on the premise that children are unique and are not miniature adults. The early part of the 20th century saw an increasing use of children in research, but little control, regulation, or studies of safety, efficacy, and ethics of such investigations. However, concern about not excluding children from the benefits of medical research has in recent years been characterized by concern for assessment of risk, ability to consent, and the proper use of children in human experimentation.

Setting and Funding Source

The nature, scope, and extent of research on children has been intimately linked to the setting and funding source of research projects. Research on children is undertaken in hospitals, academic centers, clinics, practitioners' private offices, institutions, and schools. Each setting has its own unique concerns with research

*Director, Program in Medical Ethics; Associate Professor of Pediatrics and Sociomedical Sciences (Ethics), Boston University Schools of Medicine and Public Health; Chairman, Institutional Review Board, Associate Visiting Physician (Pediatrics), Medical Ethicist, Boston City Hospital, Boston, Massachusetts

†Professor and Chairman, Department of Pediatrics, Boston University School of Medicine, Boston City Hospital, Boston, Massachusetts

design, generalizability, recruitment, retention, and need for protection of patients through consent and confidentiality. The source of funding for research on children can be supported by federal, state, or local government, or private sources such as pharmaceutical companies, corporations, or foundations. The funding source can affect not only the setting of the research but the implementation, methodology, and limits of a particular study, as well as the degree of research monitoring, regulation, and protection of subjects.

Research, Clinical Practice, and Nonvalidated Practices

Another general consideration in the history of human experimentation that has directly influenced research involving children is the difference between clinical practice, nonvalidated practice, and research. These distinctions are critical in that the definitions and goals surrounding each of these activities may vary and thus have direct impact on the welfare and protection of the patient/subject.[33, 36, 45] Research is designed to develop or contribute to generalizable knowledge.[41] Although risk to the patient will always be assessed and it is hoped that research will benefit either a particular patient, a class of patients, or society at large, research has as its primary (and often sole) concern the generation or validation of new knowledge. Clinical practice, in contrast, is designed solely to enhance the well-being of an individual who is intended as the primary (if not sole) beneficiary of the physician–patient encounter.[41] Nonvalidated practices are innovations intended to benefit the patient through new, untested, or unvalidated therapies. Such deviation from common practice in the course of rendering treatment should not be considered research unless it is structured as a scientifically and ethically valid research project. Most would recommend that significant innovations in therapy should be incorporated into a formal research project to establish safety and efficacy.[41] These distinctions are helpful in clarifying the issues of goals, risks, benefits, validity, and relevance of regulation. Research may be classified as therapeutic (research on subjects with a certain disease) or nontherapeutic (research on normal volunteers). The goal of all research, whether therapeutic or nontherapeutic, is to gain generalizable knowledge through controlled, scientifically rigorous investigation.

Ethical Use of Children in Research

The controlled, regulated, and ethical progression from the use of consenting adults to the use of adolescents, older children, younger children and, finally, infants in therapeutic research evokes little controversy. Not to allow safety and efficacy testing or controlled clinical trials in the pediatric age group would be to orphan an entire segment of the population from the potential benefits of research. Drugs found safe and efficacious in adults are not necessarily safe and efficacious in children. Not to conduct scientifically rigorous and ethically sound research would seem to violate the principles of justice and equity in society. Specific problems and diseases unique to a specific pediatric age group or population may require the use of children even without prior testing in adults. Specific ethical problems of therapeutic research in children often relate to appropriate proxy or surrogate consent, proper assessment of risks and benefits, and concerns about potential conflicts between parent and subject/child.

The use of children for nontherapeutic research has generated more controversy.[31, 34] At one extreme, Ramsey argues that children should only be used as medical subjects if the study will directly benefit the recovery of the child and thus may be considered therapeutic.[48, 49] Ramsey argues that unless a child can give a complete and informed consent, he or she should never be a subject in nontherapeutic research. Further, though such research may in fact promote generalizable knowledge, even to children as a group, such good can never outweigh the risk. The ends do not justify the means. McCormick, on the other hand, has argued that nontherapeutic research on children is ethically defensible if it involves minimal risk and holds the prospect of benefiting children as a group.[37] McCormick believes that children, as well as adults, are not only capable of participating in nontherapeutic research but also are morally obligated to participate for the good of all. Furthermore, McCormick argues that parents are the appropriate surrogates for appreciating this childhood obligation and thus for assuring a valid consent on behalf of the child as the "act is right." It is further presumed that such consent is the equivalent of a substituted judgment in that if the child were capable of consent, he or she would so consent.

Successes of Research on Children

It is important to note the remarkable successes of research on children over the past few decades. Vaccines have been developed and have proven successful in all but eradicating many previously common and often crippling diseases such as smallpox, polio, diphtheria, and tetanus. Malignancies previously considered universally fatal, such as leukemia, are now treated with increasing success. Technologic and pharmacologic innovations in cardiorespiratory support have received broad application in perinatal, neonatal, and pediatric intensive care. While much of the success of research in children has built on previous work in basic science and application to adults, extrapolation of adult data to children is fraught with difficulties. Children are not little adults. Their anatomy, physiology, metabolism, responses, and reactions to research protocols are different and therapies, which were believed to be safe and efficacious in adults, often turn out to have different safety and efficacy profiles in neonates or children. Children also have congenital, genetic, or other diseases only found in the pediatric age group, necessitating primary investigation on children.

HISTORY OF THE PROTECTION OF HUMAN SUBJECTS

While the history of research goes back thousands of years, the history of the protection of human subjects in research is perhaps less than 50 years old.[30, 32] The precipitating events that led to public policy debate and legislative regulation are dramatic. The Nazi experimentations exposed in 1949 during the Nuremberg trials had led to a proposed Universal Code of Research Ethics.[53] The cornerstone of the Nuremberg code was the informed, uncoerced, voluntary consent of the subject. Taken literally, this essential component of consent of the subject would exclude children as research subjects. In 1964, the World Medical Association's Declaration of Helsinki recognized the special population of subjects with limited capacity to consent as appropriate subjects for research but in need of special protections and adequate surrogate decision making.[58] Several research projects of the 1950s and 1960s brought a call for explicit federal regulation. A public outcry arose from such research as the Tuskegee syphilis study,[18] the injection of live cancer cells into chronically ill patients,[30] the hepatitis studies on retarded children at Willowbrook State Hospital,[30] the institution of fetal and abortus research, and the Beecher reviews of ethically suspect research.[2] In 1974, partly in response to growing concern over the ethics of human research, Congress passed P.L. 93–348, creating the National Commission for the Protection of Human Subjects in Biomedical and Behavioral Research.[43]

Final regulations for the protection of human subjects in research were promulgated in 1974 by the Department of Health, Education and Welfare (DHEW), now known as the Department of Health and Human Services (DHHS).[21] These initial regulations did not specifically address children. However, after the

National Commission recommendations of 1978, DHHS regulations governing research involving children were published.[22] Regulations relating to fetuses and pregnant women were published in 1981.[8] Finally, in 1983, a new set of regulations specifically governing children in research was published.[9]

ETHICAL UNDERPINNINGS OF RESEARCH ON CHILDREN

In 1979, the Belmont Report of the Ethical Principles and Guidelines for the Protection of Human Subjects was issued under the auspices of the National Commission for the Protection of Human Subjects in Research.[42] This report identified the ethical framework and relevant substantive principles on which procedural regulations were issued. Three basic ethical principles were elucidated as particularly relevant to the ethics of research on human subjects. The first ethical principle was that of respect for persons, which demands that autonomous, competent subjects be granted self-determination to the greatest extent possible. The procedural implementation of the respect for autonomy is the doctrine of informed consent. The principle of respect for persons would also demand that nonautonomous, incompetent subjects be afforded additional protection from harm. The second ethical principle identified was beneficence/nonmaleficence. This principle demands that subjects not only be treated with respect, but that efforts be made to ensure their well-being and, at minimum, to avoid harm. The procedural implementation of this principle demands critical assessment of the benefits and risks of research and maximizing the ratio of benefit to risk. The third ethical principle identified was distributive justice. This principle demands a consideration of fairness in distribution of the burdens and benefits of research. The implementation of this principle demands consideration of fair procedure and outcomes in the selection of research subjects.

Because children have limited cognitive capacities compared to normal adults, they must be considered a special population for the purposes of implementation of the ethical principles of research.[32] The principle of respect for persons demands that a vulnerable population such as children be afforded added protection. Insofar as adolescents are competent they should be encouraged to express their wishes through the process of informed consent. Insofar as children can register their knowledgeable agreement or disagreement with a proposed research project, they should be offered the opportunity to express their wishes through assent or dissent. Infants and small children who are incompetent to assent or dissent are respected by added protection from harm. The assessment of risk–benefit ratio required by the principle of beneficence may require the use of a surrogate parent or legally authorized representative to grant proxy consent for the vulnerable, nonautonomous child. Because of the proxy nature of consent, decisional authority of surrogates should be limited to reasonable or minimal risks unless special justification is provided. Finally, the just distribution of the burdens and benefits of research will require additional justification for the use of unconsenting, vulnerable populations. Justice requires special considerations of the potential for direct benefit to the child or at least special benefit to the class or to the condition of children as a group.

The regulatory implementation of the ethical underpinnings of research has been through the establishment of Institutional Review Boards (IRBs). These federally mandated bodies are specifically charged with the protection of human subjects through assessment of norms of research, informed consent, risk–benefit ratio, and just selection of populations such as children. Special regulatory procedures have been established for review of research with special populations. IRBs armed with their regulatory authority, substantive ethical underpinnings, procedural mechanisms for review, and broad interdisciplinary professional and lay membership, are perhaps best situated to assess and balance imperatives for research on children.[26]

REGULATIONS

Federal

Specific federal regulations governing research on minors were promulgated in 1983 by the Department of Health and Human Services.[10] The regulations recognize four possible categories into which child research participants might fall.[51] These categories include studies involving no more than minimal risk with the prospect of direct benefit to the child,[11] studies involving more than minimal risk with the prospect of direct benefit to the child,[12] studies involving more than minimal risk, with no direct benefit, but offering the prospect of "generalizable knowledge,"[13] and studies that would otherwise not receive approval that could lead to the understanding, prevention, or alleviation of a "serious problem" affecting children's health or welfare.[14]

The first category of research involving minimal risk, whether the research involves therapeutic or nontherapeutic research, does not pose great difficulty. Minimal risk as outlined by the regulations is to be understood as probability and magnitude of physical or psychological harm not exceeding that normally encountered in the daily life or routine medical or psychological examination of children. Procedures that might present minimal risk to a healthy child include urinalysis, obtaining small blood samples, ECGs, minor changes in diet or daily routine, and the use of standardized psychological or educational tests.[47] The regulations would allow such minimal risk research assuming that appropriate consent, assent, or parent's or guardian's permission is given.

Procedures that exceed the limits of minimal risk are to be assessed by the IRB on a case-by-case basis. Procedures posing greater than minimal risk might include biopsies, spinal taps, the use of drugs whose risks to children have not been established, or behavioral interventions likely to cause psychological stress.[47] Assessment of risk also must take into consideration the disease, condition, or present state of the subjects to be studied. Thus, drawing blood from children with a bleeding disorder may be seen as a greater risk than drawing blood in children with normal clotting. Similarly, obtaining blood from a child with a chronic disease accustomed to such procedures might require special consideration. Such children may consider blood drawing as either a greater or lesser stress than a normal child.

Research involving more than minimal risk may be justified if there are specific therapeutic or prophylactic benefits that may accrue to the child subject. Studies that involve only slightly more than minimal risk that offer no therapeutic benefit to the subject may still be justified, but only if the IRB determines that the "research is likely to yield knowledge vital to understanding or ameliorating the disorder or condition from which the subject suffers; the interventions involved are reasonably commensurate with the experiences in the subject's past or expected medical, dental, psychological, social or educational situation; and adequate provisions are made for soliciting the child's assent and the permission of the child's parents or guardian."[47] Research that does not fit into any applicable category of the regulation but that promises a solution to a significant and serious health problem of children may be approved by the Secretary of the DHHS after consultation with an Ethics Advisory Board and following publication and opportunity for public review and comment.

The Federal regulations also set forth specific standards and procedures for obtaining consent, assent, or permission in the child population. The regulations defining a competent, reasoned, and informed consent in the research setting is outlined in the 1981 regulations.[15] For the purposes of nonautonomous unconsenting minors the regulations define assent as a child's affirmative agreement to participate in research and permission as the agreement of a child's parent or legal guardian for the child to participate in research.

Depending on the age of consent and exceptions as determined by state law, children generally cannot give a legally valid consent on their own behalf, and the permission of a parent or guardian is required prior to participation in research. If the research intervention is nontherapeutic and the child is old enough to comprehend, assess, and appreciate the research study, the IRB can determine whether all or some of the children are capable of assent to participate. The IRB also may determine in a therapeutic protocol that the child's assent is not required. In either case, the IRB will be guided by the nature of the research and the age, maturity, status, and condition of the child/subject. Independent of solicitation of assent from a child, all children should receive in age-appropriate fashion an explanation of what will be done, how long it will take, and how uncomfortable the study will be.

Specific federal regulations exist involving research on pregnant women, fetuses, and human in vitro fertilization.[16] These legally problematic and ethically complex regulations describe research directed toward the fetus *in utero*, research involving the fetus *ex utero*, research with dead fetuses, fetal material and the placenta, research in anticipation of abortion, and research involving in vitro fertilization.

State Laws

While the federal DHHS regulations set a standard for the conduct of research in children, state law must also be complied with before embarking on a research project. Some state laws may specifically address the issue of human research with minors. Most state laws specifically address the issue of parental and minor consent.[5, 44, 54] Some state laws also address concerns over the use of institutionalized and mentally handicapped minors as research subjects.[52, 59]

In the absence of specific statutory laws regarding children in the research setting, a minimal state standard of laws pertaining to the medical treatment of children can be elucidated from statutes governing the treatment of minors in the clinical, nonresearch setting. Using state standards for the treatment of minors in the clinical realm, one may demand more rigid or restrictive postures either required by federal regulation or by the research itself.

Four state statutory considerations are relevant to the therapeutic treatment of minors when such therapy occurs to the minor's benefit.[29] The age of majority initially determines at what age there is a presumption of competence to consent which must be refuted to interfere with autonomous persons. Below the age of 18 years on the other hand, a minor is presumed incompetent for the purpose of valid consent unless one of three considerations is applicable. First, an "emancipated minor" is one who is living on his or her own, is self-supporting, and is not subject to parental control. An emancipated minor may be medically treated as an adult, and no parental permission is necessary. Most states have also enacted minor treatment statutes that provide that a child 16 years or older may be considered competent for independent medical treatment as if an adult. Second, most states also specifically allow minor treatment without parental knowledge for venereal diseases and drug/alcohol problems. Third, even in the absence of statutes, the "mature minor rule" implies that "if a young person (aged 14 or 15 years or older) understands the nature of the proposed treatment and its risks, if the physician believes that the patient can give the same degree of informed consent as an adult patient, and if the treatment does not involve very serious risks, the young person may validly consent to receiving it."[29] For the purposes of research, were a minor to be considered as mature enough to independently consent to enrollment in research to his/her own benefit, it would seem that at minimum the minor must first be considered mature by the same standards as if the therapy were standard and to be offered in the clinical sphere, and only then should involvement in research be considered further.

It also seems prudent to presume that parents should be involved in all clinical and research protocols where minors are to be subjects. The burden of proof should rest on why parents are not being involved in the consent process. In the case of research, only minimal risk procedures should be considered in mature minors, particularly in research of a nontherapeutic nature. If the treatment involves more than minimal risk, or if therapeutic research has significant risks, parents and guardians must be involved in the consent process.

States also have passed laws regarding research on fetuses, pregnant women, embryos, and even neonates.[35] One should be aware of state laws, since a researcher may be violating state statutes even while being in compliance with federal research statutes.

Case Law

There are very few legal cases involving the legal capacity of children to consent to or refuse therapy. There is even less case law involving children as research subjects. An analogy can perhaps be drawn from cases involving the rights of minors and their access to contraception.[6] Similar Supreme Court cases have held that statutes giving parents absolute veto power over an adolescent's abortion was an unconstitutional violation of the right of privacy.[3, 7] Depending on the seriousness of the medical problem, cases also have considered the adolescent's right to refuse therapies even when parents have consented, such as cases of plastic surgery.[4] Several cases have held also that for the purposes of live donors, transplantation of kidneys or bone marrow in which the donor is a minor and the recipient is a sibling, parental consent on behalf of the minor donor was granted.[19, 40] These cases reflect the evolution of the adolescent as a competent, independent decision maker. When decisions pose significant risk or are not to the direct benefit of the adolescent, courts have reflected their ambivalence through added procedural (either parental or judicial) safeguards.

FUTURE PROBLEMS AND AREAS FOR INVESTIGATION

The future problems associated with the continued use of children in research fall into three broad categories. The first area of concern involves the substantive and conceptual issues surrounding such areas as competency, risk assessment, distributive justice, and compensation for research. The second broad category in need of further analysis and development involves the procedural and regulatory issues surrounding the applicability and scope of local, state, federal, and international codes for research with children. Finally, there are specific issues surrounding the age and status of the vulnerable subpopulations of infants, children, and adolescents who may be healthy, or may have handicaps or chronic diseases. Each of these areas of future concern are themselves in need of further directed investigation, evaluation, and formal research.

SUBSTANTIVE CONCEPTUAL ISSUES

Competency to Consent

The assessment of children's competency to consent has received considerable empirical research and theoretical study over the last decade.[24, 28, 39, 55, 56, 57] The first question relating to children and consent relates to the appropriate standard for capacity, cognition, and competency. Are children developmentally similar to adults? Should children be held to the same, lower, or a higher standard of consent than adults when approached to participate in research? Is there significant difference between children and adolescents? Does the setting (hospital, clinic, research facility) change these standards? Is the clinical standard necessary or sufficient for the research setting? What weight should the child's assent, consent, or refusal play in deciding to proceed with research in the face of parental agreement or disagreement with regard to therapeutic or nontherapeutic protocols?

The classic elements necessary for informed consent include the ability to understand the nature, purpose, and procedure of research; the capability to express preferences; and the competency to consent. The area of competency has received extensive study in the adult literature.[1, 38, 50] A schematized approach to tests of competency may vary depending on the degree or sphere of competency required. A minimal standard might be the ability to express choice. This standard would be followed by increasing need for the demonstration of understanding and reasoning followed by an appreciation of the nature, extent, and probable consequences of consent and a reasonable decision that considers, weighs, and uses these elements resulting in a reasoned and informed consent. Depending on the degree or level of competency demanded and the materiality of the information to risk–benefit ratio, adults may or may not meet this standard. It is clear that children, adolescents, and adults alike may fall into various levels of competency. Adults, however, are presumed competent until proven otherwise.

Assessment of Risk and Benefit

The assessment of risk involves the prediction in terms of probability that harm will occur. In contrast, benefit is a nonprobabilistic or predictive notion that something of value will occur.[32] There are very few empiric data in children about the assessment of risk. While it is clear that different scales or standards might exist for infants as opposed to young children or adolescents, how to assess discomfort, pain, or inconvenience in these "incompetent" vulnerable populations is problematic. Within each of these age groups, certain diseases or handicapping conditions also may affect the assessment of risk and benefit. Should there be separate standards of acceptable risk for therapeutic and nontherapeutic research? Although such a discrepancy may be justified in the unconsenting incompetent child, how should one evaluate degree of risk in relation to benefit? What if the child is a member of a special vulnerable or at-risk group? What if the child is capable of meaningful assent or dissent? Does the ability to balance appropriate risk and benefit ratio exclude the possibility of randomized clinical trials in which some children will be placebo controls?

Distributive Justice

The principle of distributive justice requires consideration of the distribution of the burdens and benefits of research within society. The principle of respect for persons, with its focus on autonomy, requires informed consent as a primary means of protecting the research subject and enhancing a just and equitable distribution of research. Populations unable to provide a competent, rational, and uncoerced informed consent must a priori be considered vulnerable populations. Although orphaning such populations from reaping the benefits of research would seem inappropriate, added protections must be afforded these groups to ensure a just distribution of risks as well. As such, the burden of proof must be on why it is necessary to study a particular vulnerable group. It is obvious why such captive, restricted, and often coerced groups such as prisoners and the institutionalized should be studied only if no other competent uncoerced group could possibly serve as research subjects. Thus, institutionalized individuals should only be research subjects if the research has to do with problems associated with institutionalized individuals. This research should never be linked to privileges or the ability to stay within a facility.[30]

Children, as a vulnerable population, require added justification for participation in research protocols. Who decides what justifications are sufficient, and how and from whom consent is obtained, is problematic. Should the proxy speaking on behalf of the child vary depending on whether the research is therapeutic or nontherapeutic? What about children whose parents disagree? Is consensus necessary? What if the child is a ward of the state or in the physical or legal custody of the Department of Social Services or the Department of Youth Services? Can or should these children be participants in research? The selection of the appropriate population for study and the scientific generalizability and ethical justification for the use of vulnerable populations will require further analysis.

Compensation

Research subjects, particularly healthy adult volunteers, are often compensated for participation in research protocols through monetary payment. Such remuneration is not to be considered a benefit, but rather is compensation for time, inconvenience and, perhaps, for risk. When compensation becomes inducement or even coercion, the subject's participation will vary depending on the population and the volunteer. Particularly in the nontherapeutic realm, healthy adult subjects often volunteer out of a sense of altruism or societal obligation. While this activity may be laudatory, it is clearly superogatory and probably not a moral duty of all members of society. Can, should, or do children have similar obligations? Should children who volunteer receive compensation? If a study were very risky with no benefit, it is unlikely that children would be allowed to volunteer. However, insofar as a study involves minimal risk and no benefit, should not a child be compensated for time and inconvenience in similar fashion as an adult volunteer? If it is appropriate to compensate children, who, where, and how should they be compensated? Should parents receive any compensation for time and inconvenience when their children participate in research? How much compensation is appropriate, and what constitutes coercion or inducement in the child or adolescent population? Should adolescents be given less money than a similar adult volunteer? The significance of monetary compensation to a poor adolescent might be quite different than to a wealthy adolescent volunteer. Should this disparity be treated any differently than in the adult population? Is there a greater obligation to compensate children from research-induced injury than for adults?

REGULATORY AND PROCEDURAL ISSUES

While specific federal regulations for the use of children in research were only promulgated in 1983, when and how should they be amended or repromulgated? The DHHS regulations only cover research funded by that agency. Recently there has been an attempt to compile uniform regulations covering all federally funded research, including such diverse funding sources as the military and the Food and Drug Administration.[23] If the ethics of research are indeed universal, it would seem that similar regulations should cover not only federally funded research, but all research, whether privately or publicly funded. Indeed, it would seem necessary for regulations concerning the ethics of research to conform not only to national standards for regulation, but international as well. Such standardized and universally applicable regulations would be especially warranted when dealing with an unconsenting, vulnerable population such as children. How can one justify the acceptability of the use of children as subjects in one country but not in another? Should third-world children be considered as having vulnerability even greater than that of incompetence? Unless the aim of the research is to study children who might be poor, malnourished, and susceptible to unique infectious diseases, then it would seem unjustified to study this group of children. Whereas the same basic standards should, at minimum, apply to all children of the world, what are the limits and specific regulatory innovations needed in specific child populations?

SUBPOPULATIONS OF VULNERABLE CHILDREN

Embryos and Fetuses

Specific regulations exist concerning research on fetuses, embryos, and pregnant women.[16] As the new reproductive technologies became increasingly complex, there is considerable concern over the appropriate limits and regulation of this research. The advent of in vitro fertilization, surrogate or embryo transfer, and frozen embryos has required consideration of the moral and legal status of the embryo. Concern about research on pregnant women and the fetuses *in utero* raises questions about the balance of risk or benefit between mother and fetus. Research in abortion and the proper use of fetal tissue for research and transplant has already surfaced. Who should control this research and at what federal, state, or local level remains to be elucidated.

Infants and Neonates

The development of perinatal medicine and neonatal intensive care would not have been possible without research. The boundary between innovative practice and controlled clinical research has often been blurred in those areas. What is the proper role of large-scale randomized controlled clinical trials in this population? Can parents who have recently delivered a seriously ill infant competently consent to enrollment of their infants in a research protocol? Should infants be used for nontherapeutic research protocols? Who will follow these newborns over the ensuing 10 to 20 years to address the outcome or potential complications of a research protocol?

The Child with Physical or Developmental Disabilities

Children with physical or developmental disabilities comprise a unique at-risk population. When is it appropriate to study this population and in what setting? If those children are wards of the state, who constitutes an adequate surrogate for consent? Does this population, in spite of a parent or adequate surrogate, require a specific subject advocate or monitor? When, if ever, can these children consent to participation in research, and how much weight should their consent hold? In what ways are children suffering from psychiatric disease similar to those with physical or mental handicaps?

Adolescents

Adolescents are becoming an increasingly studied population.[29] How and when can adolescents consent to be subjects in research? Can adolescent mothers or fathers consent to enrollment of their children in research protocols? How can investigators protect confidentiality and study adolescent suicide or other self-destructive behavior? How can one study sexual activity, contraception, and abortion within the family unit and ensure confidentiality or anonymity? Is it possible to study adolescent drug use or alcoholism when such activity might be illegal or cause significant morbidity or even mortality in that adolescent or in adolescents in general? Is it possible to obtain a writ of confidentiality to protect the research records on that illegal activity from subpoena and the subsequent use in criminal prosecution? What role should parents have in adolescent research protocols? How can one differentiate the mature 13 year old from the immature 15 year old?

Children with Specific Diseases

Many children form a vulnerable subpopulation because they suffer from a specific disease. Children with cancer may be dying. When should research be undertaken on a dying population? Who decides when, after having failed several chemotherapeutic protocols, no further research is to be undertaken? What role should the parent have in the decision to continue research protocols, and what veto power should the child have? When is it inappropriate to even approach a child or family with a research protocol with minimal or negligible probability of benefit and potential or significant risk? Who are suitable candidates for transplants or other innovative therapies? How much weight should be given to the assent of a child when the alternative may be death? How much does pain and suffering or fear influence children in their decision making? Children who suffer from emergent diseases such as seizures or cardiac arrest may be vulnerable. Can research be conducted in the pediatric emergency room? Who offers consent? Is it possible to obtain consent anticipating a future emergency, or is consent possible or even necessary after the research has started under emergency conditions? Children with the acquired immunodeficiency syndrome (AIDS) form yet another vulnerable group.[25] When and how should infants or children with AIDS be studied? Can a parent who may have transmitted the virus to the child adequately serve as a surrogate for consent? When and how should randomized trials be conducted? When can research be tested on children, and who should serve as the research subject—children infected, at risk, or normal controls?

CONCLUSION

The history of children has progressed through several phases over the past centuries. While progressing from regarding children as chattels of parents to paternalism to empowerment, society has grappled with the proper balance of protection and autonomy. In the area of patient care, medicine and society have similarly balanced the protection of the rights of patients with appropriate concern for the benefits and welfare of the patient. This need to promote individuality, while imposing constraint, has been particularly difficult with children. Children as a group should not be orphaned from the benefits of research and yet, as a vulnerable population, are clearly in need of added protection. Pediatricians as experts on children are in a particularly valuable position to help balance these interests. Pediatricians are in the forefront of knowledge about what, where, when, and how childhood research should be undertaken. Pediatricians are advocates for children in general as well as advocates for an individual patient.[27] If pediatricians continue to participate in the clinical, ethical, legal, and public policy debate on children as participants in medical research, both the children and society will be exceedingly well served.

ACKNOWLEDGMENT

We would like to thank Ms. Adrienne Dillon for secretarial and editorial assistance in the preparation of this article.

REFERENCES

1. Appelbaum PS, Roth LH: Competency to consent to research. Arch Gen Psychiatry 39:951–958, 1982
2. Beecher HR: Ethics and historical research. N Engl J Med 274:1354–1360, 1966
3. Bellotti v. Baid, 424 U.S. 952 (1976)
4. Bonner v. Moran 126 F 2d 121 (D.C. Cir. 1941)
5. Cal. Health and Safety Code 26668.4 (West 1978)
6. Carey v. Population Services International, 421 U.S. 678 (1975)
7. City of Akron v. Akron Center for Reproductive Health 462 U.S. 416 (1983)
8. 45 CFR part 46, subpart B (1981)
9. 45 CFR part 46, subpart D (1983)
10. 45 CFR 46.401–46.409 (1983)
11. 45 CFR § 46.404 (1983)
12. 45 CFR § 46.405 (1983)
13. 45 CFR § 46.406 (1983)
14. 45 CFR § 46.407 (1983)
15. 45 CFR § 46.116–117 (1981)
16. 45 CFR § 46.201 (1983)
17. Cone TE: History of American Pediatrics. Boston, Little, Brown & Co, 1979, p 100
18. Curran WJ: The Tuskegee syphilis study. N Engl J Med 289:730, 1973
19. Curran WJ: A problem of consent: Kidney transplantation in minors. NYU Law Rev 34:891, 1959
20. de Mause L (ed): The History of Childhood. New York, Harper & Row, 1974, pp 1–73
21. 30 Fed. Reg. 31,786 (1978)
22. 43 Fed. Reg. 18,914 (1974)
23. June 3, 1986 Proposed Model Federal Policy, Fed. Register 51 No. 106, pp 20204–20217
24. Grisso T, Viewling L: Minors consent to treatment: A developmental perspective. Professional Psychology 9:412–427, 1978
25. Grodin M, Kaminow P, Sassower R: Ethical issues in AIDS research. Quality Rev Bull 12(10):347–352, 1986
26. Grodin M, Zaharoff B, Kaminow P: The Boston City Hospital Institutional Review Board for the Protection of Human Subjects: A 12-year audit of the IRB. Quality Rev Bull 12(3):82–86, 1986
27. Grodin M, Sassower R: Whose patient is this anyway? IRB case study. IRB: Rev Human Subjects Res 9(2):6–7, 1987
28. Grodin M, Alpert J: Informed consent and pediatric care. In Melton G, Koocher G, Saks M (eds): Children's Competence to Consent. New York, Plenum Press, 1983, pp 93–110
29. Holder AR: Minor's rights to consent to medical care. JAMA 257(54):3450, 1987
30. Katz J: Experimentation with Human Beings. New York, Russell Sage Foundation, 1972, pp 9–65, 633, 1007, and 1010
31. Leikin SL: An ethical issue in biomedical research: The involvement of minors in informed and third party consent. Clin Res 31:34–40, 1983
32. Levine RJ: Ethics and Regulation of Clinical Research, Ed 2. Baltimore, Maryland, Urban and Schwarzenberg, 1986, pp 235–250
33. Levine RJ: Research involving children: The National Commission's report. Clin Res 26:61–66, 1978
34. Lowe CU, Alexander D, Mishkin B: Nontherapeutic research on children. An ethical dilemma. J Pediatr 84(4):468–473, 1974
35. Mass Gen Laws Ann. Ch. 112 Sec. 12J (West) (1976)
36. McCarthy CR: Regulatory aspects of the distinction between research and medical practice. Rev Human Subjects Res 6(3):7–8, 1984
37. McCormick R: Proxy consent in the experimentation situation. Perspec Biol Med 18:2–20, 1974
38. Meisel A: What would it mean to be competent enough to consent or to refuse participation in research: A legal overview. Paper presented at the National Institute of Mental Health Workshop on Empirical Research with Subjects of Uncertain Competence, Rockville, Maryland, 1981

39. Melton GB, Koocher GP, Sas MJ (eds): Children's Competence to Consent. New York, Plenum Press, 1983
40. Nathan v. Farinelli Eq. No. 74–87 (Mass., July 3, 1974)
41. National Commission for the Protection of Human Subjects of Biomedical and Behavioral Research, Report and Recommendations: Research Involving Children. Washington D.C., DHEW Publication No. (OS) 77–0004, 1977
42. National Commission for the Protection of Human Subjects of Biomedical and Behavioral Research. The Belmont Report: Ethical Principles and Guidelines for the Protection of Human Subjects of Research. DHEW Publication No. (OS) 78–0012, Appendix 1, DHEW Publication No. (OS) 78–0013, Appendix II. Washington, D.C., DHEW Publication No. (OS) 78–0014, 1978
43. National Research Act, Pub. No. 93–348 (1984)
44. N.Y. Public Health Law: 2444 (McKinney 1975)
45. Pearn J: A classification of clinical pediatric research with analysis of related ethical themes. J Med Ethics 13:26–30, 1987
46. Pollock F, Maitland FF: The History of English Law, Ed 2. Washington D.C., Lawyer's Literary Club, 1859, p 436
47. President's Commission for the Study of Ethical Problems in Medicine and Biomedical and Behavioral Research, IRB Guidebook. The Office for the Protection of Research Risk, National Institutes of Health, 1984
48. Ramsey P: The Patient as Person. New Haven, Yale University Press, 1970
49. Ramsey P: Children as research subjects: A reply. Hastings Center Rep 7:40–42, 1977
50. Roth LH, Meisel A, Lidz CW: Tests of competency to consent to treatment. Am J Psychiatry 132:279–289, 1977
51. Rozovsky FA: Minors as Research Subjects in Consent to Treatment: A Practical Guide. Boston, Little, Brown & Co, 1984, pp 530–544
52. S.D. Codified Laws Ann: 27A-12–20, 1975
53. Trials of War Criminals Before the Nuremberg Military Tribunes: United States v. Karl Brandt, Vol 2. Washington, D.C., U.S. Government Printing Office, 1979, p 181
54. Va. Code: 37.1–235, 1979
55. Weithorn LA: Children's capacities to decide about participation in research. IRB, Rev. Human Subjects 5(2):1–5, 1983
56. Weithorn LA, Cambell SB: The competency of children and adolescents to make informed decisions. Child Develop 53:1589–1598, 1982
57. Weithorn LA: Developmental factors and competence to make informed treatment decisions. In Melton GB: Legal Reforms Affecting Children. Binghamton, New York, Haworth Press, 1982
58. World Medical Association: Declaration of Helsinki, 1964. In Beecher H (ed): Research and the Individual: Human Studies. Boston, Little, Brown & Company, 1970
59. Wyo Stat: 9–6–672, 1981

Children's 3
Boston City Hospital
818 Harrison Avenue
Boston, Massachusetts 02118

0031–3955/88 $0.00 + .20

Drug Use in Pregnancy: Parameters of Risk

*Ira J. Chasnoff, MD**

Although problems of substance abuse in pregnancy have received increasing attention in the medical literature since the early 1970s, there has recently been a very rapid increase in the number of articles published related to this field. The reasons for this new interest are easily understood when current statistics from the National Institute on Drug Abuse are reviewed.[14] Although patterns of abuse of alcohol, marijuana, heroin, and other substances by women of childbearing age have changed very little over the last 10 years, the incidence of cocaine use in this special population has been rising rapidly, a reflection of cocaine's increasing popularity among the general population of the United States.

Additionally, our concept of teratology has changed in that we now recognize that, although most drugs of use and abuse do not produce congenital malformations, there are definite behavioral and neurologic effects that place the neonate, infant, and child at risk for developmental abnormality.

PATTERNS OF DRUG USE

Early studies evaluating drug use by women during pregnancy revealed that around 50 to 60 per cent of women used some analgesics during pregnancy, and sedative drug use by pregnant women ranged around 25 per cent.[24] Most of the women involved in studies such as these were women who were receiving prenatal care and were obtaining many of the medications by prescription from their physicians. Use of illicit drugs rarely was considered. During a 6-month period in 1982, screening of all women enrolling at Prentice Women's Hospital and Maternity Center for routine prenatal care revealed that 3 per cent of these women had sedative–hypnotics in their urine at the time of admission to the general maternity clinic.[12] This study was performed prior to cocaine's becoming society's drug of choice. Currently, with an estimated 20 million Americans having tried cocaine at least once, and 5 million using it on a regular basis,[17] the number of pregnant

---

*Associate Professor of Pediatrics and Psychiatry, Northwestern University Medical School; Director, Perinatal Center for Chemical Dependence, Northwestern Memorial Hospital, Chicago, Illinois

cocaine users in the United States has risen rapidly, but no figures as to the actual prevalence are available.

In New York City, it was estimated that 50 per cent of all child abuse and neglect cases involved drug abuse, and if alcohol was included, substance abuse was involved in 64 per cent of child abuse cases.[28] In a survey conducted by the Child Abuse Prevention Program, Department of Health Services in Los Angeles, California, of a total of 5973 cases of child abuse reported in 1985, 538 cases (9 per cent) involved neonatal withdrawal due to maternal drug use in pregnancy. In the first 6 months of 1986, 403 of 4299 cases (9.4 per cent) of child abuse were reported due to maternal addiction during pregnancy. The patterns of drug use in this population showed a shift toward a higher frequency of cocaine use among the reported cases in the first 6 months of 1986 as compared to 1985.

In Illinois in fiscal year 1987, more than 91,000 infants and children were reported to the state child abuse hotline, a 50 per cent increase over fiscal year 1986. Of those reports, 530 were due to the finding of a drug of abuse in a neonate's urine. This represented a 77 per cent increase in such reports over a 1-year span. Even so, most cases of maternal substance abuse in pregnancy go undetected and unreported.

A study conducted in 1986 by the Illinois Department of Children and Family Services evaluated a random sample of 385 children who had become wards of the state owing to abuse or neglect and who subsequently had been placed in foster care. It was found that about half of these children came from parents or caretakers who were known or suspected substance abusers. These parents were often reluctant to accept help: 55 per cent rejected social services when offered and 68 per cent rejected substance abuse services. In addition, and perhaps most striking, 11 per cent of these children in foster care had had serious medical problems (e.g., abstinence, seizures, respiratory distress) at birth related to *in utero* exposure to substances of abuse.

ASSOCIATED RISK FACTORS

With the current shift to cocaine as one of the most common primary drugs of abuse, polydrug abuse also has become more common, with most cocaine users abusing marijuana and/or alcohol or cigarettes in addition. Thus, evaluation of risk factors for the pregnant substance abuser and her newborn must take into consideration the effects of these secondary drugs of abuse. Another mediating factor in the fetus' response to drug exposure is related to the mother's ability to metabolize and tolerate the illicit drug. This ability is determined through a variety of genetic and physiologic factors.

Numerous reviews of drug use during pregnancy show that most drugs taken by the mother during pregnancy freely cross the placenta. Drugs that act on the central nervous system are usually lipophilic and are of relatively low molecular weight, characteristics that facilitate the crossing of the substance from maternal to fetal circulation. For many sedative–hypnotic medications, there is rapid equilibration of unbound drug between the maternal and fetal circulation. Although the exact distribution of drug between maternal and fetal circulation is difficult to determine, drugs with high abuse potential (e.g., opiates, cocaine, sedative–hypnotics, alcohol, and stimulants) are found in the fetus if the mother is using or abusing these drugs.[15, 19, 20, 29]

Some drugs that accumulate in the fetus can be metabolized by the fetal liver and the placenta. The metabolites are primarily water soluble, which hinders their passage back across the placenta to the maternal circulation, where it can be excreted. Since the fetal liver is not fully developed, it is frequently difficult to anticipate the exact fate of a specific drug in the fetus. Most drugs that have been studied have a longer half-life in the fetus than in the adult.[29] This is also true in the neonate since the enzymes involved in the metabolic process of glucuronidation and oxidation are not fully developed in the fetus. In addition, the immature renal function of the newborn may delay the excretion of drugs that have been metabolized to an excretable form.

Cocaine primarily is metabolized in adults through the cholinesterase system into benzoylecgonine, with a small amount of the parent compound being broken down into norcocaine.[12] Preliminary unpublished studies at our program at Northwestern demonstrate that the more common pathway in the fetus and neonate appears to be the metabolism of cocaine into norcocaine rather than benzoylecgonine. This is most likely due to the relative deficiency or immaturity of the cholinesterase system in the fetus and neonate. Both of these primary metabolites persist in the neonate for up to 4 days after last exposure. This is significant clinically since norcocaine is a highly active metabolite and, when present, may have a strong effect on neonatal neurobehavioral status.

Multiple other factors in the environment of the pregnant substance-abusing woman, including poor nutrition, lack of prenatal care, maternal psychopathology, and the drug-seeking life-style, affect the ultimate outcome of the passively exposed infant and must be considered in the interpretation of clinical and research information.

NEONATAL OUTCOME

The fact that drugs cross the placenta and reach the fetus creates potential problems of fetal development. These problems can be manifested as congenital abnormalities, fetal growth retardation, neonatal growth retardation, and neurobehavioral abnormalities. In addition, one of the important effects of maternal drug use during pregnancy, especially use of drugs with high potential for abuse, is that dependence develops in the fetus as well as the mother. Thus, the opiate-exposed fetus will experience withdrawal when the mother is withdrawn from her drug or at term when the maternal drug use no longer provides the newborn with drugs.

Symptoms of neonatal withdrawal are often present at birth but may not reach a peak until 3 to 4 days of life or as late as 10 to 14 days after birth. The most common features of the neonatal abstinence syndrome mimic aspects of an adult withdrawing from narcotics.[16] Most significant for the neonate are the high-pitched cry, sweating, tremulousness, excoriation of the extremities, and gastrointestinal upset. Withdrawal from narcotics persists in a subacute form for 4 to 6 months after birth,[7] with a peak in symptoms at around 6 weeks of age. Abstinence symptoms in the neonate exposed to nonnarcotic drugs *in utero* have been described for phenobarbital,[3] diazepam,[1] marijuana,[18] and alcohol.[30] Although withdrawal from these substances does not appear to result in as severe a syndrome of abstinence as withdrawal from narcotics, the newborn does exhibit the irritability and restlessness, poor feeding, crying, and impaired neurobehavioral abilities that are characteristic of the neonatal abstinence syndrome.[8]

NARCOTICS

Early studies of infants delivered to heroin-using mothers showed that these infants had a higher rate of perinatal morbidity and mortality than infants in the general population. Common problems associated with heroin use during pregnancy were first trimester spontaneous abortions, premature delivery, neonatal meconium aspiration syndrome, maternal–neonatal infections (including venereal diseases), and severe neonatal withdrawal.[16, 23] Attempts to improve the outcome of these pregnancies were anchored in methadone maintenance programs in which pregnant women attended prenatal obstetric clinics and received daily methadone to replace their use of street heroin. The initial methadone maintenance programs were successful in that the more consistent medical and nutritional care provided for these women resulted in improved pregnancy outcome. However, the high doses of methadone (80–120 mg per day) produced a severe and prolonged period of abstinence for the newborn. These complications are avoided when the pregnant woman is placed on low-dose methadone maintenance, especially if the third trimester dose of methadone is less than 20 mg per day.[8]

Infants delivered to mothers who use narcotics (heroin, methadone, "Ts and blues") have a significantly lower birth weight and length and a smaller head circumference than do non–drug-exposed infants.[6] The inhibitory effects of narcotics on fetal growth, as well as the additional effects of inadequate maternal caloric and protein intake, can produce this fetal growth failure. Infants exposed to narcotics *in utero* exhibit significant impairment in their interactive abilities, making them difficult to engage and to console. Narcotic-exposed infants are more tremulous and irritable than drug-free infants, demonstrating significant and unpredictable fluctuations in their behavioral responses.[6, 8] These factors not only make these infants very difficult to comfort but also interrupt the normal processes of maternal–infant attachment that are so important to the early relationship between infant and mother.

Infants born to mothers maintained on methadone throughout pregnancy continue to be significantly smaller in weight and length compared to drug-free infants through 6 to 9 months of age but usually catch up in weight and length by 12 months of age.[6] This early stunting during a prolonged period of subacute withdrawal could be due to the direct effect of methadone on the hypothalamic–hypophyseal axis of the newborn. Following a period of slow excretion of the methadone, the plasma and tissue drug levels fall, the endocrinologic effects of the drug subside, and neonatal growth recovers. The one exception is that of head circumference measurement for the opiate-exposed infant; it does not exhibit catch-up growth. The persistent reduction in head size in these infants is of concern since small head size in young infants has been reported to be predictive of poor developmental outcome[26] and may be an indicator of the prolonged high-risk status of these infants.

Two-year developmental follow-up of narcotic-exposed infants shows that their development, measured on the Bayley Scales of Infant Development, is within the normal range.[6] Of concern, however, is the fact that the infants demonstrate a downward trend in developmental scores by 2 years of age, a phenomenon not uncommon in infants from low socioeconomic groups. This observation suggests that the infant's environment, with a lack of stimulation, has a more direct influence on 2-year development than does maternal drug use during pregnancy.

COCAINE

As in other substance-abusing populations, cocaine-addicted pregnant women have a high incidence of infectious disease complications, especially hepatitis and venereal disease. There is an increase in complications of labor and delivery in cocaine-using women so that precipitous delivery, abruptio placentae (usually occurring shortly after administration of cocaine), evidence of fetal monitor abnormalities, and fetal meconium staining are present in a significant number of pregnancies complicated by cocaine use.[19, 27] Gestational age tends to be slightly lower for cocaine-exposed infants, and neonatal birth weight, length, and head circumference smaller when compared to growth parameters for drug-free infants.[23, 31] Newborns who have been exposed to cocaine exhibit a high degree of irritability and tremulousness, with a deficiency in state control.[5, 9] The neurobehavioral changes for cocaine-exposed infants are in some areas more severe than changes noted for methadone-exposed infants.

Many of the abnormal characteristics seen in the cocaine-exposed newborn persist through at least 4 months of age.[33] When comparing motor development of cocaine-exposed infants to non–drug-exposed infants, some striking differences can be noted in muscle tone, primitive reflexes, and volitional movement patterns. Many cocaine-exposed infants feel stiff when their limbs are moved and on their backs often lie in excessively extended postures. Tremors are common, especially in their arms and hands, when they reach for objects. Generally, the cocaine-exposed infants have a more difficult time counteracting the effects of gravity and moving when supine.

Cocaine-exposed infants retain more primitive reflexes than non–drug-exposed infants. Commonly, an exaggerated positive support response is seen, characterized by stiff extension of the legs and weight bearing on the toes when held in a supported upright position. The persistence of primitive reflexes is of concern, since generally primitive reflexes are replaced by more mature movement patterns as development proceeds.

Volitional movement patterns are deficient in many cocaine-exposed infants. These infants are unable to round their buttocks off a supporting surface or kick reciprocally. The pelvic mobility needed for these movements is limited by the increased extensor muscle tone in the infant's trunk and lower extremities. By lifting their legs off the supporting surface, infants normally begin to explore their lower bodies both visually and with their hands. Accordingly, cocaine-exposed infants may miss a critical opportunity to develop body image. Well-developed body image is an important component for developing functional and efficient movement patterns within the environment.

A high rate of perinatal complications have been noted for cocaine-exposed neonates. Perinatal cerebral infarctions have occurred in infants whose mothers have used cocaine over the few days prior to delivery.[10] These perinatal cerebral infarctions are a severe example of the morbidity associated with intrauterine exposure to cocaine and are similar to intracerebral insults reported in adults who use cocaine. There is also evidence for genitourinary[11] and cardiac and central nervous system malformations[2] in infants delivered to cocaine-using mothers. Abnormalities of respiratory control, with an increase in infant apnea, have been noted in clinical studies.[4] Most published studies of cocaine's effect on pregnancy and infant outcome have focused on recognized substance-abusing populations, and little information regarding the effects of minimal cocaine use is available.

ALCOHOL

Multiple case reports and studies have confirmed the existence of the fetal alcohol syndrome.[22, 36] Unlike other forms of substance abuse, the fetal alcohol syndrome is a clinically observable entity, with specific parameters for its diagnosis. Nonetheless, there remain major areas of controversy surrounding the clinical management of the pregnant alcoholic woman and the precise assessment of the impact of alcohol use during pregnancy on the developing fetus and child.

The reported pattern of anomalies in offspring from alcoholic pregnancies is consistent in three particular parameters. These three parameters make up the primary presentation of the fetal alcohol syndrome (FAS): (1) prenatal growth deficiency in length and weight, (2) microcephaly, and (3) short palpebral fissures. Mild to moderate mental retardation is reported frequently, with average intelligence quotient (IQ) scores being around 68, although the range is quite wide. Delayed motor and language development is recognized in early infancy in most cases, and there is no improvement in developmental abilities as the child matures. Hyperactivity, hyperacusis, hypotonia, and tremulousness are commonly described in young FAS infants, and symptoms of withdrawal similar to those of narcotic abstinence in neonates have also been noted. Evaluation of infants born to alcoholic mothers has revealed that they have lower levels of arousal, poor habituation, and are more restless and irritable than drug-free infants.[25, 33]

Since the full FAS is seen in only some of the offspring of chronic alcoholic women, it is reasonable to suspect that a less severe outcome than the full syndrome may arise in other children of overtly alcoholic women and in some infants of moderate drinking women as well. In recent years, it has been recognized that some infants of frankly alcoholic mothers escape the stigmata of FAS, whereas others have only a few of the characteristics. Those infants with only partial expression are thought to display fetal alcohol effects (FAE).[13] A simple alcohol dose—response relationship is thus not the answer to the complex issues surrounding the etiology of the FAS. Recent interest focuses on the prevention of FAS or FAE in women who stop using alcohol after the first trimester of pregnancy. Such findings would speak to prevention through early pregnancy intervention.

SECONDARY DRUG USE

The association between drug or alcohol use and cigarette smoking has been repeatedly observed,[35] and the effects of cigarettes on the developing fetus must be considered in any infant being evaluated for intrauterine exposure to drugs of abuse. Smoking women have infants with significantly lower birth weight than nonsmoking women; however, no increase in neonatal mortality rate or congenital anomalies has been observed among these infants. Of interest among the many studies relating smoking and low birth weight is that none took into account that smoking itself is associated with heavier alcohol use; this could have contributed a significant portion of the variance in birth weight. Heavy use of additional substances, such as caffeine, further complicates the evaluation of drug effects on the fetus.

AIDS

In a study performed in 1982, prior to the widespread presence of acquired immunodeficiency syndrome (AIDS) in the Chicago area, infants born to intravenous drug-using mothers were found to have a more frequent rate of infections than infants of oral drug-abusing mothers or drug-free infants.[32] The number of episodes of illness was also increased among infants of intravenous-drug–addicted mothers. Some of the illnesses were the clinical manifestations resulting from exposure to specific organisms (Chlamydia pneumonia, thrush, monilia diaper rash) whereas others were caused by a spectrum of microorganisms (bronchiolitis, otitis media). Of note is the finding that the thrush in these patients was qualitatively different than the thrush usually observed in non–drug-exposed infants. It was more severe and persisted for a longer time than usual despite the use of conventional antifungal therapy. These observations suggested a possible immune defect related to intravenous opiate use. None of these infants developed severe opportunistic infections or acquired immunodeficiency syndrome (AIDS).

Recently, exposure to the human immunodeficiency virus (HIV) has become an increasingly important aspect of assessment and management of the newborn delivered to a drug-using mother. Women with a history of intravenous drug use, prostitution, or sexual intercourse with a bisexual or intravenous drug–using man should be considered at high risk for exposure. Currently, 25 per cent of the intravenous drug–using women enrolled in our program are HIV positive. Almost all infants delivered to HIV antibody–positive women will themselves be seropositive at birth, given the ease with which IgG antibodies cross the placenta. The true HIV status of an infant usually cannot be determined until 12 to 15 months of age, by which time all passively acquired maternal antibody should be absent from the infant's serum. Aside from the dysmorphologic and life-threatening infectious complications that have been reported to occur in infants with the acquired immune deficiency syndrome, these infants also exhibit poor growth and developmental delay.[21] Early studies in our program have also demonstrated impairment of mother–infant attachment and interaction, a not surprising consequence of a mother's knowing her child has a potentially fatal illness.

IMPLICATIONS FOR RISK

Little reliable information regarding long-term outcome of infants passively exposed to drugs of abuse is available. To best evaluate these children at school age, environmental factors must be taken into account. These environmental factors are not only socioeconomic but should encompass aspects of the maternal–infant relationship, including maternal psychopathology and personality. One study that did attempt to control for the caretaking environment of substance-exposed children compared these infants to those whose families began to use drugs after the birth of the children.[37] No differences were found between the *in utero*–exposed children and the children exposed to the social environment of drug-using caretakers. Further studies are needed before final conclusions can be drawn as to the long-term effects of *in utero* drug exposure on infant and child development.

The problems involved in evaluating the effects of maternal exposure to substances of abuse on the developing fetus and infant are multiple, not the least of which are the difficulties involved in following these infants over a long period. The chaotic and transient nature of the drug-seeking environment impairs the intensive followup and early intervention processes necessary to ensure maximum development by each infant. In addition, most women from substance-abusing backgrounds lack a proper model for parenting. These factors, compounded by the early neurobehavioral deficits of the drug-exposed newborns, earmark these infants to be at high risk for continuing developmental and later school problems.

A key problem in the field of substance abuse in pregnancy is a public and professional lack of knowledge of the subject. Few prospective parents recognize that their life-style, especially drug use and abuse, has a powerful impact on the outcome of their newborn infant. Information about the hazards of substance abuse during pregnancy must be presented to the public in a straightforward, nonjudgmental manner. In this way, information regarding the effects of any licit or illicit drug use during pregnancy can become part of the public consciousness.

It is easy to overlook the newborn's passive exposure to drugs of abuse, since the assessment of maternal chemical dependence tends to be insufficient in most instances. Currently, pediatricians often must rely on scanty information from the prenatal period when assessing a newborn displaying withdrawal or the neurotoxic effects of drug exposure. A study of alcoholism by Sokol et al. found that "clinicians are continuing to miss the diagnosis in at least three of every four alcohol-abusing patients. It is unlikely that there is any other obstetric diagnosis that is missed as often."[34] Today, few patients limit their abuse to alcohol and, with the current phenomenon of polydrug abuse, chemical dependence in the pregnant woman with the concomitant effects in the newborn most assuredly is one of the most frequently missed diagnoses in the perinatal period. When an untoward event in the perinatal period does occur, whether it be a perinatal cerebral infarction, unexpected premature delivery, or an unexplained accident of pregnancy such as abruptio placentae, maternal substance abuse must be placed in the differential diagnosis. The irritable newborn or one with unusual complications should be assessed with a full historical evaluation for substance exposure and, when indicated, a full toxicologic urine screen. Pediatricians have come to realize that intrauterine drug exposure has become a major cause of perinatal morbidity and mortality, and an area that can no longer be overlooked.[5]

The developmental risks imposed by the maternal use of substances of abuse are, perhaps more than many other risk factors, preventable. The first step in prevention and intervention, however, relies on the establishment in the medical and public sectors of a perception of risk. This perception should be based on education of the public as to the clear effects maternal substance abuse have on pregnancy and neonatal outcome. Secondly, the medical and psychological communities must begin to better understand risk-taking behavior and the personality and motivational factors that engender and enhance this behavior. We must delineate the measurable outcomes that best express the damage of maternal substance abuse to the child, then use the most effective means of increasing the public's recognition of this risk and influencing the individual's will to act to reduce relevant risk-taking behavior.

SUMMARY

With the increasing incidence of substance abuse in the United States, there has been a concomitant increase in the number of women becoming pregnant while using substances of abuse. The infant delivered to a drug-addicted woman is at risk for problems of growth and development as well as neonatal abstinence, and is also at increased risk of infections and exposure to HIV. The long-term outcome of these infants is influenced not only by the mother's use of illicit substances but by the frequent additional use of licit substances, such as cigarettes and alcohol. The drug-seeking environment in which many of these children are raised also may impair maximal development for these infants. In addition, many women from substance-abusing backgrounds lack a proper model for parenting and require intervention by the health care community to guide them in their roles as parents. Thus, multiple factors in the lives of these children, compounded by the early neurobehavioral deficits of drug-exposed newborns, earmark these infants to be at high risk for continuing developmental and later school problems.

REFERENCES

1. Backes CR, Cordero L: Withdrawal symptoms in the neonate from presumptive intrauterine exposure to diazepam: Report of case. JAMA 79:584, 1980

2. Bingol N, Fuchs M, Diaz V et al: Teratogenicity of cocaine in humans. J Pediatr 110:93, 1987

3. Blumenthal I, Lindsay S: Neonatal barbiturate withdrawal. Postgrad Med J 53:157, 1977

4. Chasnoff IJ: Perinatal addiction: Consequences of intrauterine exposure to opiate and nonopiate drugs. In Chasnoff IJ (ed): Drug Use in Pregnancy: Mother and Child. Boston, MTP Press Limited, 1986, p 60

5. Chasnoff IJ, Burns KA, Burns WJ: Cocaine use in pregnancy: Perinatal morbidity and mortality. Neurobehav Toxicol Teratol 9:291, 1987

6. Chasnoff IJ, Burns KA, Burns WJ et al: Prenatal drug exposure: Effects on neonatal and infant growth and development. Neurobehav Toxicol Teratol 8:357, 1986

7. Chasnoff IJ, Burns WJ: The Moro reaction: A scoring system for neonatal narcotic withdrawal. Dev Med Child Neurol 26:484, 1984

8. Chasnoff IJ, Burns WJ, Hatcher R: Polydrug- and methadone-addicted newborns: A continuum of impairment? Pediatrics 70:210, 1982

9. Chasnoff IJ, Burns WJ, Schnoll SH et al: Cocaine use in pregnancy. N Engl J Med 313:666, 1985

10. Chasnoff IJ, Bussey M, Savich R et al: Perinatal cerebral infarction and maternal cocaine use. J Pediatr 108:456, 1986

11. Chasnoff IJ, Chisum GM, Kaplan WE: Maternal cocaine use and genitourinary tract malformations. Teratology 37:201, 1988

12. Chasnoff IJ, Schnoll SH, Burns WJ et al: Maternal substance abuse during pregnancy: Effects on infant development. Neurobehav Toxicol Teratol 6:277, 1984

13. Clarren SK, Smith DW: The fetal alcohol syndrome. N Engl J Med 298:1063, 1978

14. Clayton RR: In a blizzard or just being snowed. In Kozel NJ, Adams EH (eds): Cocaine Use in Pregnancy: Epidemiologic and Clinical Perspective, NIDA Research Monograph 61. Rockville, Maryland, US Department of Health and Human Services, 1985, p 8

15. Finnegan L: Clinical effects of pharmacologic agents on pregnancy, the fetus and the neonate. Ann NY Acad Sci 281:74, 1976

16. Finnegan LP, Connaughton JF, Kron RE et al: Neonatal abstinence syndrome: Assessment and management. In Harbison RD (ed): Perinatal Addiction. New York, Spectrum Publications, 1975, p 141

17. Fishburne PM: National survey on drug abuse: Main findings: 1979 (DHHS Publication No ADM80–976). Rockville, Maryland, National Institute on Drug Abuse, 1980

18. Fried PA: Marijuana and human pregnancy. In Chasnoff IJ (ed): Drug Use in Pregnancy: Mother and Child. Boston, MTP Press, 1986, p 70

19. Goldstein A, Aronow L, Kalman SM: Principles of Drug Action: The Basis of Pharmacology. New York, John Wiley & Sons, 1974, p 198

20. Hollingsworth M: Drugs and pregnancy. Clin Obstet Gynecol 4:503, 1977

21. Iosub S, Bamji M, Stone RK et al: More on human immunodeficiency virus embryopathy. Pediatrics 80:512, 1987

22. Jones KL, Smith DW, Ulleland CW et al: Pattern of malformation in offspring of alcoholic mothers. Lancet 1:1267, 1973

23. Kandall SR: Late complications in passively addicted infants. In Rementeria JO (ed): Drug Abuse in Pregnancy and the Neonate. St. Louis, CV Mosby Co, 1977, p 116

24. Kaul AF, Harsfield JC, Osathanondh R et al: A retrospective analysis of analgesics and sedative-hypnotics in hospitalized obstetrical and gynecological patients. Drug Intell Clin Pharmacol 12:95, 1978

25. Landesman-Dwyer S, Keller RS, Streissguth AP: Naturalistic observations of newborns: Effect of maternal alcohol consumption. Alc Clin Exp Res 2:171, 1978

26. Lipper E, Lee K, Gartner LM et al: Determinants of neurobehavioral outcome in low birth weight infants. Pediatrics 67:502, 1981

27. MacGregor SN, Keith LG, Chasnoff IJ et al: Cocaine use during pregnancy: Adverse perinatal outcome. Am J Obstet Gynecol 157:686, 1987

28. Marriott M: Child abuse cases swamping New York City's family court. NY Times, 11/15/87, p 17

29. Mirkin BL: Maternal and fetal distribution of drugs in pregnancy. Clin Pharmacol Ther 14:643, 1973

30. Nichols MM: Acute alcohol withdrawal syndrome in a newborn. Am J Dis Child 113:714, 1967

31. Oro AS, Dixon SD: Perinatal cocaine and methamphetamine exposure: Maternal and neonatal correlates. J Pediatr 111:571, 1987
32. Rich KC: Immunologic function and AIDS in drug-exposed infants. In Chasnoff IJ (ed): Drug Use in Pregnancy: Mother and Child. Boston, MTP Press Limited, 1986, p 136
33. Schneider JW, Chasnoff IJ: Cocaine abuse during pregnancy: Its effects on infant motor development—a clinical perspective. Top Acute Care Trauma Rehab 2:59, 1987
34. Sokol RJ, Miller SI, Martier S: Preventing Fetal Alcohol Effects: A Practical Guide for the Ob/Gyn Physicians and Nurses. Rockville, Maryland, National Institute on Alcohol Abuse and Alcoholism, 1981
35. Streissguth AP, Barr HM, Martin DC: The effects of maternal alcohol, nicotine and caffeine use. Alcohol Clin Exp Res 4:152, 1980
36. Streissguth AP, Landesman-Dwyer S, Martin JC et al: Teratogenic effects of alcohol in humans and laboratory animals. Science 209:353, 1980
37. Wilson GW, McCreary K, Kean J et al: The development of preschool children of heroin-addicted mothers: A controlled study. Pediatrics 63:135, 1979

215 East Chicago Avenue, Suite 501
Chicago, Illinois 60611

Homeless Children—A Challenge for Pediatricians

Garth Alperstein, MB, ChB, MPH,* and Ellis Arnstein, MD†

During the past decade, homelessness has once again become a major problem in the United States. Figures as high as 3 million have been cited for the number of homeless people, nationwide.[6, 20] In New York State it is estimated that there are 50,000 homeless, of whom 85 per cent are in New York City.[21] Recent attention to this problem has revealed a changing homeless population composition; what once consisted largely of older males, now consists of increasing numbers of young men, women, and children. The fastest-growing segment of the homeless are families, most commonly single mothers with two or three children, who now comprise 40 to 45 per cent of the homeless population in New York City.[9] This article will attempt to address the health status of homeless children, delineate contributing factors, and make recommendations for methods of further identifying and remediating these problems.

Nationwide, members of families with children now represent an estimated 28 per cent of the homeless population. Denver, Detroit, Louisville, and St. Paul all reported increases in two-parent homeless families in 1985, primarily due to unemployment and underemployment. In Philadelphia, Trenton, and Yonkers, almost 50 per cent of homeless people are members of families with children. In Charleston, West Virginia, the percentage of homeless people who are women and children rose in the past year, from between 5 to 10 per cent to between 30 and 50 per cent.[3]

Another group of homeless children is composed of "runaway" and "throwaway" adolescents. Nationwide, it has been estimated that this group numbers between 250,000 and 500,000.[34] In New York City alone it is estimated that there are at least 10,000 runaway adolescents living predominantly in the streets. Over 90 per cent are from minority ethnic origin, and usually from troubled families, including mentally and physically abusive parents.[46] Runaway and throwaway adolescents are not a problem exclusive to New York City but are becoming more prevalent in most major cities across the country.

---

*Medical Consultant, Bureau for Families with Special Needs, New York City Department of Health; Attending Pediatrician, St. Luke's-Roosevelt Hospital Center, New York; Assistant Clinical Professor of Pediatrics, College of Physicians and Surgeons, Columbia University, New York, New York

†Director, Bureau for Families with Special Needs, New York City Department of Health, New York, New York

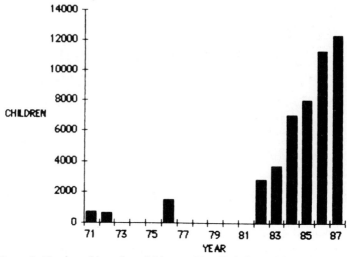

Figure 1. Number of homeless children in New York City, 1971–1987. Data from refs. 2, 27,and 28. (Numbers for years not included are not available.)

HISTORY

The problem of homelessness in New York City only began to attract public attention as a major issue in the early 1980s. Through the 1960s and 1970s the number of homeless families in New York City remained more or less stable at 600 and the number of children similarly stable at 1400.[2] During the early 1980s the numbers began to increase, and by the spring of 1984 there were 7000 homeless children.[28] By July 1987 there were 5060 homeless families with 12,303 children in New York City (Fig. 1).[29] It is noteworthy that these figures reflect only those children in the shelter system. What is not known is how many children are living in the streets, in abandoned buildings, or on the subways.

In New York City homeless families and children are predominantly sheltered in "welfare hotels," and, to a lesser degree, family centers and congregate shelters. There are over 60 welfare hotels scattered throughout the five boroughs, but with a large concentration in midtown Manhattan.

Welfare hotels are those hotels whose owners agree to accept public assistance (AFDC) payments issued to the clients by the city's welfare agency. Some of the largest of these hotels house only homeless families. Some hotels have no restrictions on length of stay, but others restrict families to less than 28 days to avoid their acquiring tenants' rights. As a result, some families move frequently within the system. Although the average length of stay for homeless families in the welfare hotels is 14 months,[29] this figure is artificially low because of the frequent movement. Some families stay as long as 5 years.

The root causes of homelessness are complex, and an in-depth analysis of them is beyond the scope of this article. Although there has been only minimal research to date on the variables contributing to homelessness, it is generally accepted that prominant factors include poverty, lack of affordable housing, gentrification of neighborhoods, deinstitutionalization of mental patients, and domestic violence. In many cities, increased unemployment (particularly affecting specific industries and specific working populations) is also a major contributing factor to homelessness.

Nationally, the worsening plight of the poor can be demonstrated by data from the U.S. Bureau of the Census. During the 1960s, the bottom 60 per cent of the

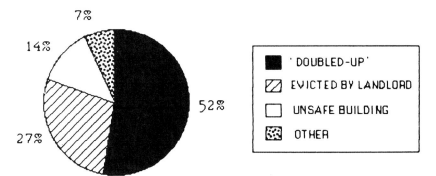

7%

14%

27%

52%

■ 'DOUBLED-UP'

▨ EVICTED BY LANDLORD

☐ UNSAFE BUILDING

▨ OTHER

Figure 2. Precipitating causes of family homelessness—New York City, 1986. (From Carraccio CL, McCormick MC, Weller SC: J Pediatr 112:982–987, 1987; with permission.)

population shared 36 per cent of total income; in 1985, that share had decreased to 32.4 per cent, the lowest recorded. According to the Federal Reserve Board, the bottom 50 per cent of the population holds only 4.5 per cent of the total net worth. In contrast, the top 2 per cent of the population holds 28 per cent of the total net worth.[42] Furthermore, the number of children ages 5 to 17 living in families that have incomes below the poverty line increased from 7.9 million in 1980 to 8.6 million in 1985. Overall, the number of people living below the poverty line increased by 13 per cent from 1980 to 1985.[24]

Another indicator of poverty, namely hunger, also appears to be on the increase. Chronic hunger and undernutrition are on the rise as a result of cutbacks by the Reagan administration in preventive programs such as food stamps, school lunches, and the Women, Infants, and Children (WIC) program. The Physicians' Task Force on Hunger in America recently calculated that 20 million people are chronically undernourished, 60 per cent of whom are children.[10]

In New York City, eviction by a primary tenant (usually a relative), or being forced to leave a "doubled-up" situation is the primary cause of homelessness for 52 per cent of homeless families (Fig. 2).[12] City officials estimate that there are 35,000 families living doubled up in public housing with friends or relatives.[26] Given that the average family size is 3.7 people (mother and 2.7 children),[30] this estimate indicates that another 129,500 people, of whom approximately 94,500 are children, may be at risk for becoming homeless in New York City public housing alone. There is no way to assess the size of the "doubled-up" population in private housing. Although these figures may not be accurate, this is clearly not a temporary or minor problem. Other reasons for seeking shelter include eviction for nonpayment of rent, fire burnout, bad housing, domestic violence, and recent arrival in New York.[12] While the situation in New York may not be typical for cities throughout the country, many of the circumstances contributing to the situation here also exist in other cities, and it may be only a matter of time before many face similar problems.

HEALTH PROBLEMS

Very little is known and even less has been published on the health status of children who, in addition to being poor, are also homeless. Since many homeless children come from families of low socioeconomic status, one might expect that health problems of these children are similar to those of other poor children. From the few studies available, however, it appears that some of the health problems of homeless children are more severe than those of poor children with homes.

There is mounting evidence that homeless children in New York City are not obtaining adequate primary care. This is clearly reflected in the high rate of delayed immunization status of these children. In a hospital-based study of 265 children living in welfare hotels, 27 per cent were either unimmunized or were significantly delayed in their immunization schedule, as opposed to 8 per cent in a comparison group of poor but domiciled children.[4] In a similar, but more recent survey of 100 homeless children in New York City, it appears that the rate of immunization delay is even higher—48 per cent.[1] With the growing homeless population, this may present a major public health problem for the City of New York. For example, during a measles epidemic in New York City in 1987, the rate of serologically confirmed cases was 410 in 100,000, as compared with 24 in 100,000 for New York City as a whole.[16] The high rate of immunization delay seen in homeless children may be due to the stresses associated with homelessness and the total disruption of their lives. The difficulties of access to health care for the poor are exacerbated by their homelessness. Homeless families also have to deal with the difficulties of finding their way around unfamiliar neighborhoods to reach health providers. Minimal financial resources often make transportation problematic and well-child care may suffer. Furthermore, already overburdened by the frequent changes in abode, by the daily searches for affordable food (some hotels do not provide refrigerators, and none allow cooking in the rooms), and by the periodic attempts to find housing, parents are unlikely to be able to manage the health care system for anything but emergency care. Similarly, homeless adolescents are less likely to use nonemergent health care providers than are domiciled youth.

Further evidence for lack of preventive care in this population is suggested by the high rate of low birth weight babies born to mothers living in the welfare hotels in New York City when compared to the rate for the city's housed poor (18 vs 8.5 per cent). This in turn has played a major role in the high infant mortality rate of 24.9 per 1000 in this group of children.[13] This rate is nearly double that of the city as a whole, although only slightly worse than the city's health district with the highest infant mortality rate.

Acute minor illness in these children often goes untreated because the parents or youth are unwilling or unable to access health care, and seek attention only when more serious consequences ensue. This results in the potential for a number of avoidable hospitalizations. In the evaluation of emergency room records of homeless children and a poor domiciled group in New York City, the rate of admission to the hospital for the homeless children was one and a half times that of the comparison group (11.6 per 1000 vs 7.5 per 1000).[4] The survey did not delineate the reasons for admission, but it is well-established that poor children are more likely to become ill, more likely to suffer adverse consequences from illness, and more likely to die than other children.[15] In addition, poor children are 75 per cent more likely to be admitted to a hospital in a given year.[15] This makes the rate of admission to hospital for homeless children even more significant.

A large number of families entering the shelter system has been reported at some time or another to Special Services for Children, the local municipal child abuse and neglect agency. Additionally, the chaotic hotel/shelter environment, demands on parents for long trips for welfare checks, for daily food shopping, and other stress factors associated with homelessness put families at higher risk for substance abuse and child abuse and neglect. In an evaluation of emergency department records at a New York City hospital serving homeless children, a rate of child abuse and neglect of 8.8 reports per 1000 children was found in the homeless group, as compared to 2.3 reports per 1000 nonhomeless children of similar socioeconomic status living in the same health districts.[4] Because this was a hospital-based and not a population-based study, however, and represents only reports by pediatricians, these figures may not reflect the true incidence of this problem.

Illicit drug use related to child abuse and neglect has become a major problem among homeless families living in the hotels. In New York City, the primary drug of choice at present is "crack" (a cheap form of cocaine that can be smoked). It is the impression of the Public Health Nurses (PHNs) from the N.Y.C. Department of Health that the longer the families remain homeless, the greater the likelihood of drug abuse.

Frank malnutrition in the form of kwashiorkor or marasmus has not been cited in the literature as a problem. In 1983, the N.Y.C. Department of Health surveyed 2100 children under the age of 12 years temporarily housed in family shelters and hotels. Fewer than 5 per cent were below the fifth percentile for height/weight ratio. However, 9 per cent had hematocrits below the fifth percentile.[38] Similar findings were described in another survey of 265 children under the age of 5 years living in welfare hotels in New York City. There was no difference in height below the fifth percentile when compared to a similar group of poor children who were not homeless (7.7 vs 7.5 per cent) and a small difference in weight below the fifth percentile (8.7 vs 6.4 per cent).[4] Although there was also no difference between the same two groups in the prevalence of iron deficiency by FEP determination (14.7 vs 14.1 per cent),[4] it is significant that the prevalence of iron deficiency in a recently studied middle-class population of children was only 3 per cent (51 of 1683 children),[47] less than one fourth that seen in the study groups. It has been documented that iron deficiency, especially in the very young, can affect cognitive development[32] and behavior,[44] which contributes to further stress in this group of children. Although very little difference in nutritional status was found between the two groups in this study, height, weight, and iron status are only gross measures of nutritional status. Furthermore, the data did not reflect a trend over time. However, it is generally impossible to eat a balanced diet on a ±$4 to $5 per person per day (includes food stamps, W.I.C. supplementation checks for an average 3 year old, and the restaurant allowance provided by the City) provided to homeless families, especially without adequate cooking facilities. In a more recent study, Acker et al. did find a significant difference for height and weight percentile distributions between homeless and domiciled children, with decreased linear growth in the homeless children.[1] In the same study, the investigators also found a significant difference in elevated FEPs between the two groups (50 per cent—homeless children vs 25 per cent—domiciled children). A prospective study looking at growth parameters over time may well reveal the development of nutritional deficiencies and more severe growth retardation for children remaining in a state of homelessness for longer periods.

Although lead poisoning has been raised as a problem for children living in temporary shelter in New York City, one study found elevated blood lead levels to be present in only 3.8 per cent of the homeless children and 1.7 per cent of a comparison domiciled group.[4] None of the children required chelation therapy. Although the prevalence of elevated lead levels was twice as great in the homeless children as in the comparison group, the prevalence of 3.7 per cent is quite low when compared to the 18.6 per cent reported for black children of parents earning less than $6000 per year in the early 1980s. However, from the same study, the percentage of children with elevated lead levels of parents earning greater than $15,000 per year was only 0.7 per cent.[25] Proposed explanations for the steady decline in lead levels over time include the decreasing use of leaded gasoline, and, to a lesser extent, elimination of lead-based paint. Elevated lead levels have been correlated with deficits in psychological and classroom performance in children[27] and pose yet another potential problem for this already jeopardized group.

Poverty, disruption of family life, homelessness, and exposure to crime and substance abuse all are associated with inappropriate social interactions and emotional problems. In a survey of 61 families living in a welfare hotel in New York City, 66 per cent reported behavioral and emotional problems in their children that developed while in the hotel. The problems they cited most often were "acting out, wild behavior, more fighting, restlessness, moodiness and frustration."[40] In a study of homeless families in Boston, nearly 50 per cent of 151 homeless children were found to have significant developmental lags, anxiety, depression, or learning difficulties.[9] Based on impressions of the Public Health Nurses and Crisis Intervention Service (CIS) workers in the hotels and teachers in schools, the scale of emotional and behavioral problems in children living in temporary shelter may well exceed those suggested to date in the literature. This is cause for grave concern and needs to be studied prospectively to obtain accurate information that could be used to generate the necessary intervention and services.

Public Health Nurses in the welfare hotels of New York City and school teachers claim that many school-aged children are not attending school, and that many of those who do attend spend much of the day sleeping in class. This is predominantly due to the choatic existence in the hotels where it is often too noisy to sleep at night. A sample of 53 homeless families surveyed revealed that 50 per cent of the children had been kept back at least one grade in school.[7] This problem may have far reaching consequences, especially as a predictor of adequate socialization and employment.

The issue of chronic illness among the homeless presents a special set of problems. A national study by the Robert Wood Johnson Foundation and Pew Memorial Trust reports that chronic illness was twice as prevalent in homeless children as in a comparable domiciled group.[45] In an unpublished survey by the N.Y.C. Department of Health of 1900 children living in the welfare hotels, 17 per cent were found to have a chronic medical problem.[38] Children with chronic illnesses often require a multidisciplinary team of health workers to provide comprehensive care. Environmental instability makes utilization of all necessary disciplines even more difficult. For example, diabetics may not have refrigeration for their insulin, and the presence of their needles, syringes, and alcohol swabs may put them at risk for assault, given the high prevalence of substance abuse in the shelters and hotels and the need for needles on the part of abusers.

The main sources of income for homeless adolescents (runaways and throwaways), especially in larger cities, include illegal substances, pornography, and prostitution. In addition to resultant psychological problems, this subgroup is at high risk for sexually transmitted diseases and diseases transmitted by sharing intravenous needles (e.g., hepatitis B and AIDS). Homeless adolescents have also been shown to have a high incidence of malnutrition, physical and sexual abuse, infectious diseases (including pneumonia), and mental health problems, including a disturbingly high rate of suicide.[26a]

Due to overcrowding, inadequate toilet facilities, and lack of knowledge of good hygiene, homeless children are also at high risk for various contagious diseases such as enteric diseases, childhood exanthems, and possibly tuberculosis. Outbreaks of Shigella dysentery[41] and measles have occurred in temporary shelters in New York City.[16]

It is evident that more information is needed to elucidate the health status of homeless children. Well-designed longitudinal studies are required to ascertain the effect of homelessness on their health. These data are of utmost importance in planning services for this disadvantaged group of children.

HEALTH CARE SERVICES

Although homeless children obviously represent only one segment of the poor population, the difficulties they encounter with health and the health care system are similar to, if not worse than, the poor population at large. Thus, it is unclear why the recently published "Health Policy Agenda for the American People" in the Journal of the American Medical Association[19] concerns itself very little, if at all, with health services for the poor and not at all with the homeless. This omission is compounded by the dearth of research and health services for homeless children.

In keeping with the varied and disorganized structure of health care services in the United States, health care for the homeless is similarly diverse, fragmented, and (in some areas) nonexistent. Nevertheless, a variety of public, private, and combined efforts have been developed to address the health needs of the various subgroups of the homeless population, including children.

In a report by the United States Conference of Mayors, health care services specifically designated for the homeless were identified in 14 of the 29 cities surveyed: Chicago, Cleveland, Detroit, Kansas City, Los Angeles, Louisville, Nashville, New York City, St. Paul, Salt Lake City, San Antonio, San Francisco, Seattle, and Washington, D.C.[8] Ten of those cities have received grants from the Health Care for the Homeless Program. This program is an example of a national effort to render health services to the homeless. Funded by the Robert Wood Johnson Foundation and Pew Memorial Trust,[14] this program provides funds to citywide coalitions of public and private agencies of 18 large U.S. cities for delivery of health services to the homeless. Program designs vary from city to city. In Denver, for example, the homeless are provided with a stable clinic site and with a mobile outreach team. In San Antonio, services are provided at existing shelters, with medical back-up from the county hospital or community clinic. In New York City three comprehensive care providers at three different locations in the city provide outreach medical and mental health, as well as social work services, at soup kitchens or nonprofit shelters. Backup services are provided by the parent provider or local hospitals. This program serves primarily single young adults. Most health services in the major cities are provided by private, nonprofit organizations. However, most cities in the United States do not have a coordinated and comprehensive system providing health care for homeless families and children. Very few city governments have made a commitment to provide its homeless population with health services. New York City is an exception, as will be described below.

New York City's Human Resources Administration (HRA), which is responsible for the City's homeless, working with the Department of Health (DOH), and the Health and Hospitals Corporation (HHC), together have developed a health management system (Fig. 3). Families enter the temporary shelter system through an Income Maintenance Center (welfare office) or an Emergency Assistance Unit (EAU). At the EAU a primary screening by HHC medical providers evaluates all family members at personal risk (e.g., pregnancy, families with newborns, immune deficiency or other chronic illnesses, etc) or those posing a risk to others (mainly contagious illnesses), to avoid placement in an inappropriate setting. Once in the system, a more in-depth secondary screening at a shelter identifies any additional health needs including immunizations. HHC has placed midlevel health providers in all the family congregate shelters to deliver routine preventive care and to treat acute illnesses. Local hospitals or health centers serve as backups to the on-site providers.

The DOH, in response to the lack of health care services for families living in the welfare hotels, established the Homeless Health Initiative (HHI) in the spring of 1986. The HHI is comprised of three components, the family health program, the environmental health unit, and the technical support unit. The family health program has placed 25 public health nurses (PHNs) and 15 community service aids (CSAs) into the largest of the hotels for case finding, health assessment, education, assistance in obtaining essential services, facilitating access to health care, and followup. Because of the high incidence of low birth weight babies born to mothers

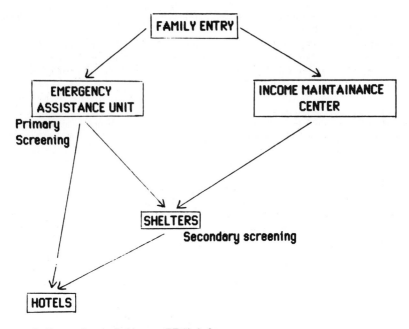

A. General population - 55 Hotels

B. Special Services - 1. 4 Hotels – focus on pregnant women
and newborns

2. 1 Hotel - contagious diseases

Figure 3. New York City temporary housing system for families.

living in the hotels and the high infant mortality rate, the PHNs pay special attention to newborns under 6 months and to pregnant women. HHC runs a special pilot project at a large hotel located near one of its hospitals to enroll pregnant women in prenatal care. A DOH counselor specially trained in substance abuse works with groups of mothers in the hotels with a high prevalence of substance abuse and assists with placement in treatment facilities. To facilitate access to health services, the DOH has initiated the development of linkages between nearby health institutions and/or clinics and all the hotels.

The environmental health unit was established to ensure protection of some homeless housed in congregate shelters from environmental hazards. Four public health sanitarians (PHSs) are responsible for inspecting the city shelters for families and single persons on a regular basis; they also conduct feasibility inspections of proposed HRA shelter sites. The PHSs also provide training and education for HRA staff.

The most recent addition to the HHI is the technical assistance unit. This unit will provide expertise in the allied fields of epidemiology and data analysis, including surveillance and monitoring of health problems of the homeless population.

In addition to municipal agencies in New York City, a variety of agencies—private, voluntary, and religious—provide both shelter and health services to the homeless. For example, a number of programs provide shelter for runaway adolescents. The American Red Cross also operates three hotels with on-site social and medical services. Several hospitals in midtown Manhattan, both voluntary and municipal (St. Vincent's, St. Luke's–Roosevelt, and Bellevue Hospitals) have developed special relationships with homeless families and children to provide them with comprehensive services. The Children's Aid Society, a private agency, provides on-site health services, a head-start program, and an after-school program at one of the larger welfare hotels, housing approximately 450 families with 1200 children. "The Door," a free clinic, provides health services and counseling on a confidential, drop-in basis to adolescents, regardless of residential status. The high quality of its work has caused "the word" of its availability and services to spread on the street. Covenant House, a residential facility that provides shelter to over 100 adolescents at a time, has on-site services and a mobile van that offers services to and does outreach for homeless youth on the streets.

LONG-TERM CONSEQUENCES

The outlook for children raised in the chaotic, severely impoverished circumstances of homelessness is rather bleak. A number of detrimental external factors faced by these children, although similar in nature to those of poor children in general, are more concentrated and intense in welfare hotels and shelters, and mitigating circumstances are correspondingly more scarce. While abuse of alcohol and other substances is not infrequent in poor communities, it rarely reaches the estimated frequency found in some welfare hotels. Some of the long-term effects of children growing up in welfare hotels may increase the rates of mental illness and substance abuse in the future. Another effect of living in these circumstances is stigmatization by the school and peers; indeed, children are sometimes labeled "hotel kids" and ostracized.

These factors predict perpetuation of the circumstances of poverty for most of these children as they grow into adulthood. In addition, one would anticipate the occurrence of an increased incidence of certain health conditions, as well as a worse-than-usual severity.[18, 22] Methods of obtaining financial support particularly for homeless adolescents include prostitution, which may contribute to higher rates of sexually transmitted diseases and the spread of AIDS.

The incidence of tuberculosis may serve as a marker of the intensity of poverty, and following a consistently downward trend for decades, has now risen over the past few years.[43] This rise has been most notable among young adult black men, the group that also predominates at New York City shelters for homeless adults. Although there is as yet no evidence to suggest spread among this population (as opposed to reactivation of latent infection by circumstances of extreme poverty or stress), this group does have contact with large numbers of both domiciled and homeless people, and this is the group that many of today's homeless children soon will enter.

Becoming homeless always involves loss, so that the occurrence of depression is to be expected. Hotel-based PHNs have noted a very high incidence of depression among temporarily housed family members (adults and children). The chaotic, relatively unsupervised environment of these hotels has contributed to a high incidence of behavior problems among children, as noted previously.

This stressful existence, along with increased illicit drug use, and mental illness and poor nutrition, can be expected to have serious short-term and long-term consequences on "physical" health as well. As noted by the data analysis of the nationwide Robert Wood Johnson–Pew Memorial Trust Health Care for the Homeless Project, the incidence of acute illness and the prevalence of chronic health problems in adults is higher than for the population in general. In addition to the expected high incidence of respiratory illness and otitis media in children, there is a high prevalence of chronic illness as well.[45] Although extensive prevalence studies do not yet exist for a variety of chronic childhood conditions among homeless children, one would expect a higher-than-average prevalence, based on income level, ethnic group, and chronic stress. In addition to a higher than expected prevalence, one also might anticipate more severe illness under these circumstances.[18, 22] Verification of these hypotheses awaits confirmation by appropriate study. Health locus of control (the degree to which individuals believe their health to be the result of self actions, actions of "powerful" others, or random events) normally tends to develop from external ("powerful" others) to internal (self) with increasing age.[33] However, the chaotic and often unpredictable life experiences that homeless children face would tend, along with chronic illness and poverty itself, to favor maintenance of an external health locus of control. An external locus is associated with less favorable outcome for a variety of chronic illnesses[11, 33, 35] and adds to the poor prognostic indicators for these youngsters.

The health care system has thus far played an inadequate role and has been too slow in meeting the health needs of homeless families and children. As evidenced by the data presented, some of the health problems are remediable by adequate high-quality preventive measures, which thus far have been lacking. Other, more complex problems, involving intervention by health and other systems (cf. hospital admission patterns, child abuse and neglect, low birth weight babies, infant mortality, and drug abuse) are also amenable to preventive programs. Although the complete solution to these problems is complex, health providers are in a strong position to effect some improvement in the health status of homeless children.

WHAT CAN BE DONE

It is clear that health status and economic status are intimately linked in a reciprocal manner. The remedies for poverty, of which homelessness represents an extreme, may require sweeping social changes. With the numbers of homeless people increasing rapidly in most major cities, city or other health institutions need to start to plan, in cooperation with state and Federal agencies, services for the homeless. An organized health care system, providing continuous care, health education, and early intervention programs, needs to be established. Not only could such a system improve the health and cognitive development of homeless children, but it may also assist their mothers by providing an opening wedge for leaving the cycle of poverty.

On the other hand, individual actions may contribute significantly toward improving the health status and the lives of homeless children. In concert with public health measures, practicing pediatricians can have a major impact in this area. The following suggestions, while based on New York City's specific problems, could easily be generalized to that of most urban, and even suburban areas:

1. Improve the health services specifically designed to address the varied needs of homeless people, such as screening procedures for immunization status. Because sheltered housing can, in some cases, itself create health risks, it is vitally important to be able to avoid the exposure of large groups of people to tuberculosis, measles, *Hemophilus influenzae* B disease, etc. Procedures designed to screen people for tuberculosis, or to bring immunization status up to date, must be applied uniformly and consistently if they are to be effective. In addition, there is a need for creative outreach programs for the traditionally hard-to-reach person, such as the mentally ill and runaway and "throwaway" adolescents.

2. Increase the availability of primary care resources, by means of providing health services on site at family shelters and by facilitating the referral of homeless people to existing primary care services that are located nearby. The success of "house calls" to sites where homeless persons gather has been documented.[36] By also promoting utilization of already-existing services, health workers may be able to foster skills that would be valuable to

homeless families after the crisis ends and housing is found. At either location, physicians and other health professionals in training could be used as health providers, giving them experience with a hard-to-reach but needy ambulatory population.[37]

3. Increase the availability of day care services for homeless families, even if used on a temporary basis. Day care would allow parents the opportunity to spend daytime hours looking for employment or housing (often difficult to do with children in tow), would provide developmentally appropriate activities for children, and would relieve the overcrowding which might predispose to abuse or neglect. Since day care standards in New York also contain specific health requirements, such as immunizations, use of these facilities would encourage the use of well-child care.

4. Improve communication with the school system, to help identify those homeless children with specific attendance or academic problems.[17] The presence of health workers at the welfare hotels, in frequent communication with the Board of Education staff, could act to encourage attendance or to resolve health issues that may be overdramatized and serve to isolate these children (e.g. head lice). Also, those children with chronic illness could be monitored more closely "at home" and at school, with an eye toward improvement.

5. Provide education, both general and public health in nature, to individual members and families who are homeless. The opportunity for parents to obtain high school diploma equivalents (while the children are in day care) would put them in a stronger position in the job market, as well as help them be better parents. And of obvious importance is the availability of public health information about AIDS, substance abuse, well-child and well-adult care, nutrition, dental health, etc.

6. Recognize substance abuse as an illness, and take appropriate measures to treat and prevent this condition. Although substance-abusers frequently commit crimes in support of their "habit," treatment slots, especially for pregnant women, are inadequate in number, and efforts to increase their number should be supported.

7. Promote research efforts designed to further the understanding of the health and psychosocial status of homeless children.

8. In recognition of the increasing problem of homeless families with children, the American Academy of Pediatrics (AAP), Chapter 2, District 3 in New York City formed a committee in May 1986 to address various health issues related to homeless children.[5] At this point in time, this is the only committee of its kind. As advocates for children, this participation by AAP members needs to be extended nationally.

9. Finally, pediatricians, through channels such as the AAP, should actively work to restore the Federal budgetary cuts in such programs as maternal–child health and preventive health services as recently advocated elsewhere.[31]

CONCLUSION

Attempting to improve the health status of a disenfranchised group in a society that frequently "blames the victim" is a difficult task.[39] This task is made even more difficult in a system that, as stated by Steven Jonas in "Homelessness and the American Way," "punishes the poor."[23] Health problems of homeless children are intimately bound to political, social, and economic conditions and to an inadequate health care system for the poor. Although some of these problems are beyond the scope of health providers, and some are probably insoluble while these children are homeless, the health status of homeless children can be improved by good preventive health care measures and by establishing a well coordinated health care system.

Unless there are major changes in the provision of health and other services to homeless children and families in the near future, the health status, especially the mental health, of homeless children will be seriously jeopardized.

REFERENCES

1. Acker P, Fierman A, Dreyer B: Health: An assessment of parameters of health-care and nutrition in homeless children (abstr). Am J Dis Child 141:388, 1987

2. A Comprehensive Plan for the Temporary and Permanent Needs of Homeless Families in New York City, January, 1984
3. A growing number of families face the crisis of homelessness. CDF The Monthly Newsletter of the Children's Defense Fund. 8(12):May 1987
4. Alperstein G, Rappaport C, Flanigan J: Health Problems of Homeless Children in New York City. Am J Public Health 78:1232–1233, 1988
5. American Academy of Pediatrics. New York Chapter 3, November, 1986
6. A Report to the Secretary on the Homeless and Emergency Shelters. Washington, D.C., U.S. Dept. of Housing and Urban Development, 1984, pp 18–19
7. A Shelter Is Not a Home. Report of the Manhattan Borough President's Task Force on Housing for Homeless Families, March, 1987
8. A Status Report on Homeless Families in America's Cities: A 29-City Survey. United States Conference of Mayors. May, 1987
9. Bassuk E, Rubin L, Lauriat AS: Characteristics of sheltered homeless families. Am J Public Health 76:1097–1101, 1986
10. Brown JL: Hunger in the U.S. Scientific American 256:37–51, February, 1987
11. Carraccio CL, McCormick MC, Weller SC: Chronic disease: Effect on health cognition and health locus of control. J Pediatr 110:982–987, 1987
12. Characteristics and Housing Histories of Families Seeking Shelter from HRA Human Resources Administration, New York City, October, 1986
13. Chavkin W, Kristal A, Seabron C et al: The Reproductive experience of women living in hotels for the homeless in New York City. NY State J Med 87:10–13, 1987
14. Clark ME et al: A flexible approach to health care services for the homeless: The National Health Care for the Homeless Program. Presented at APHA, 113th Annual Meeting, Washington, D.C., November, 1985
15. Egbuonu L, Starfield B: Child health and social status. Pediatrics 69:550–557, 1982
16. Friedman S: Personal communication, August, 1987
17. Gewirtzman R, Fodor I: The homeless child at school: from welfare hotel room to classroom. Child Welfare 66:237–245, 1987
18. Haggerty RJ: Stress and illness in children. Bull NY Acad Med 62:707–718, 1986
19. Health Policy Agenda for the American People. JAMA 257:1199–1210, 1987
20. Hombs ME, Snyder M: Homeless in America: A Forced March to Nowhere, Ed 2. Washington D.C., Community for Creative Non-Violence, 1983, p xvi
21. Homeless in New York State, vol 1. Albany, New York State Department of Social Services 1984, pp 6–8, 10
22. Johnson JH: Life Events as Stressors in Childhood and Adolescence. Beverly Hills, Sage Publications, 1986, pp 67–71
23. Jonas S: On Homelessness and the American Way. Am J Public Health 76:1084–1086, 1986
24. Life at the edge: The hard choices facing low-income American Families. Consumer Reports: 375, June, 1987
25. Mahaffey KR, Annest JL, Roberts J et al: National estimates of blood lead levels: United States, 1976–1980. Associated with selected demographic and socioeconomic factors. N Engl J Med 307:573–579, 1982
26. Main TJ: The Homeless Families of New York. Public Interest 85:3–21, 1986
26a. Meeting the Needs of Homeless Youth: A Report of the Homeless Youth Steering Committee. New York State Council on Children and Families, October, 1984
27. Needleman HL, Gunnoe C, Leviton A et al: Deficits in psychological and classroom performance of children with elevated dentine lead levels. N Engl J Med 300:689–695, 1979
28. New York City Temporary Housing Program for Families with Children, Monthly Report, Human Resources Administration, May, 1984
29. New York City Temporary Housing Program for Families with Children, Monthly Report, Human Resources Administration, July, 1987
30. No One's in Charge: Homeless Families with Children in Temporary Shelter, Citizens Committee for Children of New York, January, 1983
31. Oberg CN: Pediatrics and poverty (commentary). Pediatrics 79:567–569, 1987
32. Oski FA, Honig AS: The effects of therapy on the developmental scores of iron deficient infants. J Pediatr 92:21–25, 1978

33. Perrin EC, Schapiro E: Health locus of control of healthy children, children with chronic physical illness, and their mothers. J Pediatr 110:627–633, 1985
34. Rafferty M: The sickness that won't heal: Health care for the nation's homeless. Health PAC Bull 16:4, 20–28, 1985
35. Rappaport L, Landman G, Fenton T et al: Locus of control as predictor of compliance and outcome in treatment of encopresis. J Pediatr 109:1061–1064, 1986
36. Reuler JB, Bax MJ, Sampson JH: Physician house call services for medically needy inner-city residents. Am J Public Health 76:1131–1134, 1986
37. Rieselbach RE, Jackson TC: In support of a linkage between the funding of graduate medical education and care of the indigent. N Engl J Med 314:32–35, 1986
38. Rutherford GW: Medical status of children in family shelters and hotels: Unpublished data. NYC Department of Health, 1983
39. Ryan W: Blaming the Victim. New York, Random House, 1976
40. Seven Thousand Homeless Children: The Crisis Continues, The Third Report on Homeless Families with Children in Temporary Shelter. Citizen's Committee for Children of New York, October, 1984
41. Somerset S: Shigella outbreak, residents of the Metropolitan Respite Center, New York June, 1986 (unpublished data)
42. Thurow LC: A surge in inequality. Sci Am 256:30–37, 1987
43. Tuberculosis in New York City: The City of New York, Department of Health, Bureau of Tuberculosis, 1984
44. Webb TE, Oski FA: Behavioral status of young adolescents with iron deficiency anemia. J Spec Ed 8:153–156, 1974
45. Weber-Burdin D, Wright JD: Robert Wood Johnson Foundation and Pew Memorial Trust. Health Care for the Homeless Program, 5th report, February, 1987 (unpublished data)
46. Weinberg D: Health Needs of Homeless Adolescents ("runaways"). Unpublished report, New York City Department of Health, December, 1986
47. Yip R, Walsh KM, Goldfarb MG et al: Declining prevalence of anemia in childhood in a middle class setting: A pediatric success story. Pediatrics 80:330–334, 1987

Bureau for Families with Special Needs
111 Livingston Street, Room 2022
Brooklyn, New York 11201

Cumulative Index 1988

Volume 35

Note: Page numbers of issues and articles are in **boldface** type.

U.S. Postal Service

STATEMENT OF OWNERSHIP, MANAGEMENT AND CIRCULATION
Required by 39 U.S.C. 3685)

1A. TITLE OF PUBLICATION	1B. PUBLICATION NO.							2. DATE OF FILING
The Pediatric Clinics of North America	0	0	3	1	3	9	5	5	9-19-88

3. FREQUENCY OF ISSUE	3A. NO. OF ISSUES PUBLISHED ANNUALLY	3B. ANNUAL SUBSCRIPTION PRICE
Six Issues Annually (Feb, Apr, Jun, Aug, Oct, Dec)	6	$53.00

4. COMPLETE MAILING ADDRESS OF KNOWN OFFICE OF PUBLICATION *(Street, City, County, State and ZIP+4 Code) (Not printers)*

W.B. Saunders, Curtis Center, Independence Square W. Philadelphia, Pa 19106-3399

5. COMPLETE MAILING ADDRESS OF THE HEADQUARTERS OF GENERAL BUSINESS OFFICES OF THE PUBLISHER *(Not printer)*

W.B. Saunders, Curtis Center, Independence Square W. Philadelphia, Pa 19106-3399

6. FULL NAMES AND COMPLETE MAILING ADDRESS OF PUBLISHER, EDITOR, AND MANAGING EDITOR *(This item MUST NOT be blank)*

PUBLISHER *(Name and Complete Mailing Address)*
Joan Blumberg,
W.B. Saunders, Curtis Center, Independence Square W. Philadelphia, Pa 19106-3399

EDITOR *(Name and Complete Mailing Address)*
Mary K. Smith,
W.B. Saunders, Curtis Center, Independence Square W. Philadelphia, Pa 19106-3399

MANAGING EDITOR *(Name and Complete Mailing Address)*
Barbara Cohen-Kligerman,
W.B. Saunders, Curtis Center, Independence Square W. Philadelphia, Pa 19106-3399

7. OWNER *(If owned by a corporation, its name and address must be stated and also immediately thereunder the names and addresses of stockholders owning or holding 1 percent or more of total amount of stock. If not owned by a corporation, the names and addresses of the individual owners must be given. If owned by a partnership or other unincorporated firm, its name and address, as well as that of each individual must be given. If the publication is published by a nonprofit organization, its name and address must be stated.) (Item must be completed.)*

FULL NAME	COMPLETE MAILING ADDRESS
W.B. Saunders Inc. stock is owned	
100% by Harcourt Brace Jovanovich	
Inc.	

8. KNOWN BONDHOLDERS, MORTGAGEES, AND OTHER SECURITY HOLDERS OWNING OR HOLDING 1 PERCENT OR MORE OF TOTAL AMOUNT OF BONDS, MORTGAGES OR OTHER SECURITIES *(If there are none, so state)*

FULL NAME	COMPLETE MAILING ADDRESS
NONE	

9. FOR COMPLETION BY NONPROFIT ORGANIZATIONS AUTHORIZED TO MAIL AT SPECIAL RATES *(Section 423.12 DMM only)*
The purpose, function, and nonprofit status of this organization and the exempt status for Federal income tax purposes *(Check one)*

(1) ☐ HAS NOT CHANGED DURING PRECEDING 12 MONTHS   (2) ☐ HAS CHANGED DURING PRECEDING 12 MONTHS   *(If changed, publisher must submit explanation of change with this statement.)*

10. EXTENT AND NATURE OF CIRCULATION *(See Instructions on reverse side)*	AVERAGE NO. COPIES EACH ISSUE DURING PRECEDING 12 MONTHS	ACTUAL NO. COPIES OF SINGLE ISSUE PUBLISHED NEAREST TO FILING DATE
A. TOTAL NO. COPIES *(Net Press Run)*	33,500	33,500
B. PAID AND/OR REQUESTED CIRCULATION 1. Sales through dealers and carriers, street vendors and counter sales		
2. Mail Subscription *(Paid and/or requested)*	20,200	20,672
C. TOTAL PAID AND/OR REQUESTED CIRCULATION *(Sum of 10B1 and 10B2)*	20,200	20,672
D. FREE DISTRIBUTION BY MAIL, CARRIER OR OTHER MEANS SAMPLES, COMPLIMENTARY, AND OTHER FREE COPIES	88	87
E. TOTAL DISTRIBUTION *(Sum of C and D)*	20,288	20,759
F. COPIES NOT DISTRIBUTED 1. Office use, left over, unaccounted, spoiled after printing	13,212	12,741
2. Return from News Agents		
G. TOTAL *(Sum of E, F1 and 2—should equal net press run shown in A)*	33,500	33,500

11. I certify that the statements made by me above are correct and complete	SIGNATURE AND TITLE OF EDITOR, PUBLISHER, BUSINESS MANAGER, OR OWNER
	Lisa Kennedy, Business Manager

Changing Your Address?

Make sure your subscription changes too! When you notify us of your new address, you can help make our job easier by including an exact copy of your Clinics label number with your old address (see illustration below.) This number identifies you to our computer system and will speed the processing of your address change. Please be sure this label number accompanies your old address and your corrected address—you can send an old Clinics label with your number on it or just copy it exactly and send it to the address listed below.

We appreciate your help in our attempt to give you continuous coverage. Thank you.

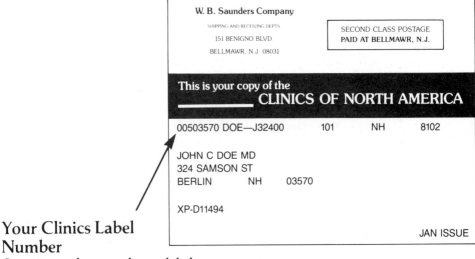

W. B. Saunders Company

SHIPPING AND RECEIVING DEPTS

151 BENIGNO BLVD

BELLMAWR, N.J. 08031

SECOND CLASS POSTAGE
PAID AT BELLMAWR, N.J.

This is your copy of the
CLINICS OF NORTH AMERICA

00503570 DOE—J32400   101   NH   8102

JOHN C DOE MD
324 SAMSON ST
BERLIN   NH   03570

XP-D11494

JAN ISSUE

Your Clinics Label Number

Copy it exactly or send your label
along with your address to:
W. B. Saunders Company, Fulfillment Services
The Curtis Center
Independence Square West, Philadelphia, PA 19106-3399.

Please allow four to six weeks for delivery of new subscriptions and for processing address changes.